Practical Psychiatric Epidemiology

Practical Psychiatric Epidemiology

SECOND EDITION

Edited by

Jayati Das-Munshi

Department of Psychological Medicine, Institute of Psychiatry,
Psychology & Neuroscience, King's College London, UK

Tamsin Ford

Department of Psychiatry, University of Cambridge, UK

Matthew Hotopf

Department of Psychological Medicine, Institute of Psychiatry,
Psychology & Neuroscience, King's College London, UK

Martin Prince

King's Global Health Institute/Health Service and Population
Research Department, Institute of Psychiatry,
Psychology and Neuroscience, King's College London, UK

Robert Stewart

Department of Psychological Medicine, Institute of Psychiatry,
Psychology & Neuroscience, King's College London, UK

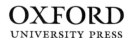

OXFORD
UNIVERSITY PRESS

OXFORD
UNIVERSITY PRESS

Great Clarendon Street, Oxford, OX2 6DP,
United Kingdom

Oxford University Press is a department of the University of Oxford.
It furthers the University's objective of excellence in research, scholarship,
and education by publishing worldwide. Oxford is a registered trade mark of
Oxford University Press in the UK and in certain other countries

First Edition published in 2003
Second Edition published in 2020
Impression: 1

Published in the United States of America by Oxford University Press
198 Madison Avenue, New York, NY 10016, United States of America

British Library Cataloguing in Publication Data
Data available

Library of Congress Control Number: 2020934184

ISBN 978–0–19–873556–4

Printed and bound by
CPI Group (UK) Ltd, Croydon, CR0 4YY

Acknowledgements

Adesewa Adelekun, Anvita Bhardwaj, Bonnie Kaiser, Rennie Qin, and Andi Schmidt for assistance in preparing the chapter 'Culture and psychiatric epidemiology'. Michael E. Dewey for assistance in preparing the chapter 'Statistical techniques in psychiatric epidemiology'. Melissa Co, Hannah Durkin, and Javid Salim for providing comments on initial drafts of the book.

Contents

Abbreviations *ix*

Contributors *xi*

1 Introduction: A 'fourth age' of psychiatric epidemiology? *1*
Jayati Das-Munshi, Tamsin Ford, Matthew Hotopf, Martin Prince, and Robert Stewart

2 Measurement in mental health *5*
Martin Prince and Kia-Chong Chua

3 Culture and psychiatric epidemiology *33*
Brandon A. Kohrt and Vikram Patel

4 Ethics and research in psychiatry: Consent, capacity, and bioethics *51*
Buddhika Lalanie Fernando and Athula Sumathipala

5 Ethics and research in psychiatry: Engagement with patients and public *71*
Stephani L. Hatch, Billy Gazard, and Diana Rose

6 Introduction to epidemiological study designs *83*
Tamsin Ford, Jayati Das-Munshi, and Martin Prince

7 Qualitative research *99*
Oana Mitrofan and Rose McCabe

8 Ecological studies *113*
Jayati Das-Munshi

9 Cross-sectional surveys *127*
Martin Prince and Jayati Das-Munshi

10 The case–control study *145*
Lisa Aschan and Matthew Hotopf

11 Cohort studies *171*
Laura Goodwin and Nicola Fear

12 Randomized controlled trials *187*
Sube Banerjee, Rod S. Taylor, and Jennifer Hellier

13 Surveillance, case registers, and big data *219*
Tamsin Ford, Robert Stewart, and Johnny Downs

14 Research synthesis: Systematic reviews and meta-analyses *237*
Marianna Purgato, Giovanni Ostuzzi, and Corrado Barbui

15 Inference 1: Chance, bias, and confounding *255*
Robert Stewart

16 Inference 2: Causation *271*
Robert Stewart

17 Critical appraisal *285*
Jo Thompson Coon and Rebecca Abbott

18 Statistical techniques in psychiatric epidemiology *303*
Lisa Aschan, Jayati Das-Munshi, Richard Hayes, Martin Prince, Marcus Richards,
Peter Schofield, and Robert Stewart

19 Genetic epidemiology: Overview *327*
Frühling Rijsdijk and Paul F. O'Reilly

20 Gene–environment interaction *343*
Craig Morgan, Marta Di Forti, and Helen L. Fisher

21 Bio-informatics and psychiatric epidemiology *359*
Nicola Voyle, Maximilian Kerz, Steven Kiddle, and Richard Dobson

22 Health economics for psychiatric epidemiology *373*
Margaret Heslin, Paul McCrone, and Daniel Chisholm

23 Life course epidemiology *389*
Marcus Richards and Rebecca Hardy

24 Evidence-based mental health policy *405*
Valentina Iemmi, Nicole Votruba, and Graham Thornicroft

25 Psychiatric epidemiology: Looking to the future *425*
Jayati Das-Munshi, Tamsin Ford, Matthew Hotopf, Martin Prince,
and Robert Stewart

Index *433*

Abbreviations

ADHA	attention deficit hyperactivity disorder	MAR	missing at random
ALSPAC	Avon Longitudinal Study of Parents and Childhood	MCA	Mental Capacity Act
		MCAR	missing completely at random
ANOVA	analysis of variance	MNAR	missing not at random
CAPSS	Child and Adolescent Psychiatry Surveillance System	MTM	multiple-treatments meta-analysis
		MZ	monozygotic
CI	confidence interval	NCCPE	National Co-ordinating Centre for Public Engagement
CIDI	Composite International Diagnostic Interview	NHS	National Health Service
CIS-R	Clinical Interview Schedule—Revised	NICE	National Institute for Health and Care Excellence
CONSORT	Consolidated Standards of Reporting Trials	NIH	National Institutes of Health
		OECD	Organization for Economic Cooperation and Development
CSA	child sexual abuse	PCA	principal components analysis
CSJCA	Centre for Social Justice and Community Action	PJAS	Parent–Child Joint Activity Scale
DALY	disability-adjusted life year	PPE	patient and public engagement
DSM	*Diagnostic and Statistical Manual of Mental Disorders*	PPI	patient and public involvement
		PTSD	post-traumatic stress disorder
DZ	dizygotic	RCT	randomized controlled trial
GMH	global mental health	ROC	receiver operating characteristic
GP	general practitioner	SCAN	Schedules for Clinical Assessment in Neuropsychiatry
GWAS	genome-wide association study		
HERON	Health Inequalities Research Network	SELPh	South East London Photography group
ICD	International Classification of Diseases and Related Health Problems	SEM	structural equation modelling
		SNA	social network analysis
		SNP	single nucleotide polymorphism
IPD	individual patient data	SR	systematic review
ITT	intention to treat	SVM	support vector machine
LD	linkage disequilibrium	WHO	World Health Organization
MacCAT-CR	MacArthur Competence Assessment Tools for Clinical Research	WMH	World Mental Health

Contributors

Rebecca Abbott
NIHR ARC South West Peninsula
(PenARC), University of Exeter Medical
School, University of Exeter, UK

Lisa Aschan
Department of Psychological Medicine,
Institute of Psychiatry, Psychology &
Neuroscience, King's College
London, UK

Sube Banerjee
Executive Dean & Professor of Dementia,
Faculty of Health, University of Plymouth,
Plymouth UK

Corrado Barbui
WHO Collaborating Centre for Research
and Training in Mental Health and
Service Evaluation, University of Verona,
Verona, Italy

Daniel Chisholm
World Health Organization, Geneva,
Switzerland

Kia-Chong Chua
Institute of Psychiatry, Psychology &
Neuroscience, King's College London, UK

Jayati Das-Munshi
Department of Psychological Medicine,
Institute of Psychiatry, Psychology &
Neuroscience, King's College London, UK

Marta Di Forti
Social, Genetic, and Developmental
Psychiatry Centre, Institute of Psychiatry,
Psychology & Neuroscience, King's
College London, UK

Richard Dobson
King's College London, UK

Johnny Downs
King's College London, UK

Nicola Fear
Department of Psychological Medicine,
King's College London, UK

Buddhika Lalanie Fernando
Institute for Research and Development,
Colombo, Sri Lanka

Helen L. Fisher
Social, Genetic, and Developmental
Psychiatry Centre, Institute of Psychiatry,
Psychology & Neuroscience, King's
College London, UK

Tamsin Ford
Department of Psychiatry,
University of Cambridge, UK

Billy Gazard
Department of Psychological Medicine,
Institute of Psychiatry, Psychology &
Neuroscience, King's College London, UK

Laura Goodwin
Department of Psychological Sciences,
University of Liverpool, UK

Rebecca Hardy
MRC Unit for Lifelong Health and Ageing
at UCL, University College London, UK

Stephani L. Hatch
Department of Psychological Medicine,
Institute of Psychiatry, Psychology &
Neuroscience, King's College London, UK

Richard Hayes
King's College London, UK

Jennifer Hellier
Department of Biostatistics and Health
Informatics, Institute of Psychiatry,
Psychology & Neuroscience, King's
College London, UK

Margaret Heslin
King's Health Economics, Institute of
Psychiatry, Psychology & Neuroscience,
King's College London, UK

Matthew Hotopf
Department of Psychological Medicine,
Institute of Psychiatry, Psychology &
Neuroscience, King's College London, UK

Valentina Iemmi
Department of Health Policy and
Department of Social Policy, London
School of Economics and Political Science,
London, UK

Maximilian Kerz
King's College London, UK

Steven Kiddle
King's College London, UK

Brandon A. Kohrt
Department of Psychiatry and Behavioral
Sciences, School of Medicine and Health
Sciences, & Department of Global Health,
Milken School of Public Health, George
Washington University, Washington,
DC, USA

Rose McCabe
City, University of London, UK

Paul McCrone
King's Health Economics, Institute of
Psychiatry, Psychology & Neuroscience,
King's College London, UK

Oana Mitrofan
Children & Young People's Mental
Health Research Collaboration,
Exeter University, UK

Craig Morgan
Health Service and Population Research
Department, Institute of Psychiatry,
Psychology & Neuroscience, King's
College London, UK

Paul F. O'Reilly
Institute of Psychiatry, Psychology &
Neuroscience, King's College London, UK

Giovanni Ostuzzi
WHO Collaborating Centre for Research
and Training in Mental Health and
Service Evaluation, University of Verona,
Verona, Italy

Vikram Patel
Department of Global Health and Social
Medicine, Harvard Medical School,
& Department of Global Health and
Population, Harvard TH Chan School of
Public Health, Boston, USA

Martin Prince
King's Global Health Institute/Health
Service and Population Research
Department, Institute of Psychiatry,
Psychology and Neuroscience, King's
College London, UK

Marianna Purgato
WHO Collaborating Centre for Research
and Training in Mental Health and
Service Evaluation, University of Verona,
Verona, Italy

Marcus Richards
MRC Unit for Lifelong Health
and Ageing at UCL, University
College London, UK

Frühling Rijsdijk
Institute of Psychiatry, Psychology &
Neuroscience, King's College London, UK

Diana Rose
Health Service and Population Research
Department, Institute of Psychiatry,
Psychology & Neuroscience, King's
College London, UK

Robert Stewart
Department of Psychological Medicine,
Institute of Psychiatry, Psychology &
Neuroscience, King's College London, UK

Peter Schofield
Department of Population Health
Sciences, Faculty of Life Sciences and
Medicine, King's College London, UK

Athula Sumathipala
Research Institute for Primary Care and
Health Sciences, School for Primary Care
Research (SPCR), Faculty of Health, Keele
University, UK

Rod S. Taylor
University of Exeter, UK

Jo Thompson Coon
NIHR ARC South West Peninsula
(PenARC), University of Exeter
Medical School, University of
Exeter, UK

Graham Thornicroft
Centre for Global Mental Health and
Centre for Implementation Science,
Institute of Psychiatry, Psychology &
Neuroscience, King's College
London, UK

Nicole Votruba
Centre for Global Mental Health and
Centre for Implementation Science,
Institute of Psychiatry, Psychology &
Neuroscience, King's College
London, UK

Nicola Voyle
King's College London, UK

Chapter 1

Introduction: A 'fourth age' of psychiatric epidemiology?

Jayati Das-Munshi, Tamsin Ford, Matthew Hotopf, Martin Prince, and Robert Stewart

At the time *Practical Psychiatric Epidemiology* was published in 2003, we had few if any thoughts of a future second edition. Back then there was very little material to provide an introduction to psychiatric epidemiology for the growing number of teaching programmes being set up on this topic—there was plenty of material on generic epidemiology, but next to nothing on the particular challenges of adapting this discipline and its methods to mental health research. The first edition served its purpose, and we thought that that would be an end to it. After all, epidemiology at its heart is simply a way of thinking about investigating health states, their risk factors, and their outcomes—a way of approaching questions of causation, finding out about populations from representative samples, measuring exposures and outcomes with minimal bias, applying statistical techniques to communicate numeric data, and considering carefully the alternative explanations for an observation before drawing inferences. How much updating would the topic really need?

Fifteen years on we are pleased to be presenting a new edition, so what has changed? In our introduction to the first edition on the development of psychiatric epidemiology we cited the three phases of methodological development proposed by Dohrenwend and Dohrenwend (1982): a first age where unstructured clinician diagnoses were used to begin to understand the prevalence and incidence of common and severe mental disorders; a second age applying semi-structured instruments and the beginnings of symptom scales for similarly descriptive applications, attempting some level of standardization; and a third age, characterized by larger-scale surveys using fully structured schedules and accompanying algorithms, with an increasing focus on analytic rather than descriptive research. At the time of preparing that introduction, we did not presume to suggest that our speciality might be entering a 'fourth age'; however, we did highlight the growth of more complex analytic designs such as historic cohort and twin studies for causal modelling, paralleled by expansion of research from high-income Western settings towards a more global coverage, and by the incorporation of biological measures and the early appreciation of gene–environment interactions. We have reproduced this introduction in the new edition as there is no reason to change the story of our specialty's emergence from mainstream epidemiology and it is always important to know where we've come from. However, while it might be still too early to define the precise onset and characteristics of a 'fourth age' of psychiatric epidemiology, it is hard to deny that the world is very different now. As an attempt to justify all the hard work of our fellow contributors to this second edition, it is worth outlining a few key features which now characterize our research environment in the early twenty-first century and which suggest that it is worth taking a fresh look at our research methods and their application in mental health.

1. Although considerable research interest and activity is now focused on novel risk factors and causal pathway modelling, the need for high-quality descriptive data has not gone away. There is no reason to suppose that the prevalence and incidence of a given mental disorder will remain constant over time, let alone its individual and societal impact. We assume, for example, that eating disorders in Western societies were once uncommon and that they have grown in prevalence with changing cultural attitudes to body size; however, we don't know this for certain because no one was carrying out mental health surveys in the nineteenth century. Time series analyses suggest, for example, that age-specific dementia incidence might be falling (although with more stable prevalence because of longer survival) (Kosteniuk et al., 2016; Prince et al., 2016), that common mental disorder prevalence is remaining relatively constant for most age groups (McManus et al., 2016), with the notable exception of young women in their late teens and earlier twenties (Sadler et al., 2018; McManus et al., 2019). In addition, certain symptoms such as insomnia and cognitive complaints have been becoming more common (Calem et al., 2012; Begum et al., 2014). Mental health research and policy frequently draw on descriptive data which are showing their age and there is as much need for traditional surveys as there ever was in the 1960s and 1970s. However, the world of data collection has changed a great deal since the days of pencil-and-paper interviews, with perhaps game-changing potential from online platforms and mobile devices.

2. The challenge of defining mental disorders is as pertinent now as it was for Kraepelin, Bleuler, and the rest of our forebears in the early twentieth century. The increasing standardization of diagnostic schedules imposes consistency in an increasingly international research field; however, the 'validity' question remains and the practice remains out of step with biological evidence challenging traditional diagnostic distinctions. As well as a return to symptom scales and a more dimensional characterization of disorder states, there is also the growing possibility of new complementary 'phenotypes' derived in real time from wearables and social media.

3. The interface between what used to be called biological and epidemiological research continues to become increasingly blurred and is likely to disappear when whole genome sequencing becomes as quick and easy as asking about occupation, social support, and life events. Likewise, the traditional distinction between 'clinical' and 'epidemiological' research has become steadily more irrelevant with the advent of 'big data' case registers derived from health records and other administrative resources. Whether a large dataset describes a clinical or community sample has little methodological relevance and doesn't really warrant different nomenclature.

4. The distinctions between psychiatric and generic epidemiology could be said to be blurring in some respects and becoming sharper in others. The need for tailored approaches to measurement in mental health and their influence on research designs is as strong as ever. On the other hand, the complex interrelationship between so-called physical and mental disorders continues to demand close integration and collaboration across traditional clinical specialties, whether this is at the level of investigating the complex bidirectional causal pathways between 'physical' and 'mental' disorder states, or articulating the broader importance of mental health in global policy (Patel et al., 2011).

5. At the interventional end of epidemiology, while the randomized controlled trial remains a mainstay, increasingly complex interventions in health service delivery are requiring new study designs and approaches, coupled with a growing awareness that research does not stop at the demonstration of effect, but needs also to consider the potentially long and tortuous pathways to implementation if new findings are to have a discernible effect on the health of populations.

If we have truly moved forwards to a new age of psychiatric epidemiology, it may turn out to be as much an integration of the past as an embrace of the future. For example, understanding and incorporating the unstructured clinical diagnosis is an important component of research using health records databases, harking back to the 'first age' reliance on routine clinical data, just as the modern case register itself can trace its ancestry directly back to the earliest asylum studies. Similarly, the need to define symptom dimensions and more informative phenotypes for addressing biological hypotheses might be said to herald a move away from 'third age' preoccupations with standardized diagnostic schedules to 'second age' semi-structured approaches. However, regardless of these historical ebbs and flows, it is reasonable to say that psychiatric epidemiology has never had a stronger potential: providing the methodological underpinning for research fields from the biological to the social, from the community to the clinic, and from description to intervention. We have sought to reflect this, through often substantial revision, and extension to the scope of the original text, describing current methods and practice in what we now recognize to be a rapidly evolving scientific discipline.

References

Begum, A., Dewey, M., Hassiotis, A., Prince, M., Wessely, S., and Stewart, R. (2014). Subjective cognitive complaints across the adult life span: a 14-year analysis of trends and associations using the 1993, 2000 and 2007 English Psychiatric Morbidity Surveys. *Psychological Medicine*, **44**, 1977–1987.

Calem, M., Bisla, J., Begum, A., Dewey, M., Bebbington, P.E., Brugha, T., et al. (2012). Increased prevalence of insomnia and changes in hypnotics use in England over 15 years: analysis of the 1993, 2000 and 2007 National Psychiatric Morbidity Surveys. *Sleep*, **35**, 377–384.

Dohrenwend, B.P. and Dohrenwend, B.S. (1982). Perspectives on the past and future of psychiatric epidemiology. The 1981 Rema Lapouse Lecture. *American Journal of Public Health*, **72**, 1271–1279.

Kosteniuk, J.G., Morgan, D.G., O'Connell, M.E., Kirk, A., Crossley, M., Teare, G.F., et al. (2016). Simultaneous temporal trends in dementia incidence and prevalence, 2005–2013: a population-based retrospective cohort study in Saskatchewan, Canada. *International Psychogeriatrics*, 28, 1643–1658.

McManus, S., Bebbington, P., Jenkins, R., and Brugha, T. (eds.) (2016). *Mental health and wellbeing in England: Adult Psychiatric Morbidity Survey 2014*. Leeds: NHS Digital.

McManus, S., Gunnell, D., Cooper, C., Bebbington, P. E., Howard, L. M., Brugha, T., Jenkins, R., Hassiotis, A., Weich, S., and Appleby, L. (2019). Prevalence of non-suicidal self-harm and service contact in England, 2000–14: repeated cross-sectional surveys of the general population. *The Lancet Psychiatry*, 6(7), 573–581.

Patel, V., Boyce, N., Collins, P.Y., Saxena, S., and Horton, R. (2011). A renewed agenda for global mental health. *Lancet*, 378, 1441–1442.

Prince, M., Ali, G.C., Guerchet, M., Prina, A.M., Albanese, E., and Wu, Y.T. (2016). Recent global trends in the prevalence and incidence of dementia, and survival with dementia. *Alzheimer's Research & Therapy*, 8, 23.

Sadler, K., Vizard, T., Ford, T., Goodman, A., Goodman, R., & McManus, S. (2018). *The Mental Health of Children and Young People in England 2017: Trends and characteristics*. Health and Social Care Information Centre: London.

Chapter 2

Measurement in mental health

Martin Prince and Kia-Chong Chua

Introduction

The science of the measurement of mental and psychological phenomena—psychometrics—is central to quantitative research in psychiatry. Without appropriate, accurate, stable, and unbiased measures, our research is doomed from the outset. Much effort has been expended over the last 50 years in the development of an array of assessments (see 'Measures for clinical use'). Most measurement strategies are based on eliciting symptoms, either by asking the participant to complete a self-report questionnaire, or by using an interviewer to question the participant. Some are long, detailed, comprehensive clinical diagnostic assessments. Others are much briefer, designed either to screen for probable cases, or as scalable measures in their own right; of a trait or dimension such as depression, neuroticism, or cognitive function, or as measures of an exposure to a possible risk factor for a disease.

Measurement of psychiatric morbidity in general, and widely applied classifications of disorders in particular, are sometimes criticized for their focus on phenomenology, course, and outcome rather than biomarkers of pathophysiological dysfunction (Cuthbert and Insel, 2013). For this very reason, psychiatry was among the first medical disciplines to develop internationally recognized operationalized diagnostic criteria. At the same time, the research interview has become progressively refined, such that the processes of eliciting, recording, and distilling symptoms into diagnoses or scalable traits are now also highly standardized. These criticisms are therefore to some extent misplaced. Thanks to the careful development and extensive validation of the better established measures in mental health research we have a much better understanding of what they do, and do not measure, and how and where they may be used most appropriately. This confidence is based on our understanding of the *validity* and *reliability* of our measures.

The *validity* of a measure refers to its accuracy as a measure of the thing that it is supposed to be measuring.

The *reliability* of a measure refers to its stability and repeatability, when, for example, measured twice, or assessed by more than one observer, when the thing that is being measured has not changed.

Validity requires reliability, but a reliable test may still not be valid. If weighing scales record a different weight every time you step on them, they will not in general be telling you the truth. However, even if they record the same weight on every measurement occasion, this may be consistently 5 kg under your true weight.

Levels of measurement

One way of classifying measures is according to the level of organization of the data that they generate. The data are coded in *variables*. In general, measures may be categorical or continuous.

Categorical variables

These may have two or more levels but describe categories to which no meaningful numerical value can be ascribed. Examples would include gender, ethnicity, and marital status (married, never married, widowed, separated, and divorced). These measures describe types rather than quantities.

1. Binary or dichotomous variables are the simplest categorical variables having only two levels, for example, exposed or unexposed, case or non-case. Examples would include gender, victim of child sexual abuse—yes/no, current International Statistical Classification of Diseases and Related Health Problems (ICD)-10 depressive episode—yes/no. Some more complex variables are reduced to binary form to simplify an analysis. For example, data on lifetime smoking habit could be reduced to a binary variable, ever smoked—yes/no.

2. Polychotomous variables may be *simple* or *ordered*.

Ordered categorical variables still describe discrete categories, but with some meaningful trend in the quantity of what is being described from level to level of the variable. Examples would include current smoking status (classified as non-smoker, 1–10 cigarettes daily, 11–20 cigarettes daily, and >20 cigarettes daily) and number of life events (classified as none, one, and two or more).

Simple categorical variables display no such trend or progression from level to level of the variable. Examples would include eye colour, country of birth, or ICD diagnostic group.

Continuous variables

These are, strictly speaking, measures of attributes or *traits* that can be indexed at any point along a scale. Thus weight can be measured as 70 kg or 70.1 kg or even more precisely as 70.09 kg. Age is another example of a continuous variable. Number of children is not a continuous variable, as only integer values are possible. Such measures generate *discrete quantitative variables*. True continuous variables should also conform to the properties of an arithmetic scale. Thus an adult who is 1.80 m tall is twice as tall as a child of 90 cm. Also they are 90 cm taller. However, somebody scoring 20 points on the Centre for Epidemiological Studies—Depression (CES-D) symptoms scale is probably not twice as depressed as somebody scoring 10 points. Likewise the difference in levels of depression between persons scoring 10 and 14, and 14 and 18 may not be the same. It should be apparent from this discussion that many 'scales' in common use in psychiatric and psychological research are neither continuous nor arithmetical, and should in fact properly be considered to be closer in character to ordered categorical variables. Sometimes these are referred to as ordinal scales.

From a technical point of view, continuous measures of dimensional traits such as depression, anxiety, neuroticism, and cognitive function offer some advantages over their dichotomous equivalents, major depression, generalized anxiety disorder, personality disorder, and dementia. These diagnoses tend to be rather rare; collapsing a continuous trait into a dichotomous diagnosis may mean that the investigators are in effect throwing away informative data; the net effect may be loss of statistical power to demonstrate an important association with a risk factor, or a real benefit of a treatment. In psychiatric genetics, for example, researchers have used endophenotypes for their linkage analyses traits that may be more directly representative of underlying neurophysiological and neurocognitive abnormalities (Greenwood et al., 2013). Trait-based methods may offer considerable advantages in terms of statistical power for identification of genes of small to moderate effect.

Domains of measurement

Measures in common use in psychiatric epidemiology can be thought of as covering six principal domains:

1. Demographic status—for example, age, gender, marital status, and household circumstances.

2. Socioeconomic status—for example, educational level, occupational class, income, wealth, debt, and employment.

3. Social circumstances—for example, social network and social support.

4. Activities, lifestyles, and behaviours—a very broad area, its contents are dictated by the focus of the research—examples would include tobacco and alcohol consumption, substance use, diet, and exercise. Some measures such as recent exposure to positive and negative life events may be particularly relevant to psychiatric research.

5. Opinions and attitudes—an area of measurement initially restricted to market research organizations, but increasingly adopted by social science, health service, and system researchers.

6. Health status—measures can be further grouped into:

   a. specific dichotomous measures of diagnoses (schizophrenia or psoriasis), or continuously distributed traits (blood pressure level, serum cholesterol, mood, anxiety, neuroticism, cognitive status),

   b. global measures, for example, subjective or objective global health assessment, disability and functioning (intrinsic capacity, activity and participation), and health-related quality of life.

   c. measures reflecting the need for, or use of health services.

Selecting a measure

A literature search is a good place to identify measures that are widely used in research practice. Typically, one quickly realizes that there are a variety of measures available for the same assessment purpose. Here, we provide a simple checklist to help with decision-making:

1. Conceptual relevance:
   - The measure should be closely conceptually related to the construct of interest for your study.
2. Comparability:
   - The measure should correspond closely to those used by studies that will serve as important benchmarks for comparing study findings.
3. Comprehensibility:
   - Is the content and response format easily understood by the target study participants and/or interviewers?
   - Are translations in local languages needed? If translated versions have been developed, did the process include forward and backward translation, expert review, cognitive interviewing, and pilot testing? See, for example, the standard recommendation of the World Health Organization (WHO) (http://www.who.int/substance_ abuse/research_tools/translation/en/).
4. Feasibility:
   - Priority should be given to key exposures and outcomes in the primary research question. It may even be necessary to consider using more than one measure for an outcome. For all other purposes (confounders, mediators, and modifiers), shorter measures may be considered to help reduce time and burden.
5. Validation studies:
   - How many validation studies have been reported? How many aspects of validity and reliability have been examined? For more details, see 'Psychometric properties'. Are these generalizable to the setting and context in which you will apply the measure?

Developing a new measure

If existing measures fail to meet each of the five criteria listed previously, then *maybe* you will need to develop your own. The decision to develop a new measure should not be taken lightly since much diligent work will be required, if your new measure is to be superior to those that already exist. The procedure for the development of scale-based measures is perhaps most clearly established (Box 2.1).

The stages in instrument development

1. *Definition of the construct*. What is the trait that is to be measured? What does it include? What does it exclude?

Box 2.1 Stages in the development of a scale

1. Definition of the construct.
2. Review of the construct definition.
3. Item drafting.
4. Item review.
5. Alpha testing (test–retest reliability, ceiling and floor effects, and internal scale consistency).
6. Beta testing (criterion or more usually concurrent validity).
7. Post-development testing.

---

2. *Review of the construct definition.* This is usually carried out both by experts in the field, and by lay persons similar to those to whom the measure will be administered. Is it clear? Does it make sense? Is it culturally appropriate?

3. *Item drafting.* Drawing up a long list of potential items felt to address the construct.

4. *Item review.* Expert and lay review of these items for content validity (do all the items address the construct? Have some aspects of the construct not been covered by the items?). Comprehensibility should be assessed, bearing in mind the range of educational levels of respondents. Poorly drafted items are discarded.

5. *Alpha testing (item reduction).* Remaining items are tested for test–retest reliability, ceiling and floor effects, and internal scale consistency. Fifty to one hundred participants usually suffice. Unreliable items, those endorsed by nearly everyone (ceiling effects) or no one (floor effects), and items that reduce internal scale consistency as evidenced by poor correlations between the item score and the total scale score are discarded. This approach, which optimizes internal consistency, derives from 'classical scale theory'. An alternative approach selects items on the basis of their item response characteristics, aiming for a scale with strong hierarchical scaling properties. An advantage of this approach is that the information content of the scale can be tailored to achieve maximum precision over a range of the trait that is of specific interest (Tasse et al., 2016).

6. *Beta testing.* In a separate sample, the surviving items, and the scale as a whole, are tested for criterion or more usually concurrent validity (see later). The internal consistency of the scale is retested, and often a factor analysis (principal components analysis) is carried out to see whether the scale is a unidimensional scale in which all items are measuring the same single underlying trait, or if two or more factors are extracted, whether the scale may effectively consist of subscales measuring related yet to some extent distinct underlying traits.

7. *Post-development testing.* Validation of a measure is never completed by its developers. Widespread use by other investigators in different settings will, over time, establish the extent and limitations of its validity.

Psychometric properties

Approaches to understanding validity and reliability have evolved considerably in the past decades, but with unequal impact across various specialist fields of mental health research, leading to different standards for 'talking and thinking about validity' (Newton and Shaw, 2013). For a historical brief, see Streiner et al. (2015). Here we aim to help readers achieve a functional understanding of these concepts. For illustration, we have used examples from the literature: the Parent–Child Joint Activity Scale (PJAS) (Kumari et al., 2000) (concurrent, convergent, discriminant, and 'known group' validity) and the EURO-D depression symptom scale (Prince et al., 1999) (construct and factorial validity).

Content validity

Content validity is a concern about whether relevant aspects of the construct to be measured have been adequately covered, and whether all items that are included in the measure are relevant to that construct. Content validity should have been addressed in the initial development of the measure (see items 1–4 in previous list). However, both the construct of interest, and the measurement context may vary somewhat from its original application. Content validity may be assessed through literature review, qualitative research (key informant interviews), and expert review, always remembering the expertise of those with direct lived experience of the construct to be studied (e.g. the target group of respondents). Particular care should be taken when the measure has been translated into another language and culture, to recheck the relevance of each item to the construct, and that the original meaning of the item has been correctly and appropriately conveyed. Vernacular expressions, for example, 'feeling blue' in a depression questionnaire, or 'as like as two peas in a pod' may be evocative in one culture but meaningless in another if concretely translated.

Construct validity

This refers to the extent to which the construct that the measure seeks to address is a real and coherent entity, and then also to the salience of the measure to that construct. It is a process in which we gather evidence on multiple aspects of the performance of a measure and its measurement characteristics to assess if we are able to make meaningful inferences to support decision-making in the context in which the measure is used. Construct validity is particularly but not exclusively relevant when there is no definitive criterion measure for the trait that is being measured, and indirect measures must be relied upon (Cronbach and Meehl, 1955). The elucidation of the trait or quality underlying the test is of central importance. Construct validity as such is not a question about how 'good' is the *measure*, but it is about the quality of our *measurements* given the use of a particular measure (Messick, 1995; Zumbo and Chan, 2014). To better understand the underlying construct, and the relationship of the measure to the construct and other more or less proximately related constructs, we need to test multiple hypotheses as described below. It is crucial to appreciate that construct validity is not binary (valid or not).

Concurrent validity

This is tested by the extent to which the new measure relates, as hypothesized, to other measures taken at the same time (hence concurrent). To see if PJAS scores have concurrent validity as a measure of parent–child joint activity, we can compare them with scores obtained from another measure that is already commonly used for this purpose. While the commonly used measure serves as the best available benchmark, this external criterion may not be the gold standard for theoretical and practical reasons. The PJAS correlated positively with a subset of six items from the nurturing subscale of the Parent Behaviour Checklist (Fox, 1994) that covered parent–child joint activities ($r = 0.56$, $p <0.001$). PJAS was also compared with the total number of parent–child joint activities, and the mean time spent in joint activities each day, assessed using the 'Yesterday's Interview' a detailed semi-structured interview to ascertain all activities conducted by the mother, with or without their child, on the previous day. Three days were selected at random for each participant. The correlation between the total number of joint activities and the PJAS score was 0.58 ($p <0.01$), and between the mean duration of joint activity and the PJAS was 0.60 ($p <0.01$). Concurrent validation helped to show that PJAS scores corresponded well with measures from existing appropriate and relevant benchmarks (Kumari et al., 2000).

Convergent validity

Convergent and divergent validity should be tested in relation to each other. A measure will be more closely related to an alternative measure of the same construct than it will be to measures of different constructs. To see if PJAS scores have convergent validity as a measure of positive parenting, we look at other outcomes that should, logically, be correlated. For instance, other empirical literature shows that low levels of parent–child positive interactions, assessed from direct observation, are associated with behaviour problems (antisocial, externalizing or disruptive behaviours) in preschool children. Given this expected relationship, we would examine whether behaviour problems are more common in children whose mothers report low levels of parent–child joint activity on the PJAS. When assessed in a population-based cross-sectional study, mean Behaviour Checklist scores increased progressively from highest to lowest quarters of the PJAS distribution. Those with low levels of joint activity were over twice as likely to have clinically significant behaviour disturbance (odds ratio 2.6; 95% confidence interval (CI) 1.4–4.8) controlling for marital status, maternal mental health, overcrowding, and dissatisfaction with housing) (Galboda-Liyanage et al., 2003).

Unlike concurrent validation, child behaviour measures do not share the same assessment objective as the PJAS but a relationship is expected for theoretical reasons. If parent–child joint activity, or the lack of it, is considered to cause an outcome (i.e. they can co-occur only after exposure to low joint activity), predictive validation could be conducted instead of convergent validation. Given evidence of convergent validity, we gain assurance that we achieved valid measurements of positive parenting since PJAS scores show an expected relationship with other pertinent factors that are present at the same time.

Divergent validity

To see if PJAS scores have divergent validity for positive parenting practices, we look at other outcomes that are logically related as in convergent validation. However, divergent validation is focused on the need to distinguish between commonly associated constructs. For instance, the Parent Behaviour Checklist nurturing subscale comprised 14 items on broader aspects of parenting such as behaviour management and help-seeking in addition to the six items that related to joint activities. The correlation coefficient for the total score on the nurturing subscale was lower ($r = 0.32$; $p = 0.03$), than for the subset of six joint activity items ($r = 0.56$; $p < 0.001$), suggesting that the PJAS is more closely aligned to the construct of parent–child joint activity than to other to some extent distinct parenting practices (Kumari et al., 2000). The assessment of divergent validity might usefully have been extended to other Parent Behaviour Checklist subscales covering discipline and developmental expectations. Divergent validity provides theoretical clarity with respect both to the precision of the measure and the distinctiveness of the construct that it purports to assess.

Known-group validity

Sometimes there is no suitable gold standard. In addition external criterion measures for concurrent validity may only be approximately related to the construct under study, or be cumbersome or impractical to assess. Under these circumstances, known-group validity can be a useful exercise, by which sensible strategies for classifying individuals in the absence of a gold standard are used. For the PJAS, five health visitors were asked to identify two groups of mothers of 3- to 4-year-old children characterized by markedly low and markedly high levels of mother–child interactions. The mean PJAS scores in the low joint activity group was 64 (standard deviation (SD) 5.1) and in the high joint activity group 72.3 (SD 8.7), with a mean difference of 8.3 points (95% CI 4.7–11.9).

Predictive validity

Predictive validity assesses the extent to which a new measure can predict future occurrences. To see if PJAS scores have predictive validity, we would need to look at other outcomes that should logically follow in time. For instance, evidence suggests that parenting interventions that enhance positive parenting skills and activities may also benefit cognitive development. Hence, we might hypothesize that higher PJAS scores, indicating more parent–child joint activities among preschoolers might independently predict better reading skills and higher SATS scores when the children are followed up to primary school age.

Unlike concurrent validation, the external criterion here differs in two ways: (1) cognitive development assessments do not share the same assessment objective as the PJAS but a relationship is expected for theoretical reasons; and (2) cognitive development (i.e. the external criterion) is measured at a later time point. We gain assurance that we achieved valid measurements of parent–child joint activity if PJAS scores show these prospective relationships. With evidence of predictive validity, the PJAS may also be useful as a prognostic tool for identifying preschool children at risk for cognitive underdevelopment.

Factorial validity (or structural validity)

Factorial validity is a test of theoretical meaning in our measurements. Using exploratory factor analysis, factorial validation starts with exploring the pattern of correlations between responses; here, we have used the example of the 12 EURO-D items. Stronger correlations among certain items suggest that these items belong to a specific topic amidst the depression-related symptoms assessed in EURO-D. Examining the content of items that belong to a family, we infer meaning from this structure to help generate a theory about what is it that we are measuring. Initial exploratory factor analysis studies showed that the 12-item EURO-D scores appear to capture two dimensions of late-life depression which could be theoretically labelled as 'affective suffering' and 'motivation' (Prince et al., 1999). Confirmatory factor analysis was subsequently used, with a priori hypotheses, to further test the presence of these two dimensions in EURO-D scores from another study conducted in six Latin American countries (Brailean et al., 2015). Taken together, these studies offered a theoretical basis for further research on individual differences in late-life depression in terms of 'affective suffering' and 'motivation'.

Diagnostic accuracy

Diagnostic accuracy can be assessed for clinical interviews that are used to generate diagnoses directly, or scale scores that are used to screen for mental disorders. In either case, to assess diagnostic accuracy we must rely on an external diagnostic criterion that is considered as an acceptable approximation to an underlying *gold standard*. This may be derived from the following:

1. A semi-structured clinical research diagnostic interview. The WHO Schedules for Clinical Assessment in Neuropsychiatry (SCAN) has been widely used.

2. A more loosely structured clinical checklist, that frees the clinician expert to ask questions appropriate to the individual assessed and/or the culture in which the assessment is conducted, and to exercise their judgement as to the clinical significance of the symptoms and signs elicited. This approach, for example, using the Comprehensive Psychopathological Rating Scale (CPRS) (Asberg et al., 1978), has been favoured particularly in the validation of diagnostic assessments based on western nosologies in non-Western or anglophone cultures (Hanlon et al., 2008; Weobong et al., 2009).

3. Routine clinical diagnoses.

Based on this external criterion, individuals are classified into two groups that are known to be cases and non-cases (i.e. depressed vs not depressed). In a validation of the Composite International Diagnostic Interview (CIDI) 2.1, diagnoses according to this fully structured lay administered diagnostic interview were compared with those using the gold standard of the SCAN (Jordanova et al., 2004). For the diagnosis of any phobic disorder, findings were as represented in Table 2.1.

Table 2.1 Diagnostic accuracy of the CIDI 2.1

CIDI 2.1	Gold standard (cases vs non-cases) (SCAN)	
	Case	Non-case
Case	22 True positive (TP)	6 False positive (FP)
Non-case	5 False negative (FN)	72 True negative (TN)

Sensitivity = TP/(TP + FN); positive predictive value (PPV) = TP/(TP + FP).
Specificity = TN/(TN + FP); negative predictive value (NPV) = TN/(TN + FN).
Accurate detection by the CIDI results in true positives (*TP*) and true negatives (*TN*). On the other hand, errors in detection result in false positives (*FP*) and false negatives (*FN*).
The *sensitivity* of the new measure is the proportion of true cases correctly identified.
The *specificity* of the new measure is the proportion of non-cases correctly identified.
The *PPV* of the new measure is the proportion of participants it identifies as cases that actually are cases according to the 'gold standard'.
The *NPV* of the new measure is the proportion of participants it identifies as non-cases that actually are non-cases according to the 'gold standard'.

Diagnostic accuracy will be high if there are:

1. high levels of *sensitivity*: the number of *cases* detected (TP) is much larger than the number of undetected *cases* (FN)

2. high levels of *specificity*: the number of *non-cases* detected (TN) is much larger than the number of *non-cases* wrongly thought to be 'cases' (FP).

As such sensitivity is expressed as a proportion (range: 0–1) of the number of *cases* we could accurately identify (TP) out of all actual *cases* (TP + FN)—*that is, the proportion of true cases accurately identified.*

Similarly, specificity is expressed as a proportion of the number of *non-cases* we could accurately identify (TN) out of all actual *non-cases* (TN + FP)—*that is, the proportion of true non-cases accurately identified.*

In the previous example, sensitivity is 22/27 = 0.81, and specificity is 72/78 = 0.92.

Without perfect sensitivity and specificity, the test will generate false positives (FP) and false negatives (FN). We would like to know how much we can trust the test. For this purpose, we shift our perspective to the rows rather than the columns of the cross-tabulation to examine positive predictive value (PPV) and negative predictive value (NPV). The CIDI will have diagnostic accuracy if there are:

1. high *PPVs*: the number of true positives (TP) is much larger than the number of false positives (FP);

2. high *NPVs*: the number of true negatives (TN) is much larger than the number of false negatives (FN)

As such PPV is expressed as the proportion (range: 0–1) of cases detected by the CIDI (TP + FP) who were cases according to the gold standard (TP).

Conversely, NPV is expressed as the proportion (range: 0–1) of all non-cases according to the CIDI (TN + FN) who were non-cases according to the gold standard (TN).

In the previous example, PPV is 22/28 = 0.79, and NPV is 72/77 = 0.94.

Unlike sensitivity and specificity, both PPV and NPV are heavily influenced by the prevalence of the condition in the test sample. If the prevalence is very low, the PPV is also likely to be low even if both sensitivity and specificity are high (Altman and Bland, 1994). The true positives from the small number of cases will be greatly exceeded by the false positives from the much larger number of non-cases. Note that in the earlier example, the test sample of primary care attendees had a relatively high prevalence of phobia, 27/105 = 25.7%.

To summarize, a question about sensitivity concerns whether the fire alarm will ring if there is a fire. A question about PPV concerns whether there is really a fire when the fire alarm is ringing. In the context of mental health measurement, a question about sensitivity would be: if a person has a mental disorder, how likely is it that they will be identified by the test? A question about PPV would be: if a person is identified by the test, how likely is it that they will have the mental disorder?

For validation of a scale-based measure for screening purposes, case and non-case groups are compared in terms of their scale scores. Here we are interested in finding a cut-off score that will help us achieve the most accurate detection of cases and non-cases. The approach is the same, but for ordinal scales, sensitivity and specificity vary depending upon the choice of cut-off score. In the example provided in Table 2.2, in a validation of the EURO-D against the gold standard of ICD-10 depressive episode from a structured clinical interview, it can be seen that as the cut-point increases, such that more depression symptoms need to be endorsed to be identified as a probable case, sensitivity falls. But at the same time specificity increases.

Youden's index is a useful summary indicator of overall test performance at a given cut point. It is calculated as (sensitivity + specificity) − 1. Hence at the 7/8 cut-point, that is (0.45 + 0.98) − 1 = 0.43. Youden's index is highest at the 4/5 cut-point, at which score sensitivity and specificity are simultaneously maximized. If one wished to favour specificity over sensitivity, one could choose the cut-point with the highest sensitivity that did not exceed specificity (5/6). If one wished to favour sensitivity over specificity, one could choose the cut-point with the highest specificity that did not exceed sensitivity (4/5).

The receiver operating characteristic (ROC) curve provides an overview of a trade-off between 'being right' and 'being wrong' (Streiner and Cairney, 2007). It is obtained by plotting 1 − specificity (on the x-axis) versus sensitivity (on the y-axis)

Table 2.2 Distribution of gold-standard (ICD-10 depressive episode) cases and non-cases by EURO-D score, and sensitivity, specificity, and Youden's indices at different possible EURO-D cut-points

EURO-D Score	ICD-10 cases	ICD-10 non-cases	Cut-point	Sensitivity	Specificity	Youden's Index
0	0 (0.0%)	977 (35.6%)	0/1	1.00	0.36	0.36
1	0 (0.0%)	548 (19.9%)	1/2	1.00	0.55	0.55
2	0 (0.0%)	378 (13.8%)	2/3	1.00	0.69	0.69
3	2 (1.4%)	305 (11.1%)	3/4	0.99	0.80	0.79
4	2 (1.4%)	203 (7.4%)	4/5	0.97	0.88	0.85
5	18 (12.5%)	170 (6.2%)	5/6	0.85	0.94	0.79
6	23 (16.0%)	88 (3.2%)	6/7	0.69	0.97	0.66
7	34 (23.6%)	35 (1.3%)	7/8	0.45	0.98	0.43
8	26 (18.1%)	24 (0.9%)	8/9	0.27	0.99	0.26
9	27 (18.8%)	13 (0.5%)	9/10	0.08	1.00	0.08
10	9 (6.3%)	6 (0.2%)	10/11	0.02	1.00	0.02
11	2 (1.4%)	1 (0.0%)	11/12	0.01	1.00	0.01
12	1 (0.7%)	0 (0.0%)				
Total	144 (100%)	2748 (100%)				

for all possible cut-points. See Figure 2.1, for an example, obtained from the data in Table 2.2. For a ROC curve, a useless test would be indicated by the diagonal green line, when the test provides no discrimination. The area under the ROC curve (AUROC) would then be 0.5. As overall discrimination improves the curve arches up and to the left, the extent to which it does so being referred to as 'gain'. A perfect test would have an AUROC of 1.0. The ROC curve also allows one to identify an optimal cut-point or cut-points, which are those closest to the top left hand corner of the curve. You will see from the ROC curve for the EURO-D, plotted from the previous tabulated data, that these are the 4/5 cut-point (1 − specificity = 0.12, sensitivity = 0.97), and 5/6 cut-point (0.06, 0.85).

The AUROC in this example is 0.97 (95% CI 0.96–0.98), suggesting excellent overall discriminability. The AUROC can be used to compare the *overall* discriminability of different screening assessments in the same population (Weobong et al., 2009) or of a particular test when used in different subpopulations or administered in different ways.

Responsiveness

To see if EURO-D scores are responsive to clinically important changes, we could evaluate changes in EURO-D scores among older adults who had a clinical intervention

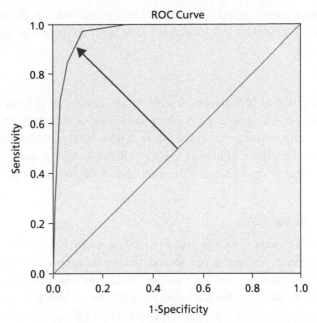

Figure 2.1 Receiver operating characteristic (ROC) curve summarizing the discriminability of the EURO-D scale against a gold standard of ICD-10 depressive episode.

known to be effective in improving depression or related outcomes. This is 'internal responsiveness'. However, it is also important to look at responsiveness related to an alternative and accepted indicator of meaningful clinical change. Hence change in EURO-D scores could be compared between older adults who were rated as clinically improved, or not clinically improved according to a structured clinical assessment designed for this purpose This is 'external responsiveness'. With evidence of responsiveness, we would gain assurance that that EURO-D scores are valid measurements of late-life depression (Hays and Hadorn, 1992). While sensitivity to differences between groups is the focus in diagnostic accuracy and known-group validation, the focus for responsiveness is sensitivity to differences over time (internal responsiveness). However, there is also a need

Table 2.3 Cross-tabulation of pairs of ratings for estimation of agreement

	Rater 2 (case)	Rater 2 (non-case)	Totals
Rater 1 (case)	a	b	a + b
Rater 1 (non-case)	c	d	c + d
Totals	a + c	b + d	a + b + c + d

to establish a meaningful anchor in term of known group differences (external responsiveness). As such these three validation processes share some similar analytic methods (Husted et al., 2000).

Reliability

Reliability is a question of what we observe *in the absence* of difference/change. If a thermometer shows different readings when there is no real change in temperature, we know that the thermometer is not reliable. In fact, we would question whether it is measuring temperature at all (i.e. construct validity). Reliable measurements are also a precondition for ability to detect small but meaningful differences/changes (i.e. sensitivity to change).

Test–retest reliability

To see if EURO-D scores have test–retest reliability, we need a repeated assessment in the absence of change. The timing of a second assessment is critical so that a meaningful change in EURO-D scores is unlikely and any difference can be attributed to random error. Among older adults with depression, their symptoms should be stable for at least a time interval of 1–2 weeks to be considered clinically significant. Hence a EURO-D assessment should be repeated within this time window for examining test–retest reliability. We would expect high levels of agreement between EURO-D scores from the initial and second assessment.

Inter-rater and inter-interviewer reliability

The use of diagnostic assessment tools like the Structured Clinical Interview for DSM disorders (SCID) requires intensive training in administration and rating so that the same diagnosis can be reached when assessed by other practitioners. Inter-rater reliability is routinely assessed during training, when those being trained practice coding of prerecorded interviews. If there are high levels of agreement between practitioners in terms of individual ratings and the final diagnosis for each interview scenario, we gain assurance that the assessment process can be conducted in a consistent manner by different practitioners. For an instance of such studies, see Lobbestael et al. (2011).

Inter-interviewer reliability is equally important, but less frequently assessed, since live interviews on the same participant need to be carried out separately by pairs of interviewers. Inter-interviewer reliability will also be affected by the ways in which the interview is conducted, and the questions asked, as well as the ratings. Note that inter-interviewer reliability will also be affected by problems with test–retest reliability, and inter-rater reliability.

When assessing reliability, we are generally interested in agreement, rather than association or correlation. If ratings are continuous instead of categorical, as would be the case for an assessment of test–retest reliability for a scale score, we would want to know if the scores on the second assessment were *the same* as the first. For this purpose, one should use intra-class correlation, a measure of agreement (Shrout and Fleiss, 1979) and Bland–Altman plots rather than simple correlation (Bland and Altman, 1986).

Categorical ratings, for example, diagnostic ratings from two practitioners (e.g. major depression: Yes/No), can be quantified using the coefficient kappa (Cohen, 1960). The first step in estimating agreement is to cross-tabulate the results of the ratings, in the form as shown in Table 2.3.

One can see that the two raters have agreed on a + d of the cases assessed. The overall observed agreement is therefore a + d/(a + b + c + d). However, this does not take into account the role of chance. Two monkeys would also have agreed with each other a certain proportion of the time.

Kappa is the agreement beyond chance, that is (observed agreement − expected agreement by chance)/1 − expected. From Table 2.2, the expected agreement by chance is calculated as follows:

The probability of agreeing on caseness by chance is the probability of being rated as a case by Rater 1 times the probability of being rated as a case by Rater 2, that is (Rater 1) a + b/(a + b + c + d) × (Rater 2) a + c/(a + b + c + d).

The probability of agreeing on non-caseness by chance is the probability of being rated as a non-case by Rater 1 times the probability of being rated as a non-case by Rater 2, that is (Rater 1) c + d/(a + b + c + d) × (Rater 2) b + d/(a + b + c + d).

The sum of the probabilities of chance agreement on caseness and agreeing on non-caseness would provide the expected agreement by chance.

The kappa coefficient is therefore a little cumbersome to calculate by hand, but most statistical software have provision for this. An alternative that is easier to calculate is the coefficient of agreement. This is expressed simply as the number of participants where both raters agree that the person assessed is a case, divided by the number where either have rated them as a case, that is a/(a + b + c).

While high levels of inter-rater reliability are desirable, we should be cautious in interpreting what constitutes a 'high' level of agreement. For instance, 70% concordance between two practitioners may be considered high when the phenomena is not easily observed (e.g. negative symptoms of psychosis), whereas 70% concordance may be considered low when rating more overt behaviours (e.g. positive symptoms of psychosis).

Note that measures of agreement, particularly kappa, are also used in validation studies, where, for example, one is looking at diagnostic concordance between one type of clinical assessment, and a gold standard.

Internal consistency

Internal consistency is a concern with whether a high EURO-D score is consistently (or reliably) reflected by every item in the presence of severe depression. Put another way, do all the items 'behave' reliably to be perceived as belonging to the same family? The lack of internal consistency will undermine measurement reliability (or precision) and hence sensitivity in EURO-D scores for discriminating individual differences in depression levels among older adults.

Internal consistency is commonly quantified with the Cronbach's alpha (Cronbach, 1951). While problems with this coefficient have long been recognized, its use continues to dominate empirical literature (Sijtsma, 2009). The specific issues are beyond the scope of this introductory material, but readers should be aware that there are better alternatives such as the omega coefficient (Zinbarg, 2006).

Measures for clinical use

This is a selection of the more rigorously constructed, best validated, and most widely used measures. The choice reflects to some extent the authors' bias towards briefer measures.

Note that some of these measures are copyrighted (e.g. GHQ and EPQ), and fees are charged for their use, although these are sometimes waived (e.g. for PhD students). For all copyrighted measures, it is essential that you seek permission to use the measure, and pay the copyright fee if required. In some cases, a public domain alternative exists (e.g. you could use the SRQ-20 instead of the GHQ). For the public domain measures, you should still, as a matter of courtesy, contact the instrument developers for permission to use their measures. They will often be able to provide you with useful advice. All WHO measures are in the public domain and copyright free, however, again you should contact the WHO Mental Health Division for the most up-to-date version of the measure (often available in a translated version suitable for use in your country).

Scalable measures with validated screening properties

Measuring psychiatric disorder

General adults (16–64)

GHQ—General Health Questionnaire

A 12- (GHQ-12), 28- (GHQ-28) or 30-item (GHQ-30) self-administered (5–10 minutes) questionnaire with a validated cut-point for identification of common mental disorder. The GHQ is copyrighted. Contact GL Assessment (formerly NFER-Nelson) for permission and information regarding copyright fees.

> Gelaye, B., Tadesse, M.G., Lohsoonthorn, V., Lertmeharit, S., Pensuksan, W.C., Sanchez, S.E., et al. (2015). Psychometric properties and factor structure of the General Health Questionnaire as a screening tool for anxiety and depressive symptoms in a multi-national study of young adults. *Journal of Affective Disorders*, 187, 197–202.
>
> Gnambs, T. and Staufenbiel, T. (2018). The structure of the General Health Questionnaire (GHQ-12): two meta-analytic factor analyses. *Health Psychology Review*, 12, 179–194.
>
> Goldberg, D.P., Gater, R., Sartorius, N., Ustun, T.B., Piccinelli, M., Gureje, O., and Rutter, C. (1997). The validity of two versions of the GHQ in the WHO study of mental illness in general health care. *Psychological Medicine*, 27, 191–197.
>
> Goldberg, G. and Williams, P. (1988). *A user's guide to the General Health Questionnaire*. Windsor: NFER-Nelson.

SRQ-20—Self Reporting Questionnaire—20

A 20-item self-administered (5–10 minutes) questionnaire with a validated cut-point for identification of common mental disorder. This is a WHO measure and therefore free of copyright charges. Very similar to the GHQ in its content, style, and properties, but a useful alternative if you wish to avoid paying licence fees.

Araya, R., Wynn, R., and Lewis, G. (1992). Comparison of two self administered psychiatric questionnaires (GHQ-12 and SRQ-20) in primary care in Chile. *Social Psychiatry & Psychiatric Epidemiology*, 27, 168–173.

Pendergast, L.L., Scharf, R.J., Rasmussen, Z.A., Seidman, J.C., Schaefer, B.A., Svensen, E., et al. (2014). Postpartum depressive symptoms across time and place: structural invariance of the Self-Reporting Questionnaire among women from the international, multi-site MAL-ED study. *Journal of Affective Disorders*, 167, 178–186.

Rasmussen, A., Ventevogel, P., Sancilio, A., Eggerman, M., and Panter-Brick, C. (2014). Comparing the validity of the self reporting questionnaire and the Afghan symptom checklist: dysphoria, aggression, and gender in transcultural assessment of mental health. *BMC Psychiatry*, 14, 206.

CIS-R—Clinical Interview Schedule—Revised

Fully structured lay interviewer or self- (computer) administered (20–30 minutes). The CIS-R can be used to screen for the presence of psychological morbidity with a scalable morbidity score, and a validated cut-point of ≥12. More recently it has been adapted to generate ICD-10 diagnoses (neurosis only) using a computerized algorithm (PROQSY). Formal training is required. Contact Glyn Lewis (glyn.lewis@ucl.ac.uk) or Martin Prince (martin.prince@kcl.ac.uk) for details.

Das-Munshi, J., Castro-Costa, E., Dewey, M.E., Nazroo, J., and Prince, M. (2014). Cross-cultural factorial validation of the Clinical Interview Schedule--Revised (CIS-R); findings from a nationally representative survey (EMPIRIC). *International Journal of Methods in Psychiatric Research*, 23, 229–244.

Head, J., Stansfeld, S.A., Ebmeier, K.P., Geddes, J.R., Allan, C.L., Lewis, G., and Kivimaki, M. (2013). Use of self-administered instruments to assess psychiatric disorders in older people: validity of the General Health Questionnaire, the Center for Epidemiologic Studies Depression Scale and the self-completion version of the revised Clinical Interview Schedule. *Psychological Medicine*, 43, 2649–2656.

Lewis, G., Pelosi, A.J., Araya, R. and Dunn, G. (1992). Measuring psychiatric disorder in the community: a standardized assessment for use by lay interviewers. *Psychological Medicine*, 22, 465–486.

Children

SDQ–Strengths and Difficulties Questionnaire

A 25-item respondent-based questionnaire with identical parent, teacher, and self-report for common difficulties with emotional symptoms, behavioural difficulties, and hyper-activity (http://www.sdqinfo.com).

Gomez, R. and Stavropoulos, V. (2017). Parent ratings of the Strengths and Difficulties Questionnaire: what is the optimum factor model? *Assessment*, 26, 1142–1153.

Goodman, R. (2001). Psychometric properties of the Strengths and Difficulties Questionnaire (SDQ). *Journal of the American Academy of Child and Adolescent Psychiatry*, 40, 1337–1345.

Stolk, Y., Kaplan, I., and Szwarc, J. (2017). Review of the strengths and difficulties questionnaire translated into languages spoken by children and adolescents of refugee background. *International Journal of Methods in Psychiatric Research*, 26, e1568.

CBCL—Child Behaviour Checklist

The CBCL comprises 118 items and has different versions for parents (CBCL), teacher (TRF Teacher Report Form), and young person (Youth Self-Report).

Achenbach, T.M. (1994). Child Behavior Checklist and related instruments. In: Maruish, M.E. (ed.) *The use of psychological testing for treatment planning and outcome assessment*, pp. 517–549. Hillsdale, NJ: Lawrence Erlbaum Associates, Inc.

Deutz, M.H.F., Vossen, H.G.M., De Haan, A.D., Dekovic, M., Van Baar, A.L., and Prinzie, P. (2018). Normative development of the Child Behavior Checklist Dysregulation Profile from early childhood to adolescence: associations with personality pathology. *Development and Psychopathology*, 30, 437–447.

Rescorla, L.A., Ghassabian, A., Ivanova, M.Y., Jaddoe, V.W., Verhulst, F.C., and Tiemeier, H. (2019). Structure, longitudinal invariance, and stability of the Child Behavior Checklist 1½–5's *Diagnostic and Statistical Manual of Mental Disorders*–Autism Spectrum Disorder scale: findings from Generation R (Rotterdam). *Autism*, 23, 223–235.

Measuring depression

CES-D—Centre for Epidemiological Studies—Depression

Self-administered (5–10 minutes).

Radloff, L.S. (1977). The CES-D scale: a self report depression scale for research in the general population. *Applied Psychological Measurement*, 1, 385–401.

Stafford, L., Judd, F., Gibson, P., Komiti, A., Quinn, M., and Mann, G.B. (2014). Comparison of the hospital anxiety and depression scale and the center for epidemiological studies depression scale for detecting depression in women with breast or gynecologic cancer. *General Hospital Psychiatry*, 36, 74–80.

ZDS—Zung depression scale

Self-administered (5–10 minutes).

Dunstan, D.A., Scott, N., and Todd, A.K. (2017). Screening for anxiety and depression: reassessing the utility of the Zung scales. *BMC Psychiatry*, 17, 329.

Romera, I., Delgado-Cohen, H., Perez, T., Caballero, L., and Gilaberte, I. (2008). Factor analysis of the Zung self-rating depression scale in a large sample of patients with major depressive disorder in primary care. *BMC Psychiatry*, 8, 4.

Zung, W.W.K. (1965). A self-rating depression scale. *Archives of General Psychiatry* 12, 62–70.

GDS—Geriatric Depression Scale (over 65s)

Self-administered (5–10 minutes).

Laudisio, A., Antonelli Incalzi, R., Gemma, A., Marzetti, E., Pozzi, G., Padua, L., et al. (2018). Definition of a Geriatric Depression Scale cutoff based upon quality of life: a population-based study. *International Journal of Geriatric Psychiatry*, 33, e58–e64.

Yesavage, J., Rose, T. and Lum, O. (1983). Development and validation of a Geriatric Depression Screening Scale: a preliminary report. *Journal of Psychiatric Research* 17, 43–49.

Chalder Fatigue Scale

Self-administered (5 minutes).

Chalder, T., Berelowitz, C., and Pawlikowska, T. (1993). Development of a fatigue scale. *Journal of Psychosomatic Research*, 37, 147–154.

Fong, T.C., Chan, J.S., Chan, C.L., Ho, R.T., Ziea, E.T., Wong, V.C., et al. (2015). Psychometric properties of the Chalder Fatigue Scale revisited: an exploratory structural equation modeling approach. *Quality of Life Research*, 24, 2273–2278.

Measuring cognitive function (and screening for dementia)

MMSE—Mini-Mental State Examination

Interviewer administered (10–15 minutes).

Creavin, S.T., Wisniewski, S., Noel-Storr, A.H., Trevelyan, C. M., Hampton, T., Rayment, D., et al. (2016). Mini-Mental State Examination (MMSE) for the detection of dementia in clinically unevaluated people aged 65 and over in community and primary care populations. *Cochrane Database of Systematic Reviews*, CD011145.

Folstein, M.F., Folstein, S.E. and McHugh, P.R. (1975). 'Mini-mental State': a practical method for grading the cognitive state of patients for the clinician. *Journal of Psychiatric Research*, 12, 189–198.

Rubright, J. D., Nandakumar, R., and Karlawish, J. (2016). Identifying an appropriate measurement modeling approach for the Mini-Mental State Examination. *Psychological Assessment*, 28, 125–233.

TICS-m—Modified Telephone Interview for Cognitive Status

Interviewer administered (over the telephone—10–15 minutes).

Brandt, J., Spencer, M. and Folstein, M. (1988). The Telephone Interview for Cognitive Status. *Neuropsychiatry, Neuropsychology and Behavioral Neurology* 1, 111–117.

Zietemann, V., Kopczak, A., Muller, C., Wollenweber, F.A., and Dichgans, M. (2017). Validation of the Telephone Interview of Cognitive Status and Telephone Montreal Cognitive Assessment against detailed cognitive testing and clinical diagnosis of mild cognitive impairment after stroke. *Stroke*, 48, 2952–2957.

CSI-D—Cognitive Screening Instrument for Dementia

Interviewer administered to participant (5–10 minutes) and informant (10 minutes).

Hall, K.S., Gao, S., Emsley, C.L., Ogunniyi, A.O., Morgan, O., and Hendrie, H.C. (2000). Community screening interview for dementia (CSI 'D'); performance in five disparate study sites. *International Journal of Geriatric Psychiatry*, 15, 521–531.

Hall, K.S., Hendrie, H.H., Brittain, H.M., Norton, J.A., Rodgers, D.D., Prince, C.S., et al. (1993). The development of a dementia screening interview in two distinct languages. *International Journal of Methods in Psychiatric Research*, 3, 1–28.

IQ-CODE—Informant Questionnaire on Cognitive Decline in the Elderly

Interviewer administered to informant (10 minutes).

Harrison, J.K., Stott, D.J., McShane, R., Noel-Storr, A.H., Swann-Price, R.S., and Quinn, T.J. (2016). Informant Questionnaire on Cognitive Decline in the Elderly (IQCODE) for the early diagnosis of dementia across a variety of healthcare settings. *Cochrane Database of Systematic Reviews*, 11, CD011333.

Jorm, A.F. (1994) A short form of the Informant Questionnaire on Cognitive Decline in the Elderly (IQCODE): development and cross-validation. *Psychological Medicine*, 24, 145–153.

Instruments generating diagnoses according to established algorithms

Assessing a comprehensive range of clinical diagnoses

General adults (16–64 years)

DIS—Diagnostic Interview Schedule

Interviewer administered (1½–2 hours).

A fully structured, lay interviewer-administered comprehensive diagnostic assessment. Used in the US ECA study, but probably of historical interest only, superseded by the CIDI (see following assessment).

> Robins, L. and Helzer, J.E. (1994). The half-life of a structured interview: the NIMH Diagnostic Interview Schedule (DIS). *International Journal of Methods in Psychiatric Research*, 4, 95–102.

CIDI—Composite International Diagnostic Interview

A fully structured, lay interviewer-administered comprehensive diagnostic assessment. A computer algorithm generates DSM-IV and/or ICD-10 diagnoses (2 hours in its full form, although shorter versions, CIDI-PC and UM-CIDI have also been developed. The neurosis modules can be administered in 20–40 minutes only). Formal training is essential. Contact the WHO for details of local training centres.

> Mitchell, P.B., Johnston, A.K., Frankland, A., Slade, T., Green, M.J., Roberts, G., et al. (2013). Bipolar disorder in a national survey using the World Mental Health Version of the Composite International Diagnostic Interview: the impact of differing diagnostic algorithms. *Acta Psychiatrica Scandinavica*, 127, 381–393.
>
> Shimoda, H., Inoue, A., Tsuno, K. & Kawakami, N. (2015). One-year test-retest reliability of a Japanese web-based version of the WHO Composite International Diagnostic Interview (CIDI) for major depression in a working population. *International Journal of Methods in Psychiatric Research*, 24, 204–212.
>
> Wittchen, H.U. (1994). Reliability and validity studies of the WHO-Composite International Diagnostic Interview (CIDI): a critical review. *Journal of Psychiatric Research*, 28, 57–84.
>
> World Health Organization (1990). *Composite International Diagnostic Interview (CIDI, Version 1.0)*. Geneva: World Health Organization.

SCAN and PSE

A semi-structured, clinician administered comprehensive diagnostic assessment. A computer algorithm generates DSM-IV and/or ICD-10 diagnoses. (1½ to 2 hours, but the neurosis modules can be administered in 20–40 minutes only). Formal training is essential. Contact the WHO for details of local training centres.

> Bech, P., Rasmussen, N.A., Olsen, L.R., Noerholm, V., and Abildgaard, W. (2001). The sensitivity and specificity of the Major Depression Inventory, using the Present State Examination as the index of diagnostic validity. *Journal of Affective Disorders*, 66, 159–164.
>
> Brugha, T.S., Jenkins, R., Taub, N., Meltzer, H., and Bebbington, P.E. (2001). A general population comparison of the Composite International Diagnostic Interview (CIDI) and the Schedules for Clinical Assessment in Neuropsychiatry (SCAN). *Psychological Medicine*, 31, 1001–1013.

WING (1983). Use and misuse of the PSE. *British Journal of Psychiatry*, 143, 111–117.

WING (1996). SCAN and the PSE tradition. *Social Psychiatry and Psychiatric Epidemiology*, 31, 50–54.

Older adults (65 and over)

GMS—Geriatric Mental State

Lay or clinician interviewer administered (25–40 minutes). A semi-structured comprehensive diagnostic assessment for older (≥65 years) participants, with a computerized algorithm to generate 'AGECAT' and ICD-10 or DSM-IV diagnoses. Formal training is necessary. Contact Martin Prince (martin.prince@kcl.ac.uk) for details of local centres.

Copeland, J.R.M., Dewey, M.E., and Griffith-Jones, H.M. (1986). A computerised psychiatric diagnostic system and case nomenclature for elderly participants: GMS and AGECAT. *Psychological Medicine*, 16, 89–99.

Prince, M., Acosta, D., Chiu, H., Copeland, J., Dewey, M., Scazufca, M., et al. (2004). Effects of education and culture on the validity of the Geriatric Mental State and its AGECAT algorithm. *British Journal of Psychiatry*, 185, 429–436.

CAMDEX

Interviewer administered to participant and informant (1 hour).

Estabrook, R., Sadler, M.E., and McGue, M. (2015). Differential item functioning in the Cambridge Mental Disorders in the Elderly (CAMDEX) Depression Scale across middle age and late life. *Psychological Assessment*, 27, 1219–1233.

Roth, M., Tym, E., Mountjoy, C.Q., Huppert, F.A., Hendrie, H., Verma, S., and Goddard, R. (1986). CAMDEX. A standardised instrument for the diagnosis of mental disorder in the elderly with special reference to the early detection of dementia. *British Journal of Psychiatry*, 149, 698–709.

Childhood psychiatric disorder

DAWBA

Development and well-being assessment for DSM-IV or ICD-10 disorders in 5–17-year-olds. Structured interview administered by computer or trained lay-interviewer, with versions for parents, teachers, and young people (http://www.dawba.com).

Goodman, A., Heiervang, E., Collishaw, S., and Goodman, R. (2011). The 'DAWBA bands' as an ordered-categorical measure of child mental health: description and validation in British and Norwegian samples. *Social Psychiatry and Psychiatric Epidemiology*, 46, 521–532.

Goodman, R., Ford, T., Richards, H., Gatward, R., and Meltzer, H. (2000) The Development and Well-Being Assessment: description and initial validation of an integrated assessment of child and adolescent psychopathology. *Journal of Child Psychology and Psychiatry*, 41, 645–655.

CAPA—Child and Adolescent Psychiatric Assessment

Semi-structured assessment administered by clinicians or lay people trained in the CAPA for 8–18-year-olds.

Angold, A., Prendergast, M., Cox, A., and Harrington, R. (1995). The Child and Adolescent Psychiatric Assessment. *Psychological Medicine*, 25, 739–753.

Wamboldt, M.Z., Wamboldt, F.S., Gavin, L., and McTaggart, S. (2001). A parent–child relationship scale derived from the Child and Adolescent Psychiatric Assessment (CAPA). *Journal of the American Academy of Child and Adolescent Psychiatry*, 40, 945–953.

DISC—Diagnostic Interview Schedule for Children

Highly structured interview for 6–17-year-olds with parent, child, and teacher versions.

Shaffer, D., Schwab-Stone, M., Fisher, P., Cohen, P., Piacentini, J., Davies, M., et al. (1993). The Diagnostic Interview Schedule for Children—revised version (DISC-R) 1. Preparation, field testing, interrater reliability and acceptability. *Journal of the American Academy of Child and Adolescent Psychiatry*, 32, 643–650.

Shaffer, D., Fisher, P., Lucas, C. P., Dulcan, M.K., and Schwab-Stone, M.E. (2000). NIMH Diagnostic Interview Schedule for Children Version IV (NIMH DISC-IV): description, differences from previous versions, and reliability of some common diagnoses. *Journal of the American Academy of Child and Adolescent Psychiatry*, 39, 28–38.

Assessing personality disorder

SAP—Standardized Assessment of Personality

Interviewer administered to informant (20–30 minutes). Formal training is required. Contact Martin Prince (martin.prince@kcl.ac.uk) for details.

Mann, A.H., Raven, P., Pilgrim, J., Khanna, S., Velayudham, A., Suresh, K.P., et al. (1999). An assessment of the Standardized Assessment of Personality as a screening instrument for the International Personality Disorder Examination: a comparison of informant and patient assessment for personality disorder. *Psychological Medicine*, 29, 985–989.

Pilgrim, J.A. and Mann, A.H. (1990). Use of the ICD-10 version of the Standardized Assessment of Personality to determine the prevalence of personality disorder in psychiatric in-patients. *Psychological Medicine*, 20, 985–992.

Pilgrim, J.A., Mellers, J.D., Boothby, H.A., and Mann, A.H. (1993). Inter-rater and temporal reliability of the Standardized Assessment of Personality and the influence of informant characteristics. *Psychological Medicine*, 23, 779–786.

Measures of other variables, relevant to mental disorder

Measuring stable traits

EPQ—Eysenck Personality Questionnaire (Neuroticism, Extroversion/ Introversion, Psychoticism)

The EPQ is copyrighted. Contact GL Assessment for permission and information regarding copyright fees.

Bowden, S.C., Saklofske, D.H., van de Vijver, F.J.R., Sudarshan, N.J., and Eysenck, S.B.G. (2016). Cross-cultural measurement invariance of the Eysenck Personality Questionnaire across 33 countries. *Personality and Individual Differences*, 103, 53–60.

Eysenck, H.J. (1959). The differentiation between normal and various neurotic groups on the Maudsley Personality Inventory. *British Journal of Psychology*, 50, 176–177.

PBI—Parental Bonding Inventory

Parker, G., Tupling, H., and Brown, L.B. (1979). A parental bonding instrument. *British Journal of Medical Psychology*, 52, 1–10.

Uehara, T., Sato, T., Sakado, K., and Someya, T. (1998). Parental Bonding Instrument and the Inventory to Diagnose Depression Lifetime version in a volunteer sample of Japanese workers. *Depression and Anxiety*, 8, 65–70.

Measuring life events

LTE—List of Threatening Events

An 11-item self-report scale. Self or interviewer administered (5–10 minutes).

Brugha, T.S., Bebbington, P., Tennant, C., and Hurry, J. (1985). The List of Threatening Experiences: a subset of 12 life event categories with considerable long-term contextual threat. *Psychological Medicine*, 15, 189–194.

Brugha, T.S. and Cragg, D. (1990). The List of Threatening Experiences: the reliability and validity of a brief life events questionnaire. *Acta Psychiatrica Scandinavica*, 82, 77–81.

Measuring social support

SPQ—Social Problems Questionnaire

Self or interviewer administered (10 minutes).

Corney, R.H. and Clare, A.W. (1985). The construction, development and testing of a self-report questionnaire to identify social problems. *Psychological. Medicine*, 15, 637–649.

CPQ—Close Persons Questionnaire

Interviewer administered (10–20 minutes).

Stansfeld, S. and Marmot, M. (1992). Deriving a survey measure of social support: the reliability and validity of the Close Persons Questionnaire. *Social Science and Medicine*, 35, 1027–1035.

Describing social network

Social Network Assessment Instrument

Self- or interviewer administered (5–10 minutes).

Wenger, G.C. (1989). Support networks in old age: constructing a typology. In: Jeffreys, M. (ed.) *Growing Old in the Twentieth Century*, pp. 166–185. London: Routledge.

Quality of Life

WHOQOL-BREF

Self-report or interviewer administered (10–15 minutes). Contact the WHO for details (e-mail: whoqol@who.ch).

Theuns, P., Hofmans, J., Mazaheri, M., Van Acker, F., and Bernheim, J.L. (2010). Cross-national comparability of the WHOQOL-BREF: a measurement invariance approach. *Quality of Life Research*, 19, 219–224.

World Health Organization (1997). *Measuring Quality of Life. The World Health Organization Quality of Life Instruments (The WHO-QOL-100 and the WHOQOL-BREF)*. WHO/MNH/PSF/97.4. Geneva: WHO.

Overall health/disablement

LHS—London Handicap Scale

Self or interviewer administered (5–10 minutes)

Harwood, R.H., Gompertz, P. and Ebrahim, S. (1994). Handicap one year after a stroke: validity of a new scale. *Journal of Neurology, Neurosurgery, and Psychiatry*, 57, 825–829.

Lo, R.S., Kwok, T.C., Cheng, J.O., Yang, H., Yuan, H.J., Harwood, R., and Woo, J. (2007). Cross-cultural validation of the London Handicap Scale and comparison of handicap perception between Chinese and UK populations. *Age and Ageing*, 36, 544–548.

SF-36—36-Item Short Form Health Survey

A 36-item self-report or interviewer administered measure of health-related quality of life (15–20 minutes). Perhaps the best validated and most widely used measure internationally. The SF-36 is copyrighted. Contact the instrument developers for permission to use.

McHorney, C.A., Ware, J.E., Lu, J.F., and Sherbourne, C.D. (1994). The MOS 36-item Short-Form Health Survey (SF-36): III. Tests of data quality, scaling assumptions, and reliability across diverse patient groups. *Medical Care*, 32, 40–66.

McHorney C.A., Ware J.E., and Raczek A.E. (1993). The MOS 36-Item Short-Form Health Survey (SF-36): II. Psychometric and clinical tests of validity in measuring physical and mental health constructs. *Medical Care*, 31, 247–263.

Su, C.T., Ng, H.S., Yang, A.L., and Lin, C.Y. (2014). Psychometric evaluation of the Short Form 36 Health Survey (SF-36) and the World Health Organization Quality of Life Scale Brief Version (WHOQOL-BREF) for patients with schizophrenia. *Psychological Assessment*, 26, 980–989.

Tucker, G., Adams, R., and Wilson, D. (2016). The case for using country-specific scoring coefficients for scoring the SF-12, with scoring implications for the SF-36. *Quality of Life Research*, 25, 267–274.

Ware, J.E., Jr. and Sherbourne, J.C. (1992). The MOS 36-item short-form health survey (SF-36). I. Conceptual framework and item selection. *Medical Care*, 30, 473–483.

SF-12—Short Form-12 (reduced version of MOS SF-36)

Self or interviewer administered (5–10 minutes). This shortened version generates simply a 'mental health component score' and a physical health component score' indicating respectively the consequences of heath impairments within these domains.

Desouky, T.F., Mora, P.A., and Howell, E.A. (2013). Measurement invariance of the SF-12 across European-American, Latina, and African-American postpartum women. *Quality of Life Research*, 22, 1135–1144.

Jenkinson, C. and Layte, R. (1998). Development and testing of the UK SF-12. *J Journal of Health Services Research and Policy*, 2, 14–18.

A fuller account of validated health measures, with particular reference to older participants, is contained in:

Braam, A.W., Copeland, J.R., Delespaul, P.A., Beekman, A.T., Como, A., Dewey, M., et al. (2014). Depression, subthreshold depression and comorbid anxiety symptoms in older Europeans: results from the EURODEP concerted action. *Journal of Affective Disorders*, 155, 266–272.

Prince, M.J., Harwood, R., Thomas, A., and Mann, A.H. (1997). Gospel Oak V. Impairment, disability and handicap as risk factors for depression in old age. *Psychological Medicine* 27, 311–321.

Practical exercises

Questions

1. A new screening questionnaire has been developed for identifying cases of schizophrenia. The method was developed, and then validated in a 'first-onset schizophrenia' service taking referrals of possible cases from primary care. The prediction provided

by the questionnaire was validated against the gold standard of SCAN diagnosis in the clinic setting. Results of the validation in this sample were as shown in Table 2.4.

Table 2.4

Test\gold standard	SCAN –ve	SCAN +ve	Totals
Test –ve	259	45	304
Test + ve	23	801	824
Totals	282	846	1128

a. What is the prevalence of schizophrenia in this sample?
b. What are the psychometric properties of the test:
   ◆ the sensitivity?
   ◆ the specificity?
   ◆ the positive predictive value (PPV)?
   ◆ the negative predictive value (NPV)?

2. The test is now tried out in the general population in the course of a national psychiatric morbidity survey. In this sample, the prevalence of schizophrenia is 0.5%. Assuming that the sensitivity and specificity of the test are the same as in the validation exercise, we would anticipate the following findings among (say) 10,000 participants (Table 2.5).

Table 2.5

Test\gold standard	Karyotyping –ve	Karyotyping +ve	Totals
Test –ve	9134	3	9137
Test + ve	816	47	863
Totals	9950	50	10,000

What is:
   a. the PPV of the test?
   b. the NPV of the test?

3. What is the relationship between PPV and prevalence (establish this for yourself empirically, if you like, by further varying prevalence in the earlier example, and keeping sensitivity and specificity constant).

4. We assumed that sensitivity and specificity would not vary as prevalence of the disorder changed in moving from the high-risk clinic referral population to the low-risk general population sample. Is this a reasonable assumption? What, if anything, do you think would be the effect of changing prevalence on sensitivity and specificity?

5. What other factors might affect the sensitivity and specificity of a test from that reported in its initial validation study?

Answers

1.
   a. 75%.
   b.
      ◆ Sensitivity: 94.7%.
      ◆ Specificity: 91.8%.
      ◆ PPV: 97.2%.
      ◆ NPV: 85.2%.

2.
   a. PPV: 5.4%
   b. NPV: 99.97%

3. As the prevalence falls the PPV falls as well. For a very rare condition, even when the test has good specificity the number of false positives overwhelms the number of true positives. This is an important point to grasp, with major implications for clinical epidemiology. Most screening (and clinical) tests only work well when the *prior probability*, that is, the probability that someone is a case before any other information (i.e. test results) is known about them, is reasonably high. This is sometimes used as a justification for having primary care doctors as 'gatekeepers' responsible for referring people to specialist clinical services. Good primary care doctors quickly and efficiently screen out likely non-cases (e.g. 'innocent' headaches) before referring those at high risk (high prior probability) to a specialist (e.g. neurologist for magnetic resonance imaging (MRI) scans to exclude brain tumour)

4. This should be a reasonable assumption. Note that sensitivity and specificity are calculated within columns of the cross tab. PPV and NPV are calculated within rows, and hence are affected by prevalence.

5. The validity coefficients of a test may vary from one setting to another, depending upon the nature of the test. Screening questionnaires may be affected by cultural or language factors, or by the characteristics of the interviewer administering the questionnaire. Tests requiring interpretation (e.g. MRI scans) may be affected by the skills of the clinician. In general, greater care is probably taken in research validation exercises, and the sensitivities and specificities from these studies may not be matched in realistic clinical practice.

References

Altman, D.G. and Bland, J.M. (1994). Diagnostic tests. 1: sensitivity and specificity. *BMJ*, **308**, 1552.

Asberg, M., Perris, C., Schalling, D., and Sedvall, G. (1978). CPRS: development and applications of a psychiatric rating scale. *Acta Psychiatrica Scandinavica*, Suppl 271, 1–69.

Bland, J.M. and Altman, D.G. (1986). Statistical methods for assessing agreement between two methods of clinical measurement. *Lancet*, **1**, 307–310.

Brailean, A., Guerra, M., Chua, K.C., Prince, M., and Prina, M.A. (2015). A multiple indicators multiple causes model of late-life depression in Latin American countries. *Journal of Affective Disorders*, 184, 129–136.

Cohen, J. (1960). A coefficient of agreement for nominal scales. *Educational and Psychological Measurement*, 20, 37–46.

Cronbach, L.E. and Meehl, P.E. (1955). Construct validity in psychological tests. *Psychological Bulletin*, 52, 281–302.

Cronbach, L.J. (1951). Coefficient alpha and the internal structure of tests. *Psychometrika*, 16, 297–334.

Cuthbert, B.N. and Insel, T.R. (2013). Toward the future of psychiatric diagnosis: the seven pillars of RDoC. *BMC Medicine*, 11, 126.

Fox, R.A. (1994). *Parent behaviour checklist*. Brandon, VT: Clinical Psychology Publishing Company.

Galboda-Liyanage, K.C., Prince, M.J., and Scott, S. (2003). Mother-child joint activity and behaviour problems of pre-school children. *Journal of Child Psychology and Psychiatry*, 44, 1037–1048.

Greenwood, T.A., Swerdlow, N.R., Gur, R.E., Cadenhead, K.S., Calkins, M.E., Dobie, D.J., et al. (2013). Genome-wide linkage analyses of 12 endophenotypes for schizophrenia from the Consortium on the Genetics of Schizophrenia. *American Journal of Geriatric Psychiatry*, 170, 521–532.

Hanlon, C., Medhin, G., Alem, A., Araya, M., Abdulahi, A., Tesfaye, M., et al. (2008). Measuring common mental disorders in women in Ethiopia: Reliability and construct validity of the comprehensive psychopathological rating scale. *Social Psychiatry and Psychiatric Epidemiology*, 43, 653–659.

Hays, R.D. and Hadorn, D. (1992). Responsiveness to change: an aspect of validity, not a separate dimension. *Quality of Life Research*, 1, 73–75.

Husted, J.A., Cook, R.J., Farewell, V.T., and Gladman, D.D. (2000). Methods for assessing responsiveness: a critical review and recommendations. *Journal of Clinical Epidemiology*, 53, 459–468.

Jordanova, V., Wickramesinghe, C., Gerada, C., and Prince, M. (2004). Validation of two survey diagnostic interviews among primary care attendees: a comparison of CIS-R and CIDI with SCAN ICD-10 diagnostic categories. *Psychological Medicine*, 34, 1013–1024.

Kumari, G.L., Prince, M., and Scott, S. (2000). The development and validation of the Parent–Child Joint Activity Scale (PJAS). *International Journal of Methods in Psychiatric Research*, 8, 219–227.

Lobbestael, J., Leurgans, M., and Arntz, A. (2011). Inter-rater reliability of the Structured Clinical Interview for DSM-IV Axis I Disorders (SCID I) and Axis II Disorders (SCID II). *Clinical Psychology & Psychotherapy*, 18, 75–79.

Messick, S. (1995). Validity of psychological assessment: validation of inferences from persons' responses and performances as scientific enquiry into score meaning. *American Psychologist*, 50, 749.

Newton, P.E. and Shaw, S.D. (2013). Standards for talking and thinking about validity. *Psychological Methods*, 18, 301–319.

Prince, M.J., Reischies, F., Beekman, A.T.F., Fuhrer, R., Hooijer, C., Kivela, S., et al. (1999). The development of the EURO-D scale—a European Union initiative to compare symptoms of depression in 14 European centres. *British Journal of Psychiatry*, 174, 330–338.

Shrout, P.E. and Fleiss, J.L. (1979). Intraclass correlations: uses in assessing rater reliability. *Psychological Bulletin*, 86, 420–428.

Sijtsma, K. (2009). On the use, the misuse, and the very limited usefulness of Cronbach's Alpha. *Psychometrika*, 74, 107–120.

Streiner, D.L. and Cairney, J. (2007). What's under the ROC? An introduction to receiver operating characteristics curves. *Canadian Journal of Psychiatry*, 52, 121–128.

Streiner, D.L., Norman, G.R., and Cairney, J. (2015). *Health measurement scales: a practical guide to their development and use.* Oxford: Oxford University Press.

Tasse, M.J., Schalock, R.L., Thissen, D., Balboni, G., Bersani, H.H., Jr., Borthwick-Duffy, S.A., et al. (2016). Development and standardization of the Diagnostic Adaptive Behavior Scale: application of item response theory to the assessment of adaptive behavior. *American Journal on Intellectual and Developmental Disabilities,* 121, 79–94.

Weobong, B., Akpalu, B., Doku, V., Owusu-Agyei, S., Hurt, L., Kirkwood, B., and Prince, M. (2009). The comparative validity of screening scales for postnatal common mental disorder in Kintampo, Ghana. *Journal of Affective Disorders,* 113, 109–117.

Zinbarg, R.E. (2006). Estimating generalizability to a latent variable common to all of a scale's indicators: a comparison of estimators for ωh. *Applied Psychological Measurement* 30, 121–144.

Zumbo, B.D. and Chan, E.K.H. (2014). *Validity and validation in social, behavioural, and health sciences.* New York: Springer International Publishing.

Chapter 3

Culture and psychiatric epidemiology

Brandon A. Kohrt and Vikram Patel

Introduction

Cross-cultural studies of schizophrenia, suicide, and other neuropsychiatric conditions illustrate the challenges in interpreting the role of culture and the importance of conceptualizing culture clearly when designing and implementing psychiatric epidemiology studies (Box 3.1). Culture shapes the meaning and social experience of mental illness (Kleinman, 1988), influences the types of exposures to factors that cause mental illness and moderates the relationship between risks and mental health outcomes. Cultural variations in describing, disclosing, and categorizing suffering are also sources of potential bias in epidemiological research (Flaherty et al., 1988). If we acknowledge that culture plays a key role in influencing the epidemiology of psychiatric disorders, then by definition, cultural issues in measurement and research are relevant in every epidemiological investigation. The concepts and methods described in this chapter provide a guide for both *what* to ask in relation to culture and psychiatric epidemiology and *how* to ask about it in a manner that reduces cross-cultural bias. This chapter reviews historical periods and key concepts that have shaped approaches to culture and mental health. The applications of culture to psychiatric epidemiology are outlined, including the need for multicultural, multidisciplinary research teams. The chapter concludes with a practical exercise to design and implement a study of culture and mental health.

Definitions of culture and relevance to mental health

Culture is often poorly defined in research studies. In population health, it is frequently invoked as a 'black box' to broadly refer to unexplained variance in a study (Hruschka, 2009). Definitions of culture have been reviewed to identify common elements that could be operationalized and measured in epidemiological research. These elements are 'values, beliefs, knowledge, norms, and practices and the notion that that these are shared among a specific set of people' (Hruschka and Hadley, 2008, p. 947). Beliefs refer to conscious psychological processes. Norms are behaviours maintained by social sanctioning and affective responses. Values are valences placed on beliefs, knowledge, and norms that lead to engagement in or avoidance of behaviours.

Box 3.1 Challenges in cross-national and cross-cultural studies of schizophrenia

The International Pilot Study of Schizophrenia (IPSS) was a World Health Organization (WHO) initiative to compare the prevalence and outcomes of schizophrenia across nations (Sartorius et al., 1972). The IPSS and subsequent replication studies presented a paradox: persons with schizophrenia in low- and middle-income countries appeared to have better prognoses than persons in high-income countries, despite greater availability of psychiatric services in the latter (Hopper and Wanderling, 2000; Harrison et al., 2001). Some researchers have suggested that these findings result from cultural differences in expressed emotion, attribution of mental illness, family care, social inclusion, and content of hallucinations (Leff et al., 1987; Kulhara and Chakrabarti, 2001; Larøi et al., 2014). However, methodological shortcomings including lack of testable cultural hypotheses and failure to distinguish between culture and health context limited the validity and generalizability of these findings (Patel et al., 2006). Moreover, follow-up studies have demonstrated poor prognosis in low- and middle-income countries (Thara et al., 1994). Recent studies also have demonstrated that Western-based instruments may miss schizophrenia diagnoses in different cultures. In an Ethiopian population, the Composite International Diagnostic Interview (CIDI) failed to identify cases of schizophrenia. However, when using a cultural concept of distress (*marata*), researchers were able to identify persons with schizophrenia and other severe mental illness (Shibre et al., 2010). *These limitations in cross-national studies highlight the need for rigorous approaches to operationalize culture, distinguish between culture and context, and account for cultural differences in the assessment.*

Differentiating culture from other social and contextual labels

When defining culture, it is equally important to clarify what is *not* culture. Culture should not be conflated with ecology or other aspects of context, which may be in transaction with culture but are separate phenomena (Hruschka and Hadley, 2008). For example, though neighbourhood composition, city layout, and social hierarchies are all shaped by culture, they should be studied as separate variables accordingly. Public health researchers, social epidemiologists, and anthropologists have critiqued public health research for conflating culture with contextual factors such as poverty, lack of access to resources, barriers to education, and experiences of marginalization and discrimination (Krieger, 2005; Marmot et al., 2008; Metzl and Hansen, 2014). A key contextual factor is the health system. Putative differences in healthcare outcomes are influenced strongly by health systems factors, such as differential access to and quality of healthcare based on race and ethnicity (Physicians for Human Rights, 2003). Health systems design, priorities, and funding are shaped by the cultural beliefs, norms, and preferences of groups in power (Baer et al., 2003). Therefore, studies need to evaluate both context (e.g. poverty and health system structures) and cultural elements that shape context (e.g. economic values and consumption norms).

Similarly, culture shapes the distribution and impact of social determinants of health. Social determinants of health are social and economic factors impacting prevalence and severity of mental disorders, such as poverty, income inequality, interpersonal and collective violence, and forced migration (Lund et al., 2018). For example, culture shapes the values that determine whether a small percentage of the population can control the majority of societies wealth, i.e., the level of income inequality. Similarly, culture shapes whether gender-based violence or collective violence against certain ethnic, religious, or political groups is acceptable.

Another pitfall in culture and epidemiology research is confusing cross-cultural studies with cross-national studies. *Cross-cultural studies* refer to those that compare mental health symptom presentation, prognosis, treatment seeking, or other factors *between groups that differ based on values, beliefs, knowledge, norms, and practices*. In contrast, *cross-national studies* compare mental health prevalence, prognosis, or other factors across different countries. Because values, beliefs, knowledge, norms, and practices can be as variable within as between nations, it is not accurate to assume that cross-national differences are synonymous with cultural differences. To describe different cultural groups, there needs to be demonstration that groups, which could be nationalities, differ based on specific values, beliefs, and the other components of culture that co-vary with mental health outcomes.

Conflating culture with race, ethnicity, and language is a pitfall that often results in misleading research outcomes and unfounded public health or clinical recommendations. Membership in a racial or ethnic group does not guarantee shared norms, beliefs, and practices. The *Lancet* Commission on Culture and Health states, 'Culture ... does not equate solely with ethnic identity, nor does it merely refer to groups of people who share the same racial heritage' (Napier et al., 2014, p. 1609). Racial categories increasingly are understood as social constructs rather than biological categories. There is greater genetic heterogeneity in traits that influence health and behaviour *within* rather than *between* racial groups (Brown and Armelagos, 2001). Presumed biological differences in health outcomes (so-called racial differences) are largely the result of differences in socioeconomic status and experiences of racism rather than in genetics (Gravlee et al., 2009). Therefore, researchers need to specify their definition of cultural categories and clarify how the categorization is not only based on race, census ethnicity classifications, or political groupings.

Cultural concepts can be used to improve psychiatric genetic research (see Chapter 20). In a gene-by-environment-*by-culture* comparison, Kim and colleagues (2010) examined a three-way interaction of culture (defined as ethnicity) finding that the same oxytocin genotype predicted the degree of social support seeking in American and Korean American samples but not in a Korean sample, suggesting the genotype reflects environmental sensitivity to culturally normative behaviour when distressed. In another study, a

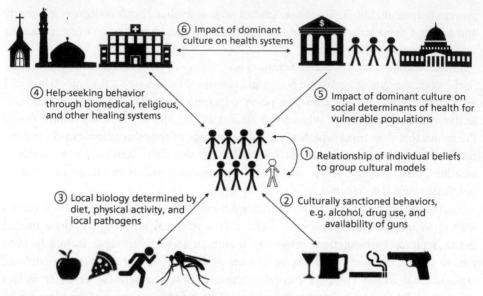

Figure 3.1 Pathways for the interaction of culture and mental health.

single nucleotide polymorphism that interacts with child maltreatment to predict post-traumatic stress disorder in some cultural groups, defined as different populations, e.g., African-descent, European-descent, Asian, and South Asian, was found to associate with depression in other populations (Kohrt et al., 2015).

Cultural pathways and mental health

Based on the understanding that culture refers to shared values, beliefs, knowledge, norms, and practices, we can consider examples that would be appropriate to refer to as cultural or cross-cultural studies of mental health (Figure 3.1).

Historical overview of culture and mental health

Comparative psychiatry

Emile Kraepelin, a German physician, developed the categorization system of mental illness that is now the central framework for psychiatry. He founded the field of *comparative psychiatry* (German: *vergleichende Psychiatrie*) to study if mental illness in places around the world differed from those in Europe (Jilek, 1995). Comparative psychiatry was characterized by the dichotomy of form and content, with *form* referring to universal features in pathology of mental disorders and *content* to the experiential (cultural) processes that shape how disorders manifest in a particular context. For example, dementia praecox (now schizophrenia) had a comparable form across populations studied, but the content of the disorder varied. Kraepelin stated that all clinical features of dementia praecox were present in Javanese (i.e. the form was consistent), but agitated behaviour was more common, auditory hallucinations played a minor role, and delusions were not systematized (i.e. the content differed) (Jilek, 1995). A criticism of comparative psychiatry is that the lack of attention to personal, familial, and cultural meanings attributed to the experience of mental illness (Kleinman, 1988).

Universalist–relativist approaches

In the mid-twentieth century, some psychiatrists and anthropologists began emphasizing cultural uniqueness and challenging the application of psychiatric labels in non-Western groups. This established two different lenses for examining mental health: a *universalist* lens in which a generalizable framework (often assumed to be biomedicine) is applied across all populations and a *relativist* approach in which mental illness is viewed from the specific categorizations of the local culture. Within the field of medical anthropology, these two perspectives are identified as emic versus etic perspectives, based on linguistic classifications of phonemic versus phonetic (Hahn, 1995). *Emic* distinctions are relevant within a cultural group whereas *etic* distinctions are putatively categories universally applied across populations. In mental health, the *Diagnostic and Statistical Manual of Mental Disorders (DSM)* or International Classification of Disease (ICD) categories are often used as the etic categorization systems.

There is now a large body of literature indicating similitudes in emic categories of psychological distress. A systematic review identified 138 publications mentioning 'thinking too much', with examples from every populated continent including terms such as *kufungisisa* (Zimbabwe), *reflechi twòp* (Haiti), *pensando mucho* (Nicaragua), and *kut careen* (Cambodia) (Kaiser et al., 2015). Across cultures, 'thinking too much' is characterized by ruminative, intrusive, and anxious thoughts that, if prolonged, result in a range of physical and psychological complaints. Moreover, coping mechanisms share commonalities across cultures, for example, controlling or suppressing thoughts, distraction, and engaging in social activities, all of which overlap with evidence-based psychological treatments.

The new cross-cultural psychiatry

The new cross-cultural psychiatry began in the late 1970s with Arthur Kleinman's work critiquing the lack of social context in psychiatry and the misapplication of Western diagnostic labels. A major contribution was the concept of *category fallacy*, which is a critique of the assumption that symptoms and behaviours have comparable personal and social meaning regardless of cultural context (Kleinman, 1988). This highlights the pitfall of solely using etic perspectives. The new cross-cultural psychiatry increased attention on the social origins of suffering, stigma, and morality, including the role of health systems in shaping trajectories of suffering. A goal of the new cross-cultural psychiatry was to understand the social origins of distress and how individuals, families, and societies addressed this distress. The new cross-cultural psychiatry also focused on how biomedical treatments and public health efforts could have unintended effects that worsened rather than improved patient and family well-being.

Box 3.2 Instruments to assess explanatory models

The *Short Explanatory Model Interview* (SEMI). The SEMI is an interview derived from Kleinman's explanatory model concept that aims to elicit a person's view about his/her illness. The advantages of this interview are its simple, open-ended format and brevity, which enable it to be incorporated as part of ongoing epidemiological studies. This interview provides contextual information on symptoms by eliciting patients' views about causes or outcomes (Lloyd et al., 1998).

The *Explanatory Model Interview Catalogue* (EMIC) is a comprehensive interview to document patterns of distress, perceived causes, treatment preferences, and general illness beliefs (Weiss, 1997). The EMIC generates both quantitative and qualitative data. The EMIC has been used globally on a wide variety of illnesses.

The *McGill Illness Narrative Interview* (MINI) is a semi-structured interview protocol for eliciting symptom experience, illness narratives, and help seeking. It facilitates production of multiple narratives: a basic narrative account structured by contiguity, a prototype narrative centred on previous experiences, and an explanatory model narrative organized by causes and mechanisms (Groleau et al., 2006). The MINI has been used in studies of depression, medically unexplained symptoms, non-epileptic seizures, and severe mental illness.

Another contribution was the *explanatory model*, which highlights the role of personal and social meaning in experiences of illness (Box 3.2). Explanatory models have been incorporated in psychiatric clinical care, such as through the Cultural Formulation Interview, which is a component of the *DSM-5* (Lewis-Fernandez et al., 2015).

Global mental health

Global mental health (GMH) is characterized by four key principles: (1) mixed methods approaches such as epidemiology combined with ethnographic and other qualitative approaches; (2) participatory methods in which local communities participate in the research process through priority-setting activities and guiding care development and implementation; (3) multidisciplinary approaches, exemplified by endeavours that bring together clinicians, public health researchers, epidemiologists, economists, and policy researchers; and (4) emphasis on knowledge uptake and dissemination in which the primary objective is increased access to evidence-based services around the world (Patel et al., 2014).

GMH is based on the principles of *health systems research*, which is an approach to elucidate how health systems develop, the actors involved, and the impact of health systems on population health (Varkevisser et al., 1991). Therefore, GMH can be a powerful tool to elucidate gaps in policies, planning, and implementation, and to uncover potential cultural biases that underlie such shortcomings. GMH addresses the confounding factors of the health system while generating practical solutions for public health problems in the community. Epidemiological research practices that project astronomical prevalence rates of mental illness without attention to demonstrating affordable solutions are unlikely to influence health policy.

GMH builds on new cross-cultural psychiatry's attention to social determinants of health. GMH recognizes that health is profoundly influenced by the complex interaction of numerous social, political, economic, and historical factors and goes further to offer pragmatic models for studying and intervening to improve mental health. GMH's approach to culture and mental health is important because it acknowledges the cross-country homogeneity of health systems. For example, even though urban Asian and African settings have substantial 'cultural' differences, they may share many health system characteristics allowing research in one setting to better inform health services in the other. In contrast, urban and rural Asian settings, even though 'culturally' related, may actually differ greatly in their health systems. Moreover, there is increasing evidence for the role of common practice elements in psychological treatments that are effective across a wide range of cultural contexts (Murray et al., 2014). GMH employs combined emic–etic approaches to assess mental health problems and to adapt interventions so that they can have optimal benefit for populations and minimize risk of stigma or other unintended consequences (Patel et al., 2011; Chowdhary et al., 2014). GMH also takes cultural issues into account when considering the most effective avenues for disseminating evidence. Cultural issues play a key role in who has access to and authority for knowledge dissemination and uptake, such as through Community Advisory Boards (see Chapter 24 on evidence-based mental health policy for participatory approaches for equitable and ethical dissemination).

Applications to psychiatric epidemiology

Understanding culture will influence both *what* is measured in epidemiological studies and *how* these measurements are made. This section addresses both of these areas, including ways to reduce measurement bias in cross-cultural mental health research. Major sources of bias include failures to (1) verify the cross-cultural equivalence of measurement instruments for mental health, (2) distinguish cultural groups from national or regional groups, and (3) integrate culture into statistical models and analyses. Methodological differences are important contributors of inter-study variability in cross-national studies, such as accounting for 28% of variability in depression rates as evidenced in a 2009 meta-analysis (Steel et al., 2009). These issues point toward the need for a rigorous approach to the measurement of culture and its influences on assessing mental health.

Measurement of cultural variables

A primary challenge is to address the meaning of a 'cultural group'. It is crucial that researchers clarify when categories are based on self-identification, nationality, linguistic proficiency, census groupings, or medical record categories. The Group for Advancement of Psychiatry committee on cultural psychiatry created reporting guidelines for culture in research, especially epidemiological studies that make claims on how culture accounts for explanatory power, moderating effects, and other processes (Lewis-Fernández et al., 2013). In addition, the Systematic Assessment of Quality in Observational Research (SAQOR) has been adopted for reporting culture aspects of psychiatric epidemiology (Kohrt et al., 2014).

An improvement upon limiting culture to an ethnic or racial label is to measure specific beliefs, norms, and values (Hruschka and Hadley, 2008). This facilitates hypothesis testing and can provide actionable results for interventions. *Cultural consonance modelling* is a method to quantitatively identify sets of values, preferences, and so on and the degree to which a person endorses these beliefs (Dressler, 2012). Another approach, *social network analysis* (SNA), examines group membership and quantifies connections an individual has to different groups and linkages among groups (Scott, 2012). In a globalizing world, this is beneficial as it does not presume association with only one cultural group. It can be used to analyse face-to-face networks and connections via social media, telephone, and other forms of non-proximity communication. SNA has been used to examine cultural group influences on smoking and drug use, obesity, and mood (Ennett et al., 2006; Fowler and Christakis, 2008). SNA can facilitate hypothesis-driven epidemiology on acculturation and health because it allows modelling of how health burdens change with migration, globalization, and other movements of people and ideas (Broesch and Hadley, 2012).

There is no perfect solution for measuring culture, and approaches should vary based on the study needs. Ultimately, the key is for epidemiological studies to report how culture, race, or ethnicity were categorized and the rationale, implications, and limitations associated with such categorizations (Lewis-Fernández et al., 2013).

Measurement of symptoms and diagnoses

There are two general approaches to measuring mental health. In one, the starting point is biomedical psychiatric categories based on *DSM* or ICD criteria. The other is to develop a novel scale with locally salient categories of distress (Figure 3.2). Each approach has benefits and drawbacks (Weaver and Kaiser, 2015). When adapting Western-developed psychiatric tools for cross-cultural comparison of biomedical psychiatric categories, the objective is *measurement invariance*, which assumes that 'individuals who are identical on the construct being measured, but are from different populations, have the same probability of achieving any given score on a test' (Millsap and Kwok, 2004, p. 93). Content, semantic, technical, criterion, and conceptual equivalence are needed to achieve measurement invariance (Flaherty et al., 1988) (see Chapter 2).

A qualitative *transcultural translation and adaptation process* has been developed that draws on the above-mentioned equivalences to optimize cross-cultural measurement invariance for adults (Van Ommeren et al., 1999) and has been adapted for children and adolescents (Kohrt et al., 2011). Qualitative research methods are used to evaluate each item on five criteria: comprehensibility, acceptability, relevance, response set issues, and completeness (Box 3.3). Using these principles, the tool goes through the following steps: (1)

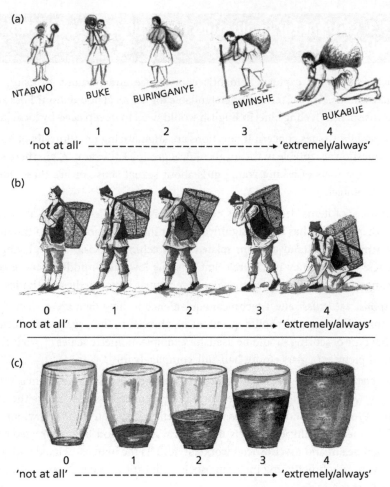

Figure 3.2 Pictorial response sets. (a) Pictorial response scale for function impairment used in Rwanda. (b) A basket scale developed for assessment of emotional severity among children in Nepal. The scale was rejected after piloting with children in focus groups because children endorsed the scale in the opposite direction that developers intended. The developers had expected children to identify the boy with a full basket as having the greatest severity of a negative mood. However, children identified option '0' (empty basket) as 'sad' or 'lazy' because the boy had no bricks in his basket and would therefore earn no money compared with '4' (full basket), which was associated with happiness and other positive emotions because of high earning potential with a large number of bricks. (c) Water glass scale used to assess emotional severity in Nepal. A similar water glass scale was implemented successfully with the Afghan Symptom Checklist.

Adapted with permission from Bolton, P., Tang, A. M. An alternative approach to cross-cultural function assessment. *Social Psychiatry and Psychiatric Epidemiology*, 37(11): 537–554. https://doi.org/10.1007/s00127-002-0580-5. Copyright © 2002, Steinkopff Verlag; *BMC Psychiatry*, 11, 127, Kohrt BA, Jordans MJD, Wietse AT et al., Validation of cross-cultural child mental health and psychosocial research instruments: adapting the Depression Self-Rating Scale and Child PTSD Symptom Scale in Nepal. © Kohrt et al; licensee BioMed Central Ltd. 2011. This article is published under license to BioMed Central Ltd. This is an Open Access article distributed under the terms of the Creative Commons Attribution License (http://creativecommons.org/licenses/by/2.0).

Box 3.3 Criteria for evaluating transcultural translation and adaptation

- *Comprehensibility* captures semantic equivalence and pertains to using appropriate idioms. Are the terms understandable for the local population? For example, idioms such as 'feeling blue' in English would need to be replaced by local idioms.

- *Acceptability* issues concern if questions are stigmatizing or culturally offensive. Is the question acceptable in the local cultural group? For example, are there socially acceptable ways of asking young girls about sexual abuse or are these questions unacceptable?

- *Relevance* of items demonstrates content equivalence. Relevance is a measure of whether the item has locally significant meaning. For example, even though children may understand an item related to 'watching television' or 'playing video games,' the item may not be relevant in some low- and middle-income country settings where rural children may not have regular access to these activities.

- *Response set issues* reflect technical equivalence in how data are collected across cultures. For example, should questions be phrased in the negative or affirmative? What type of scoring should be used, for example, numeric scales (1 = a little, 7 = a lot) or pictures (a glass empty, half-full, completely full)?

- *Completeness* combines semantic, criterion, and conceptual equivalence, thus capturing whether a question relates to the same concepts and ideas as the original item. Probes may include 'Does the item reflect a symptom or behaviour related to the mental health constructs in the local culture and is it addressed by local mental health and psychosocial workers?' and 'Is the item associated with impairment in daily functioning including social, education, occupational, and physical functioning?'

translation by a bilingual team, (2) review by mental health professionals, (3) focus group discussion with target beneficiaries, (4) blind back translation, (5) cognitive interviewing, and (6) validation study (Box 3.4). During the process, the concepts of comprehensibility, acceptability, relevance, technical issues, and completeness are documented on the 'transcultural translation monitoring form' (Box 3.5).

Measurement with locally developed tools

An alternative to cultural adaptation and validation of existing mental health tools is to develop local tools from the ground up. These tools have the advantage of being more relevant to the target population and to treatment goals. Locally developed tools have been used in Zimbabwe (Shona Symptom Questionnaire) (Patel et al., 1997), Uganda (Acholi Psychosocial Assessment Instrument) (Betancourt et al., 2009), Haiti (Kreyòl Distress

Box 3.4 Transcultural translation, adaptation, and validation process for psychiatric instruments

1. A group of *bilingual, indigenous translators* develop an initial translation for each item. The team should have expertise in linguistics, anthropology, and mental health. On the translation monitoring form, they document the preliminary translation and include a lexical back translation. For each item, they make comments regarding word choice and modifications in light of the five criteria: comprehensibility, acceptability, relevance, response set issues, and completeness.

2. *Mental health professionals* then review the translation monitoring form and make recommendations for additional modifications. They provide their own comments regarding the five criteria. At the end of this step, the research team revises items so that the items can then be used in focus groups with target beneficiaries.

3. *Focus group discussions* are used to evaluate each item. Focus group discussion should consist of participants who represent the target beneficiary group. For example, they may be uneducated, monolingual, local lay people. The focus group facilitator then documents how the participants appraise each item in terms of the five criteria and records alternative translations.

4. A bilingual indigenous translator who is unfamiliar with the original version then produces a *blind back translation* into the original language of the tool. After the focus group discussion, the research team revises the items in the target language then gives the tool to a bilingual translator who produces a back translation which the team reviews using the five criteria and further modifies the tool.

5. The tool is pilot tested through *cognitive interviewing*. A small qualitative sample are administered the tool and asked how they interpret each item, why they give the answers they provide, and to point out any areas of confusion in terms of comprehensibility, acceptability, and technical issues (Willis, 2005). The team revises the tool based on the cognitive interviews.

6. A *validation study* should then be conducted comparing the tool performance with a clinical structured interview or other external criterion. See Chapter 2 for details.

Source data from Van Ommeren, M. et al. Preparing instruments for transcultural research: use of the translation monitoring form with Nepali-speaking Bhutanese refugees. *Transcultural Psychiatry*, 36(3), 285–301, Sage Publications.

Idioms Screener) (Kaiser et al., 2013), and many other settings. A range of approaches can be used to develop these tools, and the use of multiple approaches could reduce the risk of bias. After a local scale is developed, it still needs to go through the same validation steps as outlined for cultural adaptation of existing instruments to assure comprehensibility, acceptability, relevance, and completeness (Van Ommeren et al., 1999) (also see

Box 3.5 Transcultural translation monitoring form

Tool: Item number:
Item in original language:
Translation of item:
Lexical back translation:

Comprehensibility (semantic equivalence)

Is the item understandable in the language known to the local population? Please comment on any difficulties. *Are local idioms used that the local population will understand?*

+ Translators' view:

+ Professionals' view:

+ Focus group results:

+ Back translation comments:

+ Cognitive interview results:

Acceptability (semantic and content equivalence)

Would certain respondents be uncomfortable to respond honestly to this question? Please explain. *Are questions acceptable by local moral and religious standards?*

+ Translators' view:

+ Professionals' view:

+ Focus group results:

+ Back translation comments:

+ Cognitive interview results:

Relevance (content equivalence)

Is this question relevant in the local culture? If not, please explain. *Is the question related the same mental health issues being addressed? Is the question locally appropriate based on lifestyle and behaviour?*

+ Translators' view:

+ Professionals' view:

+ Focus group results:

+ Back translation comments:

+ Cognitive interview results:

Response set (technical equivalence)

Will respondents answer in a similar manner across cultural groups, across literacy differences? *What is the best method of assessment for this question: numerical scale, pictures, or something else?*

- Translators' view:
- Professionals' view:
- Focus group results:
- Back translation comments:
- Cognitive interview results:

Completeness (semantic, criterion, and conceptual equivalence)

Would the translated item relate back to the same concepts and ideas as the original? If not, please explain. *Does the question address an area of life related to daily functioning, if so how –as an impairment in daily functioning or an improvement in daily functioning?*

- Translators' view:
- Professionals' view:
- Focus group results:
- Back translation comments:
- Cognitive interview results:

Adapted with permission from Van Ommeren, M. et al. Preparing instruments for transcultural research: use of the translation monitoring form with Nepali-speaking Bhutanese refugees. *Transcultural Psychiatry*, 36(3), 285–301. Copyright © 1999, © SAGE Publications. DOI: https://doi.org/10.1177/136346159903600304.

Chapter 2 for further details). Locally developed instruments should be evaluated for psychometric properties such as inter-rater reliability, test–retest reliability, and internal reliability. Locally developed instruments can be especially useful for evaluating treatment outcomes because they include symptoms most salient to the intervention participants (Hinton et al., 2009).

Combined emic–etic assessment approaches

Combining use of etic and emic measures can provide useful insights into culture and mental health and have a positive impact on improving research and mental health services. In Zimbabwe, when emic evaluations (Shona Symptom Questionnaire and evaluation by traditional medical practitioner or primary care nurses) were compared with etic ones (Revised Clinical Interview Schedule), high levels of concordance in classification of respondents as having a mental illness or not were observed suggesting convergence between emic and etic measures of common mental disorders (Patel and Mann, 1997). In Sri Lanka, comparisons between the two approaches have demonstrated that locally developed tools can explain variance in mental health outcomes above and beyond adapted Western tools (Jayawickreme et al., 2012). In Nepal, an algorithm using the Patient Health Questionnaire (PHQ-9) and locally developed screeners for idioms of distress reduced the number of patients requiring administration of the PHQ-9 by 50%, reduced false positives by 18%, and correctly identified 88% of patients with depression (Kohrt et al., 2016).

Conclusion

The epidemiology of mental disorders and their treatments in different cultures and health systems provides an important opportunity for unravelling aetiological factors underlying mental disorders and for discovering effective treatments. Although psychiatric symptoms can be elicited across cultures, taxonomies may differ considerably. Instruments developed in one culture may be used in others, but greater emphasis must be placed on their adaptation to ensure equivalence. Use of cultural frameworks is crucial to optimize utilization and outcomes of culturally adapted psychological treatments and other mental health interventions. Study designs need to incorporate a range of health system variables to ensure the findings are relevant to local health policy. Research must be planned in collaboration with potential users and consider a range of dissemination strategies. These principles form the basis for the growth of a truly international psychiatric epidemiology.

Practice exercise

You wish to conduct an epidemiological investigation to determine the number of people with dementia in a multicultural community in a low-income country. Develop a study design. Consider the following issues:

1. How would you develop the study proposal itself (i.e. who, for what purpose, and with whom would you consult)?
2. What variables (and why) would you consider important to measure?
3. How would you ensure the validity of the interview you used for the diagnosis of dementia?
4. What are the ethical issues you would consider?
5. How, and to whom, would the study findings be disseminated?

Further reading

Janes, C., Stall, R., and Gifford, S.M. (eds.) (2012). *Anthropology and epidemiology: interdisciplinary approaches to the study of health and disease*. Dordrecht: Springer.

Trostle, J.A. (2005). *Epidemiology and culture*. New York: Cambridge University Press.

Wakefield, J.C. and Demazeux, S. (eds.) (2015). *Sadness or depression?: International perspectives on the depression epidemic and its meaning*. Dordrecht: Springer.

References

Baer, H.A., Singer, M., and Susser, I. (2003). *Medical anthropology and the world system.* Westport, CT: Praeger.

Betancourt, T., Bass, J., Borisova, I., Neugebauer, R., Speelman, L., Onyango, G., et al. (2009). Assessing local instrument reliability and validity: a field-based example from northern Uganda. *Social Psychiatry and Psychiatric Epidemiology,* **44,** 685–692.

Broesch, J. and Hadley, C. (2012). Putting culture back into acculturation: identifying and overcoming gaps in the definition and measurement of acculturation. *The Social Science Journal,* **49,** 375–385.

Brown, R.A. and Armelagos, G.J. (2001). Apportionment of racial diversity: s review. *Evolutionary Anthropology,* **10,** 34–40.

Chowdhary, N., Jotheeswaran, A., Nadkarni, A., Hollon, S., King, M., Jordans, M., et al. (2014). The methods and outcomes of cultural adaptations of psychological treatments for depressive disorders: a systematic review. *Psychological Medicine,* **44,** 1131–1146.

Dressler, W.W. (2012). Cultural consonance: linking culture, the individual and health. *Preventive Medicine,* **55,** 390–393.

Ennett, S.T., Bauman, K.E., Hussong, A., Faris, R., Foshee, V.A., Cai, L., et al. (2006). The peer context of adolescent substance use: findings from Social Network Analysis. *Journal of Research on Adolescence,* **16,** 159–186.

Flaherty, J.A., Gaviria, F.M., Pathak, D., Mitchell, T., Wintrob, R., Richman, J.A., et al. (1988). Developing instruments for cross-cultural psychiatric research. *Journal of Nervous & Mental Disease,* **176,** 257–263.

Fowler, J.H. and Christakis, N.A. (2008). Dynamic spread of happiness in a large social network: longitudinal analysis over 20 years in the Framingham Heart Study. *BMJ,* 337:a2338.

Gravlee, C.C., Non, A.L., and Mulligan, C.J. (2009). Genetic ancestry, social classification, and racial inequalities in blood pressure in Southeastern Puerto Rico. *PLoS ONE,* **4,** e6821.

Groleau, D., Young, A., and Kirmayer, L.J. (2006). The McGill Illness Narrative Interview (MINI): an interview schedule to elicit meanings and modes of reasoning related to illness experience. *Transcultural Psychiatry,* **43,** 671–691.

Hahn, R.A. (1995). *Sickness and healing: an anthropological perspective.* New Haven, CT: Yale University Press.

Harrison, G., Hopper, K., Craig, T., Laska, E., Siegel, C., Wanderling, J., et al. (2001). Recovery from psychotic illness: a 15- and 25-year international follow-up study. *British Journal of Psychiatry,* **178,** 506–517.

Hinton, D.E., Hofmann, S.G., Pollack, M.H., and Otto, M.W. (2009). Mechanisms of efficacy of CBT for Cambodian refugees with PTSD: improvement in emotion regulation and orthostatic blood pressure response. *CNS Neuroscience & Therapeutics,* **15,** 255–263.

Hopper, K. and Wanderling, J. (2000). Revisiting the developed versus developing country distinction in course and outcome in schizophrenia: results from ISoS, the WHO collaborative followup project. International Study of Schizophrenia. *Schizophrenia Bulletin,* **26,** 835–846.

Hruschka, D.J. (2009). Culture as an explanation in population health. *Annals of Human Biology,* **36,** 235–247.

Hruschka, D.J. and Hadley, C. (2008). A glossary of culture in epidemiology. *Journal of Epidemiology & Community Health,* **62,** 947–951.

Jayawickreme, N., Jayawickreme, E., Atanasov, P., Goonasekera, M.A., and Foa, E.B. (2012). Are culturally specific measures of trauma-related anxiety and depression needed? The case of Sri Lanka. *Psychological Assessment,* **24,** 791–800.

Jilek, W.G. (1995). Emil Kraepelin and comparative sociocultural psychiatry. *European Archives of Psychiatry and Clinical Neuroscience*, 245, 231–238.

Kaiser, B.N., Haroz, E.E., Kohrt, B.A., Bolton, P.A., Bass, J.K., and Hinton, D.E. (2015). "Thinking too much": a systematic review of a common idiom of distress. *Social Science & Medicine*, 147, 170–183.

Kaiser, B.N., Kohrt, B.A., Keys, H.M., Khoury, N.M., and Brewster, A.-R.T. (2013). Strategies for assessing mental health in Haiti: local instrument development and transcultural translation. *Transcultural Psychiatry*, 50, 532–558.

Kim, H.S., Sherman, D.K., Sasaki, J.Y., Xu, J., Chu, T.Q., Ryu, C., et al. (2010). Culture, distress, and oxytocin receptor polymorphism (OXTR) interact to influence emotional support seeking. *Proceedings of the National Academy of Sciences of the United States of America*, 107, 15717–15721.

Kleinman, A. (1988). *Rethinking psychiatry: from cultural category to personal experience*. New York: Free Press, Collier Macmillan.

Kohrt, B.A., Jordans, M.J., Tol, W.A., Luitel, N.P., Maharjan, S.M., and Upadhaya, N. (2011). Validation of cross-cultural child mental health and psychosocial research instruments: adapting the Depression Self-Rating Scale and Child PTSD Symptom Scale in Nepal. *BMC Psychiatry*, 11, e127.

Kohrt, B.A., Luitel, N.P., Acharya, P., and Jordans, M.J.D. (2016). Detection of depression in low resource settings: validation of the Patient Health Questionnaire (PHQ-9) and cultural concepts of distress in Nepal. *BMC Psychiatry*, 16, e58.

Kohrt, B.A., Rasmussen, A., Kaiser, B.N., Haroz, E.E., Maharjan, S.M., Mutamba, B.B., et al. (2014). Cultural concepts of distress and psychiatric disorders: literature review and research recommendations for global mental health epidemiology. *International Journal of Epidemiology*, 43, 365–406.

Kohrt, B.A., Worthman, C.M., Ressler, K.J., Mercer, K.B., Upadhaya, N., Koirala, S., et al. (2015). Cross-cultural gene–environment interactions in depression, post-traumatic stress disorder, and the cortisol awakening response: FKBP5 polymorphisms and childhood trauma in South Asia. *International Review of Psychiatry*, 27, 180–196.

Krieger, N. (2005). Stormy weather: race, gene expression, and the science of health disparities. *American Journal of Public Health*, 95, 2155–2160.

Kulhara, P. and Chakrabarti, S. (2001). Culture and schizophrenia and other psychotic disorders. *Psychiatric Clinics of North America*, 24, 449–464.

Larøi, F., Luhrmann, T.M., Bell, V., Christian, W.A., Deshpande, S., Fernyhough, C., et al. (2014). Culture and hallucinations: overview and future directions. *Schizophrenia Bulletin*, 40, S213–S220.

Leff, J., Wig, N.N., Ghosh, A., Bedi, H., Menon, D.K., Kuipers, L., et al. (1987). Expressed emotion and schizophrenia in north India. III. Influence of relatives' expressed emotion on the course of schizophrenia in Chandigarh. *British Journal of Psychiatry*, 151, 166–173.

Lewis-Fernandez, R., Aggarwal, N.K., Hinton, L., Hinton, D.E., and Kirmayer, L.J. (2015). *DSM-5 Handbook on the Cultural Formulation Interview*. Washington, DC: American Psychiatric Association.

Lewis-Fernández, R., Raggio, G.A., Gorritz, M., Duan, N., Marcus, S., Cabassa, L.J., et al. (2013). GAP-REACH: a checklist to assess comprehensive reporting of race, ethnicity, and culture in psychiatric publications. *The Journal of Nervous and Mental Disease*, 201, 860–871.

Lloyd, K.R., Jacob, K.S., Patel, V., St Louis, L., Bhugra, D., and Mann, A.H. (1998). The development of the Short Explanatory Model Interview (SEMI) and its use among primary-care attenders with common mental disorders. *Psychological Medicine*, 28, 1231–1237.

Lund, C., Brooke-Sumner, C., Baingana, F., Baron, E.C., Breuer, E., Chandra, P., … Saxena, S. (2018). Social determinants of mental disorders and the Sustainable Development Goals: a systematic review of reviews. *The Lancet Psychiatry*, 5(4), 357–369.

Marmot, M., Friel, S., Bell, R., Houweling, T.A.J., and Taylor, S. (2008). Closing the gap in a generation: health equity through action on the social determinants of health. *Lancet*, 372, 1661–1669.

Metzl, J.M. and Hansen, H. (2014). Structural competency: theorizing a new medical engagement with stigma and inequality. *Social Science & Medicine*, 103, 126–133.

Millsap, R.E. and Kwok, O.-M. (2004). Evaluating the impact of partial factorial invariance on selection in two populations. *Psychological Methods*, 9, 93–115.

Murray, L.K., Dorsey, S., Haroz, E., Lee, C., Alsiary, M.M., Haydary, A., et al. (2014). A common elements treatment approach for adult mental health problems in low- and middle-income countries. *Cognitive and Behavioral Practice*, 21, 111–123.

Napier, A.D., Ancarno, C., Butler, B., Calabrese, J., Chater, A., Chatterjee, H., et al. (2014). Culture and health. *Lancet*, 384, 1607–1639.

Patel, V., Chowdhary, N., Rahman, A., and Verdeli, H. (2011). Improving access to psychological treatments: lessons from developing countries. *Behaviour Research & Therapy*, 49, 523–528.

Patel, V., Cohen, A., Thara, R., and Gureje, O. (2006). Is the outcome of schizophrenia really better in developing countries? *Revista Brasileira de Psiquiatria*, 28, 149–152.

Patel, V. and Mann, A. (1997). Etic and emic criteria for non-psychotic mental disorder: a study of the CISR and care provider assessment in Harare. *Social Psychiatry & Psychiatric Epidemiology*, 32, 84–89.

Patel, V., Minas, H., Cohen, A., and Prince, M. (2014). *Global mental health: principles and practice*. Oxford: Oxford University Press.

Patel, V., Simunyu, E., Gwanzura, F., Lewis, G., and Mann, A. (1997). The Shona Symptom Questionnaire: the development of an indigenous measure of common mental disorders in Harare. *Acta Psychiatrica Scandinavica*, 95, 469–475.

Physicians for Human Rights (2003). *The right to equal treatment: an action plan to end racial and ethnic disparities in clinical diagnosis and treatment in the United States*. Boston, MA: Physicians for Human Rights.

Sartorius, N., Shapiro, R., Kimura, M., and Barrett, K. (1972). WHO international pilot study of schizophrenia. *Psychological Medicine*, 2, 422–425.

Scott, J. (2012). *Social network analysis*. Thousand Oaks, CA: SAGE Publications.

Shibre, T., Teferra, S., Morgan, C., and Alem, A. (2010). Exploring the apparent absence of psychosis amongst the Borana pastoralist community of Southern Ethiopia. A mixed method follow-up study. *World Psychiatry*, 9, 98–102.

Steel, Z., Chey, T., Silove, D., Marnane, C., Bryant, R.A., and Van Ommeren, M. (2009). Association of torture and other potentially traumatic events with mental health outcomes among populations exposed to mass conflict and displacement: a systematic review and meta-analysis. *JAMA*, 302, 537–549.

Thara, R., Henrietta, M., Joseph, A., Rajkumar, S., and Eaton, W.W. (1994). Ten-year course of schizophrenia—the Madras longitudinal study. *Acta Psychiatrica Scandinavica*, 90, 329–336.

Van Ommeren, M., Sharma, B., Thapa, S., Makaju, R., Prasain, D., Bhattaria, R., et al. (1999). Preparing instruments for transcultural research: use of the translation monitoring form with Nepali-speaking Bhutanese. *Transcultural Psychiatry*, 36, 285–301.

Varkevisser, C.M., Brownlee, A., and Pathmanathan, I. (1991). *Designing and conducting health systems research projects: data analysis and report writing*. Ottawa: IDRC.

Weaver, L.J. and Kaiser, B.N. (2015). Developing and testing locally derived mental health scales: examples from North India and Haiti. *Field Methods*, 27, 115–130.

Weiss, M.G. (1997). Explanatory Model Interview Catalogue (EMIC): framework for comparative study of illness. *Transcultural Psychiatry* 34, 235–263.

Willis, G.B. (2005). *Cognitive interviewing: a tool for improving questionnaire design*. Thousand Oaks, CA: Sage Publications, Inc.

Chapter 4

Ethics and research in psychiatry: Consent, capacity, and bioethics

Buddhika Lalanie Fernando and Athula Sumathipala

Introduction

Ethics is a friend of research. In fact, ethics is the best friend of research since it is a supportive but critical friend (Ives, 2018). Ethics enables enhancing the scientific value and rigour of research while ensuring that such scientific value is not adulterated by the exploitation of human beings in carrying out the research. It is said that 'the moral test of government is in how it treats those at the dawn of life, children; those in the twilight of life, the elderly; and those in the shadows of life, the sick, the needy and the handicapped' (Humphrey, 1977). The same applies to scientific research. Scientific rigour must be most vigorously applied and ethical concerns most conscientiously addressed when carrying out research involving those with the reduced ability to protect themselves.

In research situations involving a certain amount of risk, conventional wisdom allows that informed consent from the research participant suffices to alleviate ethical concerns about harm or exploitation. This is because individual autonomy has gained primacy as the decisive factor in the researcher–research participant relationship. It is generally considered that a person has the right to weigh the risks against the benefits of a particular issue and to decide if they want to take on the associated risks; the only moral compulsion on the researcher is to be conscientious about disclosing all the relevant factors to the potential participant, ensuring comprehension, and that consent to research is given without undue duress.

Carrying out research among people with mental disorders, regardless of whether the research is conducted in the context of mental health services, the population, or in the community, needs to be approached with extra caution due to the inherent dilemma in psychiatric research: the positive duty not to cause harm to a vulnerable individual versus the negative duty not to deny them the potential benefits of the research. In this situation, consent from the participant does not always provide the customary moral and legal authority since cognitive deficits in certain people with mental disorders may impair the ability to clearly understand the risks of the research versus the benefits to be gained. As discussed in detail further on in the chapter, a person can provide valid consent to participate in research only when it is given after they have received full disclosure of the key relevant facts and it has been established that they have the capacity to consent—that is, the ability to fully understand, appreciate, reason, and communicate. It is also essential that the consent is provided voluntarily, without coercion.

Prescriptive laws and regulations that could help in a situation where a person does not have full capacity to provide consent do not exist in most countries. In their absence, researchers often operate an informal 'sliding scale' approach. Consent considerations are more rigorously addressed when the validity of the consent may be questionable—to alleviate ethical concerns regarding the participation of those who have or may have mental health problems.

In this chapter, we discuss the factors necessary to obtain valid consent from the participant: full disclosure of key relevant facts, comprehension, the person's capacity to consent, and the consent being given voluntarily. Next, we examine the tools of assessment available to assess capacity to consent, and lastly, we look at what can be done when it is not possible to obtain valid consent from the participant for research, but it may be in their best interests to participate in the research. The emphasis in current literature and practice is mainly on the consent process, and on the primacy of autonomy, though some recent discussions on moral philosophy have been critical of this model. We consider the question of the minimum criteria necessary to make an autonomous decision, and the qualitative nature of the assessment of the capacity to give consent. We examine the role of beneficence as a guiding principle in psychiatric ethics, especially in cases where the capacity of that person to give consent is uncertain. Pellegrino and Thomasma (1987) have described merely giving such a person the facts and ask them to make a decision as 'a form of moral abandonment'. While the freedom to make one's own decisions should be respected, there is an argument that consent should not be the sole criterion in determining participation in psychiatric research, given the concerns related to ensuring that people with mental disorders have the capacity to make a truly autonomous decision. This is not advocacy for hard paternalism, but rather emphasizes the subjugation of the researcher's/physician's self-interest (of having the person participate in the research) to the best interests of the participant.

The ethical responsibility of the researcher is to ensure that concern for the best interests of the potential research participant increases in inverse proportion to the level of competence the latter displays. Where there is unambiguous decision-making capacity, and where no therapeutic misconception exists (failure to appreciate the difference between scientific experiment and clinical treatment), autonomy of the potential research participant can and must be respected. The type of research to be carried out, (therapeutic versus non-therapeutic research), also directly impacts the benchmark for beneficence, that is, capacity for consent and informed consent would generally be required for non-therapeutic research, whereas beneficence should be the guiding principle for therapeutic research. In brief, capacity to consent and informed consent is necessary in psychiatric research; however, even if consent has been given, the researchers' obligation must extend to beyond 'mere respect for a person's choices' and they need to 'ensure that the subject receives all possible benefits and avoids all possible harms from participating in the research' (Gostin, 1991).

In this chapter we aim to equip readers with the necessary attitude and skills to view and accommodate ethics as part and parcel of clinical and population research in psychiatry, ensuring best practices during the consent process, and adherence to the highest standards. We highlight contemporary thinking on consent and capacity. The overall aim is to guide investigators to fulfil their moral obligation of producing new knowledge through research, while protecting the rights and welfare of the research participants.

Ethics, bioethics, and psychiatric research

Ethics in the broadest sense refers to moral rights and wrongs, and involves systematizing, defending, and recommending concepts of right and wrong behaviour (Stevenson, 2010). In the new era of genetics, biotechnology, and in the face of new infectious diseases and environmental degradation, bioethics can be defined as the ethics of all aspects of life (for a detailed definition of bioethics, see Benatar (2006)). Ethics is linked intimately with attitudes, beliefs, and human relationships which involve consideration of power, driving the link between ethics, power, injustice, and the hierarchy created by the power differential (for a discussion of power differentials in ethical situations, see Gibson et al. (2014)). The objective of biomedical research is to develop generalizable knowledge to improve health and/or increase the understanding of human biology/functioning, and behaviour (Emanuel et al., 2000). Even with a beneficent objective, research has the potential to inflict harm, and to treat participants as mere 'subjects' and as a means to an end. The role of ethics, therefore, is to ensure that participants are treated with dignity and respect while they contribute to the social good, and to find the 'least harmful' ways to do research. Ethics aims to protect participants from harm that could potentially be caused by science and experimentation and to promote their welfare. However, it is a given that ethics can and should also promote good science (Sumathipala and Fernando, 2014).

Clinical ethics deal with the relationship between patients and doctors/healthcare providers, whereas research ethics deal with that between research participants and researchers. Our focus here is specifically consent to research, the capacity to give consent, and the ethical considerations thereof. Further details on the broader subject of ethics in mental health research and trials, particularly in low- and middle-income country settings are provided elsewhere (Sumathipala and Fernando, 2014).

Ethical research in psychiatry and other specialties: the same difference

Emanuel and colleagues (2000) identified seven specific features that make clinical research ethical, emphasizing that informed consent is neither necessary nor sufficient to make clinical research ethical. They specify that, in order to be considered ethical, research must have social or scientific value, scientific validity, a fair selection of research participants, a favourable risk–benefit ratio, informed consent, independent review, and respect for the participants, including protection of their privacy, having their well-being monitored, and giving them the ability to withdraw from research (Box 4.1).

Box 4.1 What makes clinical research ethical?

1. Social or scientific value.
2. Scientific validity.
3. Fair selection of research participants.
4. A favourable risk–benefit ratio.
5. Informed consent.
6. Independent review.
7. Respect for research participants.

Source data from Emanuel, E.J., et al. (2000). What makes clinical research ethical? *JAMA*, 283, 2701–2711.

These requirements apply to research in psychiatry as to other branches of medicine, and their application should enable ethical conduct of psychiatric research. The question is whether there are additional risks specific to psychiatric research that warrant increased safeguards? Vaz and Srinivasan (2014) voice this concern by stating that 'the ethical principles are the same, but the challenges and ethical dilemmas may be different or more complex in psychiatric research'.

The dilemma arises from two distinct sources, neither of which applies uniquely to psychiatric research. Firstly, ethical issues arise when certain study designs in psychiatric research (such as the use of placebos, challenge, and washout study designs) pose additional risks to the research participants given the nature of their condition. Treatments such as electroconvulsive therapy also pose additional risks to patients, and may need a greater level of justification of necessity if they are to be examined in a research context. Secondly, ethical concerns arise from the difficulty of ensuring that the person with mental health issues providing the consent for research does in fact have the cognitive capacity to provide a valid consent, with as full an understanding as would be usual in other branches of medicine.

It has been pointed out that a blanket exclusion of persons with mental disorders from research would, in itself, be unethical, as all persons have a right to 'the best treatment, and to participate in research and to contribute to the establishment of best treatments' (Vaz and Srinivasan, 2014). The position statement issued by the UK Royal College of Psychiatrists (2011) states that 'it is untrue and stigmatizing to assume that all psychiatric research entails greater risk and has less potential benefit than in other areas of medicine', and the US National Institutes of Health (NIH) (2009) in its paper on conducting research involving individuals with questionable capacity to consent states that 'excluding persons who may have impaired consent capacity from participation in such research can significantly delay attempts to answer important scientific questions that could lead to new treatments and better diagnostic, predictive, and preventive strategies'.

Procedural elements of obtaining a valid consent for research

Informed consent, as discussed in this chapter, does not refer to the ability to provide consent to treatment, but to the ability to provide consent to participate in research. The distinction is important because treatment is of direct potential benefit to the person with mental health issues whereas participation in research may or may not be of direct benefit to the participant. Confusion over this distinction, on the part of the potential participant, would constitute therapeutic misconception.

Van Staden (2015) states that the categorical approach to incapacity, where a patient was considered unable to give a valid consent merely due to their reported disease condition (e.g. dementia or psychosis) without a clinical assessment of their ability at the time of concern (Appelbaum, 2007), is being gradually replaced by a more functional approach. A functional approach requires the clinical assessment of the capacity to give consent to the specific process or intervention under consideration, and appreciates that capacity may vary according to the complexity of the process considered, the nature of the process followed to obtain consent, and according to the tools used to assess capacity. Christopher and Dunn (2015) analysed empirical research available on the capacity of people with serious mental illnesses (schizophrenia, major depression, and bipolar disorder) to provide valid informed consent to research and concluded that psychiatric illness does not necessarily equate to impaired capacity. Although serious mental illness was a risk factor, cognitive function was the most consistent predictor of decisional ability. Appreciation of risk and potential of being subject to coercion or undue influence was similar to that in the general population. They also found that therapeutic misconception was prevalent (not necessarily at a greater level than for other diseases) and that enhanced consent procedures could mitigate impairments in decision-making ability.

We shall now consider the current recognized good practice for obtaining valid consent for research from a person who may potentially have impaired cognitive abilities. First, we discuss the key elements required for valid consent, the extent of information disclosure required, the instruments available to assess capacity, and then, the non-cognitive elements of a valid consent—consent given of free will without coercion. Finally, we present and discuss options to be considered when the person does not have capacity to consent (Figure 4.1).

The requirements for valid consent

The basic requirements for a valid consent for psychiatric research require verifying the participant's capacity to consent after a suitable assessment of cognitive and non-cognitive factors (such as voluntarism). The full disclosure of all key relevant factors and verification of comprehension should precede obtaining consent. Emanuel (2000) succinctly explains what is necessary for informed consent:

> To provide informed consent, individuals must be accurately informed of the purpose, methods, risks, benefits, and alternatives to research; understand this information and its bearing on their own clinical situation; and make a voluntary and un-coerced decision whether to participate.

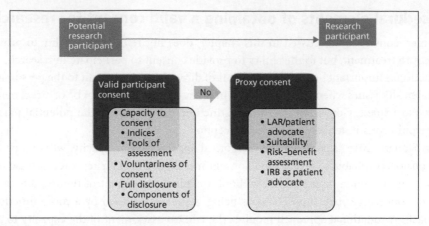

Figure 4.1 Consent procedures. IRB, Institutional Review Board; LAR, legally acceptable representative.

In the UK, the Mental Capacity Act (MCA) 2005 (Legislation.gov.uk, 2005), and its accompanying Code of Practice (Department for Constitutional Affairs, 2007) detail the requirements for deciding whether a patient has the capacity to give valid consent, and the circumstances under which a decision can be taken in the person's best interests when the person does not have the capacity to give a valid consent (Box 4.2). Capacity refers to the person's ability to make a *particular decision* at the time it needs to be made, when they have been given all the relevant information necessary to make the decision and all necessary information on alternatives, if there is a choice available. According to the MCA, a person lacks capacity 'if they have a disability, condition or trauma that affects the way

---

Box 4.2 Five statutory principles underpin the legal requirements in the Mental Capacity Act 2005

1. Assume a person has decision-making capacity unless it is proven to be otherwise.

2. Do not treat a person as unable to make a decision, unless all practicable steps to help him/her to do so have been taken without success.

3. Do not treat a person as unable to make a decision merely because he/she makes an unwise decision.

4. Any act done or decision made on behalf of a person who lacks capacity must be done/made in his/her best interests.

5. Treatment and care provided or decisions made on behalf of the person who lacks capacity must be the least restrictive of their basic rights and freedoms.

England and Wales, Department of Health (2005).

their mind or brain works' and 'they are unable to make a specific decision at the time it needs to be made' (Department for Constitutional Affairs, 2007).

Capacity to consent: indices of capacity to consent

There are several key components to the capacity to give a valid consent—comprehension, appreciation, reasoning, and communication—discussed as early as in 1988 by Appelbaum and Grisso as the four related skills of communicating a choice, understanding relevant information, appreciating the current situation and its consequences, and manipulating information rationally. Competence in each of these areas is required. The MacArthur Competence Assessment Tool for Clinical Research (MacCAT-CR), developed by the same authors, is the most frequently cited tool for capacity assessment. It looks at the same four dimensions of decision-making—termed as understanding, appreciation, reasoning, and expressing a choice (Appelbaum and Grisso, 2001).

Comprehension which refers to understanding, with a deep, full realization of the matter at hand, is a key aspect of the informed consent process. This has been strongly emphasized in guidelines and recommendations for ethical conduct in scientific research (e.g. National Bioethics Advisory Commission, 2001; CIOMS, 2002; Nuffield Council on Bioethics, 2002, 2005). Even with the use of a person's preferred language, it is often difficult for people to understand information included on consent forms used in biomedical or behavioural research (Ogloff and Otto, 1991; Goldstein et al., 1996; Davis et al., 1998; Raich et al., 2001; Marshall 2007). Clear plain language and the right balance of information, not too much or not too little, are important in this regard. Indemnity-driven consent forms may be long and will not necessarily facilitate comprehension (Lindegger and Richter, 2000).

Information transmission is traditionally viewed as a one-way process, whereas it is best conceptualized as bidirectional. Providing information alone is therefore not sufficient. Participants' comprehension must be ensured and assessed. We emphasize the need to distinguish between informed consent and understood consent, and hence the need to ensure participants' understanding of the research. Bhutta (2004) stresses the need to ensure true comprehension and voluntary participation, while providing an excellent critique on areas of controversy and ambiguity, as well as of problems arising with the application of guidelines for obtaining informed consent for research in low-resourced settings. Involvement of community representatives well in advance is one mechanism that can help this process. To achieve this, there is today heavy emphasis on public and patient involvement, engagement, and participation (PPIE) in the design and conduct of research, for example, in the UK. Ethical issues that arise in psychiatric research when considered in the context of engagement with patients and the general public are discussed in detail in Chapter 5—'Ethics and research in psychiatry: engagement with patients and public'.

Appreciation relates to a person's current perception about the research they are asked to participate in, the consequences of participation, and the potential risks of participation. It overlaps with comprehension, and could be described as 'how an individual uses their understanding of diagnostic and treatment information, and relates this to their own personal circumstances and belief systems' (Lamont et al., 2013). This is similar to what the MCA 2005 in England and Wales considers as 'using and weighing information' in the key abilities required for capacity to consent (understanding, retaining, and communicating being the other key factors) (Legislation.gov.uk, 2005). Assessing appreciation is not straightforward and different assessment tools use different mechanisms ranging from assessing the doubts a person has about the factual information given to them, to assessing the person's opinion about the potential results of the proposed research or the potential extent of harm perceived by the person (Dunn et al., 2006).

Reasoning refers to the ability of a person to process information rationally and arrive at a decision, in this case whether to participate in the research or not. Reasoning is again an abstract concept that is hard to assess, and current methods used for the assessment of reasoning include assessing the ability to identify risk, benefits, assessing insight and judgement, and assessing the underlying values that influence decision-making (Gupta and Kharawala, 2012).

Communication refers not only to the ability of the participant to communicate with the researcher on general terms but the specific ability to communicate a reasoned choice regarding the matter in question, and the reasoning behind that decision.

Information disclosure needs to be comprehensive

Consent is considered to be 'informed' when it is given by a person who understands the purpose and the nature of the research, what participating in the study requires the person to do, the risks involved, and what benefits are intended to result from the study (Gupta and Kharawala, 2012). The concept of informed consent was developed to promote individual autonomy and to encourage rational decision-making. Acknowledging the difficulty of prescribing a list of specific information necessary to be given in each different case, the MCA 2005 (England and Wales) recommends giving the person access to all the information they need to make an informed decision that does not miss out important information; it also cautions against giving too much detail, which could confuse the person. Risks, benefits, foreseeable consequences of making the decision and the consequences of remaining undecided, the options available, if any, the effects the decision might have on the person and those close to them, and in some cases access to advice from another unbiased third party are all requirements under the MCA (Department for Constitutional Affairs, 2007). Given the wide availability of literature on the process of informed consent, we do not discuss the process of informed consent here, but list the elements of comprehensive information disclosure in Box 4.3.

Capacity to consent: tools and instruments for assessing capacity to consent

The fluid nature of the cognitive capacity of persons with psychiatric disorders has led to the creation of assessment tools to assess cognitive capacity, in an attempt to standardize and bring consistency to the evaluation process. There are around 20 different instruments

Box 4.3 Elements of comprehensive information disclosure

1. Aims, purpose, and duration of the research.
2. Methods: randomization, placebo, blinding, etc.
3. Practical aspects (e.g. counselling, tests, visits, use, storage of tissue samples).
4. Potential risks (e.g. trial-related discrimination).
5. Expected benefits (e.g. counselling).
6. The right to withdraw.
7. Compensation for research-related injury.
8. Confidentiality (and limits if any).
9. Personal implications.

currently in use and most of these are structured to assess the indices of cognitive capacity previously discussed, usually through interviews (structured/semi-structured) and hypothetical vignettes (for a detailed list of instruments used in capacity assessment, see Lamont et al. (2013)). The Evaluation to Sign Consent (ESC), one of the first tools used to assess the ability of a person to provide valid consent, is a five-item questionnaire which attempts to evaluate the person's factual comprehension about the research (Moser et al., 2002). The most comprehensive of these tools is the 20-page questionnaire in the MacArthur Competence Assessment Tools for Clinical Research (MacCAT-CR) (Appelbaum and Grisso, 2001), which is sometimes deemed too time-consuming and as setting too high a bar for a positive assessment (DeRenzo et al., 1998).

It must be noted that tools and instruments for assessing capacity to consent are only as good as the people using the tools, since their qualitative nature means the assessment involves judgement calls by the clinician/researcher. It is therefore essential that staff receive adequate training and gain in-depth understanding and experience of the issues involved. The MCA, for example, specifies that the final decision about someone's capacity must be made by the person intending to make the decision or carry out the action on behalf of the person who lacks capacity, not the professional who may be there only in an advisory capacity (Legislation.gov.uk, 2005).

The MCA sets out a two-stage test of capacity where stage 1 of the test requires proof that the person suspected of lacking capacity has an impairment of the mind or the brain, including some form of mental illness, dementia, significant learning disabilities, long-term effects of brain damage, conditions that cause confusion, drowsiness, or loss of consciousness, delirium, concussion following a head injury, or the symptoms of alcohol or drug use. Stage 2 assesses if the impairment or disturbance means that the person is unable to make a specific decision at that point in time—defining a person who is unable to make a decision as someone who cannot understand the relevant information, retain that information in their mind, use or weigh that information as part of the decision-making process, or communicate the decision.

Assessing non-cognitive elements influencing the validity of consent—voluntariness of consent

It is also necessary to assess certain non-cognitive features such as the voluntariness of the consent, its nature, and its extent. Participants' consent must be given free of coercion (threat of negative sanction) or undue influence to participate (excessive incentives could pressure a person to consent against his/her better judgement). Special care must be taken with participants who are considered vulnerable and therefore constrained in their ability to make free choices. Researchers can promote participants' freedom by adequate assessment of the specific vulnerability factors, and offsetting these, for example, by education to offset lack of familiarity with research. Avoiding undue incentives to offset impoverishment being a factor in consent is an important factor to be considered. Providing participants with ways to voice concerns, monitoring the impact of participation and reminding participants of the right to withdraw are also crucial.

Consent for research in cases where capacity to consent is absent

If cognitive capacity assessment reveals that the potential research participant cannot provide valid consent, such a person should be involved in the research only under certain specific circumstances.

The guiding principle in carrying out any act or taking any decision on behalf of a person who does not have capacity is that the act must be done or the decision taken in the best interests of that person. In the UK, the only exceptions to this requirement are in relation to research and where there is an advance decision to refuse treatment.

In England and Wales, the MCA 2005 applies to all research that is not a clinical trial, where there are plans to involve persons who lack capacity to consent for research that would require consent under usual circumstances. The Clinical Trials Regulation (European Union (EU) No. 536/2014) (European Commission, 2014) comes into application in 2020 (postponed from 2019) with consistent rules for conducting clinical trials throughout the EU and will replace the Clinical Trials Directive (2001/20/EC) which is currently in effect (European Medicines Agency, n.d.).

In a clear example of where legislation can act pre-emptively to protect vulnerable persons, the MCA 2005 provides strict and clear guidelines on when a person who lacks capacity can be involved in research. Research covered by the MCA (i.e. research other than clinical trials) can involve persons lacking capacity to consent to research only if the project has approval from a research ethics committee recognized by the Secretary of State/Welsh Assembly (as applicable); in addition, the researchers should consider the views of carers and other relevant parties, treat the person's interests as more important than the interests of science and society, and respect the objections of the person during the research. A research ethics committee can approve a project involving people who lack capacity to consent to research only if:

1. the research is linked to the impairing condition that affects the incapacitated person or the treatment thereof

2. it is reasonably clear that the research is less effective if only competent persons are included

   and, either

3. the research has some chance of benefiting the incapacitated person and the benefit is proportionate to the burden caused by taking part in the research

   or

4. the aim of research is to provide knowledge about the cause of, treatment/care of people with the same or a similar condition, in which case

   a. the risk to the incapacitated person must be negligible.

   b. there is no significant interference with the privacy or freedom of action of the person.

   c. nothing unduly invasive or restrictive is carried out on the person.

The EU Clinical Trials Regulation due to come into effect in 2020 imposes similar conditions. In addition to meeting all the criteria applicable for research involving people with the capacity to consent, it requires research involving incapacitated people to meet broadly the MCA 2005 criteria detailed earlier, though worded slightly differently, and in addition requires:

1. informed consent from a legal representative

2. incapacitated persons to receive the information in a way that is within their capacity to understand

3. no incentives or financial inducements are given to the incapacitated person or their legal representatives.

Use of surrogate decision makers to provide proxy consent is the most common prevailing practice, both where there is no legal/regulatory guidance and in jurisdictions such as the EU with clear guidance. All EU states allow a surrogate to make a decision in case of incapacitated patients and differ only in who the surrogate can be (Lemaire et al., 2005). Evidence on the use of surrogates is mixed. There is some evidence to support that people are willing to grant leeway to their surrogates, and that this willingness was either sustained or increased after democratic deliberation, suggesting that the attitude toward leeway is a reliable opinion (Scott et al., 2013). Eliciting a person's current preferences about future research participation should also involve eliciting his or her leeway preferences. Torke and colleagues (2008) discuss another important point, the need of surrogate decision makers to use substituted judgement, that is, a best estimate of what the person would choose if they could, as opposed to best interest judgement, that is, a choice made based on community norms and what the surrogate believes to be in the best interest of that person. However, empirical research also shows the weakness of sub-stituted judgement given the propensity of individuals to change their mind over time, surrogates finding it difficult to predict the decision the incapacitated person would have made, and the strong preference for autonomy that those with the potential to have im-paired capacity themselves display (Roberts et al., 2000; Torke et al., 2008). Accordingly, Anderson and Mukhergee (2007) consider that a surrogate decision maker should not be used as a 'catch-all solution' where there is doubt about decisional capacity and that a surrogate should be used only as a last resort.

An advance directive, a living will which gives durable power of attorney to a surrogate decision-maker, remains in effect during the incompetency of the person making it. In England and Wales, the MCA 2005 introduced 'advance care planning,' giving a person the right to make decisions about their healthcare treatment in the future, for a time when they may no longer have the capacity to make such decisions for themselves. However, this is not necessarily a formal process with a legally binding effect, and can simply refer to discussing and communicating values and preferences, to inform, but not bind, future decision-making.

An advance directive for research has been proposed that could allow cognitively impaired adults to be enrolled in research only when they complete a formal research advance directive while competent (Tri-Council Working Group, 1997; Maryland Attorney General's Working Group, 1998; National Bioethics Advisory Commission, 1998; New York State Advisory Work Group, 1998). However, Muthappan and col-leagues (2005) argue that allowing cognitively impaired adults to participate in research only with a formal advance directive could block important research. Their conclusions were based on a study of 2371 adults admitted as inpatients to the NIH Clinical Center in Bethesda, Maryland, US. Only 11% of adult inpatients completed a research advance directive. The authors suggest more flexible approaches should be considered to protect these individuals.

An ombudsman, an independent person used either to obtain the consent or to be an observer when the consent is taken by the researchers, was proposed by Sumathipala and Siribaddana (2004). The concept of a third-person decision maker is not an entirely a novel concept, for example, under the MCA, the 'Independent Mental Capacity Advocate' performs a similar role in the absence of next of kin, in issues involving clinical research. However, issues such as how to find a truly independent person, the financial implica-tions of such a structure, confidentiality, obligations, and liabilities of the independent observer could operate as implementation barriers to this practice. The *tri-partite consent process* proposes oversight of consent by three professionals, with 'distinct domains of responsibility and expertise' to address the issue of recruitment conflict in any research context (Posever and Chelmow, 2001). The first step is assessment by the prospective participant's treatment team of whether the person is suitable to be approached for a study (initial consent). The second step is an independent assessment of their decision-making capacity (capacity to consent), capacity review, and the third step is a designated patient advocate to review the research with the prospective participant (advocate review). If all three recommended steps are carried out over a span of more than one day, and all steps provide a satisfactory review, then it is considered that the person is capable of giving informed voluntary consent. The challenge is the availability of human resources for such an elaborate and comprehensive consent process.

Continued consent refers to the process where capacity to consent is reassessed if there is any reason to consider that the capacity of the person to give a valid consent to research is now in question.

Capacity in children

When research involves both the sensitive topic of mental health and research subjects who lack capacity because of their developmental stage, the ethical issues become more complex still. However, children and young people can and should be involved in all stages of research as well as being participants (INVOLVE, 2016). The legal and ethical framework that governs research with children and other vulnerable groups will vary between countries and over time, so it is essential that researchers familiarize themselves with their local requirements when planning their work. Most countries will have a chronological age at which a young person is considered to be adult and therefore has the capacity to provide informed consent for research participation, unless it can be demonstrated otherwise. In the UK, this is 16 years of age, although refusals of treatment between 16 and 18 years of age are often overturned, particularly when related to mental health (Ford and Kessel, 2001).

Gillick competence refers to the decision that a child who is younger than 16 years has the capacity to consent, and the resultant Fraser guidelines have been used in healthcare but also research situations where gaining parental consent may be difficult, such as universal interventions or surveys in secondary schools (*Gillick* v *West Norfolk & Wisbech Area Health Authority*, 1985). For example, a cluster randomized trial of mindfulness (Kuyken et al., 2017) and a similar trial of Mental Health First Aid (Kidger et al., 2016), both in secondary schools, employed consent from pupils while parents were informed and provided time to opt their child out, if they wished.

Under the legal age of majority, children can provide 'assent' and it is good practice to ensure that the purpose and nature of the research is explained to them in an age-appropriate manner. This often requires the preparation of different information sheets for different age groups, and active involvement of children and young people in the development of these materials will ensure that they are optimally effective (INVOLVE, 2016). Failure to do so can undermine the quality of the data collected, and anxiety or reluctance should be treated as a withdrawal of consent on that occasion or for that data point (Spriggs, 2010).

Research into child mental health commonly benefits from multiple informants about each child, which can raise issues about who can provide consent for what (Singh, 2017). Similar issues arise with the use of proxies and secondary informants for vulnerable adults. Once young people are legally considered an adult (16 years in the UK), they are the primary informant and their consent is required to approach others, such as parents or teachers. For younger children, the parent, or adult with parental responsibility in the case of children who are looked after, is the primary informant. Cluster randomized trials can raise particular issues that require a clear protocol to ensure that all are clear about who is approached to consent about which aspects of the study. For example, if a cluster randomized controlled trial is studying a universal intervention in schools, the head teacher consents to the school's involvement in the research. Teachers consent for their own participation and often the involvement of their class or lessons while parents and/or young people consent for their involvement in the *research*, but they cannot alter their school's involvement in the research study. It is important to plan with the school for what happens for children who are opted out when the research and/or the intervention is taking place (Ford et al., 2013; Kidger et al., 2016; Kuyken et al., 2017). Similarly, it is important that standardized operating procedures ensure that teachers nominated to take part by their head teacher are allowed sufficient autonomy to provide valid consent (Ford et al., 2013; Kidger et al., 2016; Kuyken et al., 2017), as are practitioners in a clinical situation (Ford et al., 2013).

Protecting the best interests of vulnerable research participants

Beneficence as a principle has over the past 40 years been relegated to the background as autonomy gained ascendancy as the defining moral principle, primarily due to concerns of paternalism. Even the most ardent advocates of autonomy, however, admit that soft paternalism becomes morally appropriate where the choices of a person cannot be considered that person's own in a meaningful, sufficiently robust sense; in such cases, the moral duty to protect a person against the potentially harmful consequences of his/her choices gains primacy over promoting autonomy (Radoilska, 2015).

The difficulties in establishing the validity of informed consent and the lack of an internationally accepted standard mean that we must look beyond autonomy to ensure ethical recruitment of vulnerable participants. In countries that do not have regulation/legal frameworks to guide the issue, we propose the simple process shown in Figure 4.2, where there is an additional step before assessing capacity to give consent. This ensures benefit to the person and avoids harm, through an assessment of whether the participant can directly benefit from being a part of the research study.

Where there is no therapeutic benefit to the participant, that is, the research is non-therapeutic, rather than assessing capacity to consent, the next question to be considered is if the proposed research can be carried out with non-vulnerable persons, where there is no ambiguity about the capacity to give consent to research. If that is the case, there is no moral justification in extracting a potentially invalid consent from a person with questionable cognitive capacity, and such persons should be excluded from the proposed research. There should be no question of proxy/surrogate consent in such a case, as there must be no assuming or imposing of altruism on the part of another (Pellegrino and Thomasma, 1987).

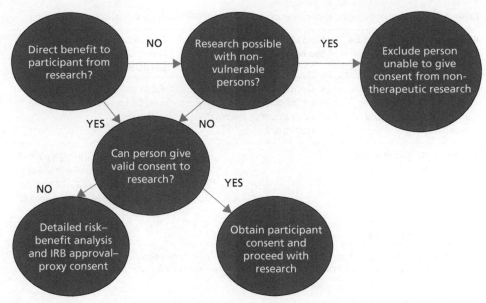

Figure 4.2 Recruiting persons into research where capacity to consent is doubtful—consider benefit to the participant in the absence of a legal/quasi-legal framework for guidance.

If the research is indeed therapeutic, that could justify the risk of undertaking the proposed research. In such a case, the next step would be the assessment of capacity to give consent to research. Where there is unambiguous, voluntary consent to research, the participant can join the research study. Where the proposed research participant lacks capacity to provide valid consent, but the researcher believes with a high degree of certainty that the participant can benefit from the research, the ethical dilemma arises. And this is where the model of beneficence comes in, superseding both autonomy and paternalism.

Beneficence as a guiding principle in psychiatric research ethics

The lowest level of beneficence is non-maleficence, and to avoid harm to potentially vulnerable persons is a basic minimum requirement for a clinician/researcher. The ascending spectrum of moral requirements progresses from the duty to remove/limit the possibility of harm, to restrict individual autonomy so as to prevent harm to the individual/society, and lastly to prevent harm/do good to the individual at some risk to the benefactor. This last level of beneficence is not one that is usually legally required, but one that the medical profession generally undertakes as a duty.

The beneficence model proposed by Pellegrino and Thomasma (1987) was developed for use in clinical practice. The model, comprising six major features, can be simplified and adapted to research contexts. First, the aim of research should be beneficent, with three specific features: the research participant's interests should take precedence over those of the researcher, harm should be avoided, and the primary obligation on the researcher is

Table 4.1 Beneficence model in deciding on research participation by vulnerable populations

Aim of research should be beneficent	Consider current condition of the research participant	Consensus between researcher and research participants
◆ Interests of the research participant should take precedence over those of the researcher	◆ Decisions should not be based on previous history or situation of the research participant	◆ Consensus on the processes to be carried out during the research
◆ Primary obligation of the researcher is to act in the best interest of the participant		◆ Best achieved through patient and public involvement in the research design at the earliest possible stage of the research process
◆ Avoid harm to participants		

Source data from Pellegrino, E.D. and Thomasma, D.C. (1987). The conflict between Autonomy and Beneficence in Medical Ethics: Proposal for a Resolution. *Journal of Contemporary Health Law & Policy, 3*, 23–46.

to act in the best interest of the participant rather than to promote autonomy or to act paternalistically. Second, the current condition of the research participant is what needs to considered. Third, there should be consensus between the researchers and the research participants on the processes to be carried out, and this is best achieved through patient and public involvement in the research design, at the earliest possible stage in the process (Table 4.1).

Under the beneficence model the researcher has the greater moral responsibility as the person with the greater information and power. They must be a person of moral integrity, and must accept moral ambiguity and ethical dilemmas as inherent features of research to be resolved through ethical reasoning.

References

Anderson, K.K. and Mukherjee, S.D. (2007). The need for additional safeguards in the informed consent process in schizophrenia research. *Journal of Medical Ethics, 33*, 647–650.

Appelbaum, P.S. (2007). Assessment of patients' competence to consent to treatment. *New England Journal of Medicine, 357*, 1634–1640.

Appelbaum, P.S. and Grisso, T. (1988). Assessing patients' capacities to consent to treatment. *New England Journal of Medicine, 319*, 1635–1638.

Appelbaum, P.S. and Grisso, T. (2001). *MacArthur competence assessment tool for clinical research (MacCAT-CR)*. Sarasota, FL: Professional Resource Press/Professional Resource Exchange.

Benatar, D. (2006). Bioethics and health and human rights: a critical view. *Journal of Medical Ethics, 32*, 17–20.

Bhutta, Z.A. (2004). Beyond informed consent. *Bulletin of the World Health Organization, 82*, 771–777.

Christopher, P.P. and Dunn, L.B. (2015). Informed consent, capacity and voluntarism. In: Sadler, J.Z., Van Staden, C.W., and Fulford, K.W.M. (eds.). *Oxford handbook of psychiatric ethics*, pp 945–957. Oxford: Oxford University Press.

CIOMS (2002). *International ethical guidelines for biomedical research involving human subjects.* Geneva: Council for International Organizations of Medical Sciences.

Davis, T.C., Holcombe, R.F., Berkel, H.J., Pramanik, S., and Divers, S.G. (1998). Informed consent for clinical trials: a comparative study of standard versus simplified forms. *Journal of the National Cancer Institute*, **90**, 668–674.

Department for Constitutional Affairs (2007). Mental Capacity Act 2005: Code of Practice.https://assets.publishing.service.gov.uk/government/uploads/system/uploads/attachment_data/file/497253/Mental-capacity-act-code-of-practice.pdf

DeRenzo, E.G., Conley, R.R., and Love, R. (1998). Assessment of capacity to give consent to research participation: state of the art and beyond. *Journal of Healthcare and Policy*, **1**, 66–87.

Dunn, L.B., Nowrangi, M.A., Palmer, B.W., Jeste, D.V., and Saks, E.R. (2006). Assessing decisional capacity for clinical research or treatment: a review of instruments. *American Journal of Psychiatry*, **163**, 1323–1334.

Emanuel, E.J., Wendler, D., and Grady, C. (2000). What makes clinical research ethical? *JAMA*, **283**, 2701–2711.

European Commission (2014). Regulation (EU) No 536/2014 of the European Parliament and of the Council of 16 April 2014 on clinical trials on medicinal products for human use, and repealing Directive 2001/20/EC. https://ec.europa.eu/health//sites/health/files/files/eudralex/vol-1/reg_2014_536/reg_2014_536_en.pdf

European Medicines Agency (n.d.). Clinical trial regulation. http://www.ema.europa.eu/ema/index.jsp?curl=pages/regulation/general/general_content_000629.jsp

Ford, T. and Kessel, A. (2001). Feeling the way: childhood mental illness and consent to admission and treatment. *British Journal of Psychiatry*, **179**, 384–386.

Ford, T.J., Last, A., Henley, W., Norman, S., Guglani, S., Kelesidi, K., et al. (2013). Can diagnostic assessment be used as a useful adjunct to clinical assessment in child and adolescent mental health services? A randomised controlled trial of disclosure of the Development and Well-Being Assessment to practitioners. *Social Psychiatry and Psychiatric Epidemiology*, **48**, 583–593.

Gibson, C., Medeiros, K.E., Giorgini, V., Mecca, J.T., Devenport, L.D., Connelly, S., and Mumford, M.D. (2014). A qualitative analysis of power differentials in ethical situations in academia. *Ethics & Behaviour*, **24**, 311–325.

Gillick v West Norfolk & Wisbech Area Health Authority, UKHL 7 (17 October 1985). http://www.bailii.org/uk/cases/UKHL/1985/7.html

Goldstein, A.O., Frasier, P., Curtis, P., Reid, A., and Kreher, N.E. (1996). Consent form readability in university-sponsored research. *Journal of Family Practice*, **42**, 606–611.

Gostin, L. (1991). Ethical principles for the conduct of human subject research: population-based research and ethics. *Law, Medicine & Healthcare*, **19**, 3–4.

Gupta, U.C. and Kharawala, S. (2012). Informed consent in psychiatry clinical research: a conceptual review of issues, challenges, and recommendations. *Perspectives in Clinical Research*, **3**, 8–15.

Humphrey, H.H. (1977). [Speech given on the occasion of the Health, Education and Welfare building's being named for him.] http://quotes.yourdictionary.com/author/hubert-humphrey/65231

INVOLVE (2016). Top tips for involving young people in research. http://www.invo.org.uk/wp-content/uploads/2016/01/involvingcyp-tips-keyissues-January2016.pdf

Ives J (1 June 2018). Presentation at Keele University, UK.

Kidger, J., Evans, R., Tilling, K., Hollingworth, W., Campbell, R., Ford, T., et al. (2016). Protocol for a cluster randomised controlled trial of an intervention to improve the mental health support and training available to secondary school teachers—the WISE (Wellbeing in Secondary Education) study. *BMC Public Health*, **16**, 1–13.

Kuyken, W., Nuthall, E., Byford, S., Crane, C., Dalgleish, T., Ford, T. et al. (2017). The effectiveness and cost-effectiveness of a mindfulness training programme in schools compared with normal school provision (MYRIAD): study protocol for a randomised controlled trial. *Trials*, **18**, 194.

Lamont, S., Jeon, Y.H., and Chiarella, M. (2013). Assessing patient capacity to consent to treatment: an integrative review of instruments and tools. *Journal of Clinical Nursing*, **22**, 2387–2403.

Legislation.gov.uk (2005). Mental Capacity Act 2005. http://www.legislation.gov.uk/ukpga/2005/9/contents

Lemaire, F., Bion J, Blanco J, Damas P, Druml C, Falke K, et al. (2005). The European Union directive on clinical research: present status of implementation in EU member states' legislations with regard to the incompetent patient. *Intensive Care Medicine*, **31**, 476–479.

Lindegger, G. and Richter, L. (2000). HIV vaccine trials: critical issues in informed consent. *South African Journal of Science*, **96**, 313–318.

Marshall, P.A. (2007). *Ethical challenges in study design and informed consent for health research in resource-poor settings*. Special Topics in Social, Economic and Behavioural (SEB) Research report series; No. 5 TDR/SDR/SEB/ST/07.1. Geneva: World Health Organization. http://apps.who.int/iris/bitstream/10665/43622/1/9789241563383_eng.pdf

Maryland Attorney General's Working Group (1998). *Final Report on Research Involving Decisionally Impaired Subjects*. Baltimore, MD: Office of the Maryland Attorney General.

Moser, D., Schultz, S.K., Arndt, S., Benjamin, M.L., Fleming, F.W., Brems, C.S., et al. (2002). Capacity to provide informed consent for participation in schizophrenia and HIV research. *American Journal of Psychiatry*, **159**, 1201–1207.

Muthappan, P., Forster, H., and Wendler, D. (2005). Research advance directives: protection or obstacle? *American Journal Psychiatry*, **162**, 2389–2391.

National Bioethics Advisory Commission (1998). *Research involving mental disorders that may affect decision-making capacity*. Rockville, MD: National Bioethics Advisory Commission.

National Bioethics Advisory Commission Group (2001). *Ethical and policy issues in international research: clinical trials in developing countries*. Bethesda, MD: National Bioethics Advisory Commission.

National Institutes of Health (2009). Research involving individuals with questionable capacity to consent: points to consider. http://grants.nih.gov/grants/policy/questionablecapacity.htm

New York State Advisory Work Group (1998). *Recommendations on the oversight of human subjects research involving the protected classes*. Albany, NY: State of New York Department of Health.

Nuffield Council on Bioethics (2002). *The ethics of research related to healthcare in developing countries*. London: Nuffield Council on Bioethics.

Nuffield Council on Bioethics (2005). *The ethics of research related to healthcare in developing countries: a follow-up Discussion Paper*. London: Nuffield Council on Bioethics.

Ogloff, J.R. and Otto, R.K. (1991). Are research participants truly informed? Readability of informed consent forms used in research. *Ethics & Behaviour*, **1**, 239–252.

Pellegrino, E.D. and Thomasma, D.C. (1987). The conflict between autonomy and beneficence in medical ethics: proposal for a resolution. *Journal of Contemporary Health Law & Policy*, **3**, 23–46.

Posever, T.A. and Chelmow, T. (2001). Informed consent for research in schizophrenia. *IRB: Ethics and Human Research*, **23**, 10–15.

Radoilska, L. (2015). Autonomy in psychiatric ethics. In Sadler, J.Z., Van Staden, C.W., and Fulford, K.W.M. (eds.). *Oxford handbook of psychiatric ethics*, pp. 354–371. Oxford: Oxford University Press.

Raich, P.C., Plomer, K.D., and Coyne, C.A. (2001). Literacy, comprehension and informed consent in clinical research. *Cancer Investigation*, **19**, 437–445.

Roberts, L.W., Warner, T.D., and Brody, J.L. (2000). Perspectives of patients with schizophrenia and psychiatrists regarding ethically important aspects of research participation. *American Journal of Psychiatry*, **157**, 67–74.

Royal College of Psychiatrists (2011). Ethics of psychiatric research. Position statement PS 02/2011. https://www.rcpsych.ac.uk/pdf/PS02_2011.pdf

Scott, K.Y.H., Kim, H.M., Ryan, K.A., Appelbaum, P.S., Knopman, D.S., Damschroder, L., and De Vries, R. (2013). How important is 'accuracy' of surrogate decision-making for research participation? *PLoS One*, **8**, e54790.

Singh, I. (2017). Commentary: what makes a life go well? Moral functioning and quality of life measurement in neurodevelopmental disorders—reflections on Jonsson et al. (2017). *Journal of Child Psychology and Psychiatry*, **58**, 470–473.

Spriggs, M. (2010). *Understanding consent in research involving children: the ethical issues. A handbook for human research ethics committees and researchers*. Melbourne: Children's Bioethics Centre, University of Melbourne. https://www.vu.edu.au/sites/default/files/research/pdfs/ethics-children-handbook.pdf

Stevenson, A. (ed.) (2010). *Oxford dictionary of English*. Oxford: Oxford University Press.

Sumathipala, A. and Fernando, B.L. (2014). Ethical issues in global mental health trials. In: Thornicroft, G. and Patel, V. (eds.). *Global mental health trials*, pp. 123–137. Oxford: Oxford University Press.

Sumathipala, A. and Siribaddana, S. (2004). Revisiting freely given informed consent. Role of an ombudsman. *American Journal of Bioethics*, **4**, W1–W7.

Torke, M.A., Alexander, G.C., and Lantos, J. (2008). Substituted judgment: the limitations of autonomy in surrogate decision making. *Journal of General Internal Medicine*, **23**, 1514–1517.

Tri-Council Working Group (1997). *Code of conduct for research involving humans: final report of the Tri-Council Working Group*. Vancouver: Canada, Centre for Applied Ethics.

Van Staden, C.W. (2015). Informed consent to treatment. In: Sadler, J.Z., Van Staden, C.W., and Fulford, K.W.M. (eds.). *Oxford handbook of psychiatric ethics*, pp. 1129–1142. Oxford: Oxford University Press.

Vaz, M. and Srinivasan, K. (2014). Ethical challenges & dilemmas for medical health professionals doing psychiatric research. *Indian Journal of Medical Research*, **139**, 191–193.

Chapter 5

Ethics and research in psychiatry: Engagement with patients and public

Stephani L. Hatch, Billy Gazard, and Diana Rose

Introduction

This chapter explores the ethical issues that arise in psychiatric research in relation to engagement with patients and the general public. Over the past decade, there has been a significant shift in psychiatric and other medical research that places an emphasis on the engagement and involvement of patients and the public. This shift has resulted in changes in the expectations of the way research is conducted and disseminated, specifically regarding the level of scientific knowledge that should be accessible to service users and the public. In emphasizing public understanding of science or 'knowledge transfer', researchers have been more likely to consider participatory research approaches, which in theory should include the sharing of power and resources, as well as collective action towards mutually beneficial outcomes (National Co-ordinating Centre for Public Engagement (NCCPE), 2012). However, there is little attention given to how this approach is being practised in psychiatric research or how the relevant ethical safeguards expected in all research are being addressed (Hughes, 2008).

This chapter will begin by making the distinction between patient and public engagement (PPE) and patient and public involvement (PPI). This will be followed by a discussion of basic ethical principles as they relate to engagement, and examples of how PPE is situated within psychiatric research agendas, particularly as it relates to participatory action approaches. The chapter will conclude with three brief case studies of engagement approaches in psychiatric research with discussion of ethical issues that may arise in different types of engagement.

Defining patient and public engagement

This chapter primarily focuses on PPE, but it should be considered in the context of being one of two distinct approaches that are often entrenched and expected in research programmes. The more commonly considered approach is PPI. PPI is defined as action that promotes direct participatory approaches in research, the importance and value of service user experiences in improving treatments and services, and increased accountability

Box 5.1 Defining engagement and involvement

Patient and public engagement

Informing, consulting, and collaborating with the public.

Patient and public involvement

Direct participatory approaches in research, incorporating and valuing service users' experiences in improving treatments and services, and increased accountability among researchers.

among researchers (Boaz et al., 2016). In comparison, PPE is centred on informing, consulting, and collaborating with the public (NCCPE, 2012) (Box 5.1). It generally operates on the premise that there is a need to ensure a dialogue or debate between scientists, researchers, and public audiences with a commitment to a more socially responsible research approach. Further, PPE is described as having a strong focus on educating the public about science and building trust in scientific activities (Wynne, 2006; Boaz et al., 2016). Notably, PPE also creates an important opportunity for reciprocity and accountability on the part of researchers.

Ethical principles in relation to engagement

This section considers basic ethical principles as they relate to engagement with patients and the public in the context of research. As outlined in guidance documents such as the Helsinki Declaration (Human and Fluss, 2001), the basic ethical principles include *beneficence, non-maleficence, protection of autonomy*, and *justice* (Box 5.2). The principles of ethical conduct in research are intended to provide guidance for the development and process of all research activity, which is regulated by governing bodies primary located within educational and health systems. The premise of this process is that shared values are adopted by researchers. However, in practice this is achieved to varying degrees.

While ethical guidance is widely available for what is traditionally considered within the boundaries of research, there is limited information that specifically guides researchers in

Box 5.2 Basic ethical principles

- Beneficence
- Non-maleficence
- Protection of autonomy
- Justice.

related research activities, such as PPE. The UK NCCPE provides general guidelines regarding ethical principles and practice in PPE (Centre for Social Justice and Community Action (CSJCA) and NCCPE, 2012). As previously noted, activities related to PPE raise issues regarding basic ethical principles and more specifically, concerning mutual respect, democratic participation, equality and inclusion, transparency, systems of accountability, and reciprocity that deserve further consideration (Nowotny et al., 2001; Boaz et al., 2016). However, many of these issues are not currently acknowledged or addressed by existing institutional ethical conduct requirements in PPE and across all research (Pickersgill, 2011).

Beneficence and non-maleficence

Beneficence is considered alongside non-maleficence to refer to the principle of promoting good while actively trying to maximize benefits over harm, with researchers seeking to address an exposure to harm (Gillon, 1994). In psychiatric research, a common ethical consideration relates to direct risk of psychological stress, humiliation, or other negative consequences of the research and how these risks will be addressed by the researcher should they occur. In relation to engagement, questions arise regarding the communication of benefits and risks. For example, exposure to sensitive topics in PPE and what will be done to address any distress caused by PPE is not monitored by most researchers or oversight committees. More broadly, the assumptions researchers make about how and to what extent patients and the public want to be engaged and made aware may limit possible benefits. Moreover, it has been noted that the language of ethical guidelines (e.g. the US Belmont Report) referring to *maximizing possible benefits* places considerable emphasis on research priorities being defined in conjunction with service users and community members (Department of Health, Education and Welfare, 2000; Brydon-Miller, 2008). It is this joint process of defining research agendas and priorities that can take place in the context of engagement.

Determining how benefit can be realized in the context of research requires consideration of notions of trust and reciprocity. The maintenance and restoration of public trust is not an unfamiliar issue in psychiatric research (Wynne, 2006). Trust or the lack thereof, has the potential to have both positive and negative impacts on communities. When need is solely defined from the perspective of the researchers acting solely in the interest of collecting data without reciprocity, trust tends to erode over time at both individual and community levels (Pittaway et al., 2010). A lack of trust hinders research in a number of ways. Noted concerns of community members range from a lack of feedback from researchers (e.g. promised reports, newsletters) to expected exploitation based on past experiences with researchers who 'fly in and out' of communities with little or no consideration for the social, political, or economic consequences of their presence (Pittaway et al., 2010; DuBois et al., 2011). This can be reinforced by PPE that only focuses on transient and temporary involvement of service user groups and communities. Including and valuing engagement approaches in research does have the ability to create opportunities for community level action and improvements.

PPE has a capacity to challenge structures of power and knowledge, including access to knowledge. As with PPI, PPE often involves the participation of key stakeholders, particularly those historically excluded from decision-making about research (e.g. patients and community members). However, how researchers define a stakeholders group to contribute to a research project has implications for whose views are valued and what is considered valued knowledge. PPE is an opportunity to develop relationships and exchanges within research that are based on an acknowledgement that the generation of information and knowledge are not an inherent right of the academic to produce. This is likely to be complicated by researchers reporting engagement as a positive activity and simultaneously expressing negative attitudes and actions that resist sharing the generation of scientific knowledge (Boaz et al., 2016; Staley et al., 2014). This is perhaps most evident in the failure of many researchers to engage on a basic level (e.g. obtaining feedback on data interpretation where appropriate or disseminating findings) with service users, the public, and wider communities.

Autonomy

The principle of autonomy primarily considers the protection and respect of an individual's ability to make decisions, confidentiality, and communication with research participants. Within the process of conducting research, issues of diminished autonomy are addressed in the process of informed consent. Because PPE often involves the collection of information that may not traditionally be considered data but contributes to the overall research process, consideration should be given to whether or not the consent requirement should be extended to individuals, groups, or organizations involved in engagement. For example, confidentiality and anonymity may receive less consideration when research teams disseminate information through multiple outlets (e.g. presentations, visuals, and social media) (CSJCA and NCCPE, 2012). The use of social media is heavily encouraged as a mode for engaging larger and wider audiences, but little consideration is given to ensuring and maintaining confidentiality when disclosing the identity of individuals, groups, organizations, and locations of engagement activities. Moreover, the purpose and use of information generated through PPE is also likely to change over the course of the research. As a result, repeated review and negotiation of individual or collective consent may also be necessary, as well as transparency about the planned use of information generated through PPE (CSJCA and NCCPE, 2012).

Ensuring autonomy is also predicated upon the type and method of communication in research. Researchers should aim to present knowledge that is complete and accurate, and reflective of the ways in which the research was conducted, the ethical regulations governing a project, and its potential impact on the individual and society (Pickersgill, 2011). Autonomy is more likely to be preserved when communication is central to engagement, beginning with public understanding of science and knowledge about research methods and related ethical issues. Fundamentally, researchers should seek to avoid deception and ambiguity in communication and engagement with patients and the public. While health researchers are required to include a general statement of no direct benefit of research when seeking consent, how knowledge is managed and deception is avoided in dissemination and engagement is less clear.

Justice for human participants

Notions of justice obligate researchers to consider equality, respect for people's rights, and legal justice. In the context of ethics, justice is considered from organizational, professional, and societal perspectives. From an organizational perspective, the practice of research is primarily guided by a shared understanding of ethical principles, and this is upheld by ethics committees within academic and health institutions. Ethics committees operate on these principles and assess the practice of research through specific requirements, including, but not limited to, informed consent; coercion or pressure to participate; assessments of risks and benefits; the inclusion and exclusion of participants; and data handling and protections (Brydon-Miller, 2008). Despite an increasing number of funding bodies emphasizing and in some cases requiring PPE, questions about who regulates engagement activities or how they should be regulated remain unaddressed in institutional processes.

Related to participation in the construction of knowledge, discussed previously, justice concerns equality and inclusion in PPE. Engagement is an avenue through which more disempowered or marginalized groups can contribute and challenge existing systems of power. This involves not only encouraging groups representing a wide range of social statuses and identities (e.g. race, ethnicity, sexual orientation, disability, education, gender, and age) but actively enabling these groups to participate. There are practical considerations, such as accessibility of physical spaces and information, but also more complex social processes, such as challenging stigmatizing and discriminatory attitudes and behaviours.

Patient and public engagement in psychiatric research agendas

This section provides examples of a broad psychiatric research agenda that tends to benefit from participatory approaches and PPE. In addition, three PPE case studies are presented to provide examples of the types of ethical issues that may arise in networks, programme or project partnership.

There are two types of psychiatric research agendas where participatory approaches in general and PPE more specifically are particularly relevant. Translational psychiatric research, that is, it aims to translate clinical research to benefits for patients and health systems, inherently suggests that it is applied. Translational approaches in psychiatric research not only generate new knowledge, but also have the ultimate goal of offering new or improved treatments and services. The potential for increasing the benefits of psychiatric research is likely to be more sustainable when people have the opportunity to be active agents of change rather than simply the subjects of inquiry. Another area of psychiatric research that is well suited for participatory approaches is inequalities in mental health and health service use, particularly since its focus is centred on excluded or marginalized groups (Beresford, 2007). Given the potential for the latter research focus to reinforce the exclusion of certain groups, researchers working in this area of psychiatric research should be proactive about addressing inclusion and diversity from initial development stages through to dissemination beyond the end of the project. Beyond these ethical considerations, participatory approaches all have engagement as a fundamental principle. This is manifested in many forms and levels of engagement vary. At the very least, developing a dissemination plan at the start of a research project is likely to be more effective than waiting until the research has concluded. In participatory research approaches, sharing research findings can begin at any point of the data analysis. However, researchers have to be prepared for positive and negative influences of their work. For example, identifying inequalities in access to protective resources for mental health or disparities within mental health services may have deleterious effects on individuals and communities. Thus, the NCCPE suggests that discussions and negotiations with stakeholders about which information should be shared, methods and formats for dissemination, and preferred outcomes and possible negative impacts should be integral throughout the research process (CSJCA and NCCPE, 2012). Finally, authorship and acknowledgements should be openly discussed with engagement partners in advance of any activities or dissemination.

Case studies: PPE approaches and related ethical considerations

This section presents three brief case studies of engagement approaches in psychiatric research. Each case study describes engagement networks and activities with examples that will aid researchers to consider the types of ethical issues that may arise and how they may be addressed.

Case study 1: Health Inequalities Research Network (HERON)

Brief description
HERON was developed to formalize and sustain a network of people involved in action and research in mental health-related inequalities. The network consists of public members, students, voluntary sector advocates, healthcare practitioners, researchers, and service users. The basic principle of the network is to develop and promote the interaction of health practitioners and researchers with community members and representatives in order to have a more collaborative approach to addressing inequalities. The main aims of the network are as follows: (1) to provide a forum in which health practitioners, researchers, and community members can collectively share their experiences and information in order to further understand the problems affecting health; (2) to empower individuals within their neighbourhoods and communities by providing a forum to voice their opinions and contribute to a dialogue on health inequalities; (3) to highlight health inequalities through a variety of media and work towards reducing these inequalities. HERON is an international network, but primarily operates at a local level through the work of a dedicated group of volunteers who help to maintain community group ties,

as well as organize and run events. HERON uses a range of approaches to engage and interact with its members and the wider community.

Ethical issues emerging

Ethical issues in the engagement activities emerged in the process of engaging and disseminating information to wide range of stakeholders and were generally unanticipated by event coordinators. Their experiences with considering and dealing with ethical issues predominantly occurred within the context of university research. There was little consideration of how access to language, knowledge construction, and physical spaces (i.e. location of events) may impact engagement experiences. This issue arose in two particular types of HERON engagement activities.

The HERON Research Road Show travelled to libraries and other public spaces to disseminate locally relevant research findings and generate discussions about the findings from the South East London Community Health (SELCoH) study, an urban mental health study of a household population in the London boroughs of Southwark and Lambeth. During these events, it emerged in the interactions with the public and from feedback during the event that what we meant by 'health inequalities' was not as widely understood as we had anticipated and key messages were unclear. As a result, we had to rethink the accessibility of the knowledge that we were disseminating, as well as the presentation of printed and online materials. As a result, authors of SELCoH research papers were instructed to write short lay summaries of research papers to be made available on our website. We also had further discussions about different communication styles and strategies that may be more appropriate for the audiences that we were engaging.

During HERON's events involving visual and performance art collaborations with students and young service users from local schools and community organizations, concerns came up in relation to who was involved in knowledge generation, how people access spaces, and consent. In preparation for one event, we spent several months devoting time to building relationships and trust between academic researchers, students, and young service users. We considered the potential vulnerability of the young service users and were conscious of potential ethical issues that may arise as a result of them sharing their experiences of discrimination and stigma through narratives and art. However, we had not realized that the students felt excluded from an opportunity to share their experiences or that they felt vulnerable in ways that we had not considered. The accessibility of space was an issue in the next step of the project which involved having the students come to the university for a project meeting; this idea was met with great resistance by the students. The students, many from social and economically disadvantaged backgrounds, viewed the university as an intimidating and inaccessible space. To resolve this, the HERON team decided to add a meeting at their school to continue to work on building their trust. After working with an ethnically and socioeconomically diverse group of university students and researchers, the students showed interest in coming to the university. We also changed the planned format from a meeting to an interactive workshop that would allow the students to use their knowledge in the arts in discussions of examples of how mental health and the arts can be interrelated. As a result, we created an opportunity for the students to participate in similar ways to the young service users and re-evaluated possible ethical issues. At the end of this process, visual and performance art pieces were shared in a public exhibition. While we had gained consent for participation in the project, we had not considered additional consent for the reproduction of images of the art produced in our efforts to communicate the impact of the event. To try to better anticipate similar issues and address these points in future projects, we have had to form a more formal HERON planning group which includes a student representative.

Learning points

- Academics researchers need to modify their communication styles and avoid jargon.
- All event partners may be in a position of vulnerability.
- Attention should be given to how physical spaces represent power and exclusion.
- Building trust may take more time than anticipated.
- Consider issues of confidentiality and consent for all outputs, visual as well as written.

Case study 2: South East London Photography group (SELPh)

Brief description

SELPh is a community photography project run as a voluntary collaboration between researchers, mental health practitioners, and community members with experience of mental illness. It offers people with recent experience of mental illness an opportunity to take photographs and use them to reflect on their experiences in a group setting. The aim of the project is to improve mental well-being, promote recovery, and build social support networks for people recovering from mental illness using innovative participatory photography methods. Members have the opportunity to talk about their everyday experiences in a group setting, represent themselves, voice their opinions to contribute to a dialogue on health and well-being, and tackle the stigma that surrounds mental illness through group exhibitions at local public art galleries. Each member is loaned a digital camera so that they can take pictures around a chosen theme each week. During the sessions, members discuss their pictures in small groups and present their favourite image to the group at the end of the session. Facilitators gently guide discussion towards reflection and interpretation and away from more technical aspects of photography. Members are encouraged to reflect and comment as much as possible. At the end of the process, the group organizes a public exhibition to showcase their work.

Ethical issues emerging

SELPh was formed with the intention of a collaborative approach to generating discussion around experiences of mental health using the photovoice method, which was developed within the framework of CBPR (Wang and Burris, 1997). While founding members of the group formed a protocol based on ethical approaches to PPE as a guideline, ethical issues emerged as the project developed.

One of the key ongoing ethical issues was the sharing of power between all stakeholders and balancing the dynamics of the group. At the introductory session, ground rules were set by group members to ensure equality in group dynamics and that every group member's voice was heard. Facilitators and group members had to continually monitor and ensure that no one person, particularly facilitators, was dominating the group discourse and that everybody felt comfortable to contribute to group conversation. Group members were involved in all decision-making, including goals and expected outcomes of the project. This was particularly important in terms of exploring how mental illness impacts everyday life and group members' concerns around representations of mental illness in public exhibitions. Group members navigated discussions concerning confidentiality, anonymity, the potential harm and benefit of such representations in public exhibitions, and their involvement in this process.

Building trust between researchers and health practitioners with group members was particularly salient in this project. Group members expressed concern about previous treatment from researchers and health practitioners and were cautious in being fully involved in the process at the early stages. Only through attention to balancing power dynamics and transparency of intentions were facilitators able to gain trust and form productive relationships. Paramount to maintaining trust is the concept of autonomy and consent. Group members continue to have ownership over their photographs and accompanying narratives and individual consent is continually negotiated for their collective use.

One of the most difficult ethical issues with PPE is developing strategies for participation on an ongoing basis. Group members have become members of the steering committee and gone on to become facilitators while SELPh has also collaborated with other projects to involve group members in other PPE projects involved in mental health research. This has involved providing access to training and added another layer to the collaborative process of the project.

Learning points

- Develop tailored protocol for ethical considerations.
- Ensure balanced power dynamics between all stakeholders.
- Build trust with communities in PPE projects.
- Transparency and informed consent are needed for all outputs.
- Importance of maintaining ongoing relationships with communities.

Case study 3: involvement of service users in Biomedical Research Centre (BRC) structure

Brief description

This project involved increased participation in the governance structures of our Maudsley BRC for Mental Health. There was already a BRC Service User Advisory Group (SUAG) which advised at the early stage of research proposals thus ensuring service user engagement in shaping research at its initial stages. To further embed this group, two projects were undertaken. First, members of the SUAG began to sit on research Steering Groups and also took up positions on governance structures, such as 'Cluster Boards' which are the 'first level' of governance in the organization. To facilitate this there were regular meetings between representatives and Deputy Cluster Leads as well as the salaried service user researchers who facilitated the SUAG. Second, a series of research priority setting meetings were convened at local mental health service user groups in the Trust catchment area and then fed back to the Executive of the BRC (Robotham et al., 2016). The aim of both these endeavours was to embed service user perspectives more thoroughly in the BRC.

Ethical issues emerging

SUAG representatives said that both Steering Groups and Cluster Boards were 'business meetings' where it was difficult to have a voice. Papers often were not ready in advance and the impression was that decisions were already settled by professional members before the meeting. At worst, representatives felt not only that they were sidelined but that the discussions 'objectified' mental health issues which they themselves might have experienced. These issues were discussed in professional diagnostic terms and not approached as human problems. For the priority-setting workshops, there were difficulties in reaching excluded communities such as people from black and ethnic minority communities and older people. We did secure a small grant specifically to run workshops with these groups. The workshops will be a blend of dissemination of BRC work and priority setting from the perspectives of these groups. To see how successful these changes have been, we are now conducting an ethnography.

Learning points

- Mental health professionals need to be more flexible in their language.
- Mental health professionals must not objectify service users.
- Strategies are needed for reaching excluded groups.
- We must realize that conventional methods may make no sense to these groups.

Case study websites

HERON: https://heronnetwork.com/

South East London Photography group (SELPh): https://selphgroup.com/

Maudsley Biomedical Research Centre (BRC): http://www.maudsleybrc.nihr.ac.uk/

BRC Service User Advisory Group: http://www.maudsleybrc.nihr.ac.uk/patients-public/support-for-researchers/

References

Beresford, P. (2007). User involvement, research and health inequalities: developing new directions. *Health and Social Care in the Community*, **15**, 306–312.

Boaz, A., Biri, D., and McKevitt, C. (2016). Rethinking the relationship between science and society: has there been a shift in attitudes to patient and public involvement and public engagement in science in the United Kingdom? *Health Expectations*, **19**, 592–601.

Brydon-Miller, M. (2008). Ethics and action research: deepening our commitment to principles of social justice and redefining systems of democratic practice. In: Reason, P. and Bradbury, H. (eds.). *The SAGE handbook of action research participative inquiry and practice*, pp. 199–210. London: Sage.

Centre for Social Justice and Community Action (CSJCA), Durham University and National Coordinating Centre for Public Engagement (NCCPE) (2012). *Community-based participatory research: a guide to ethical principles and practice, national coordinating centre for public engagement*. Bristol: NCCPE http://www.publicengagement.ac.uk/how-we-help/our-publications/community-based-participatory-research-guide-to-ethical-principle

Department of Health, Education and Welfare (2000). Belmont report: ethical principles and guidelines for the protection of human subjects of research. In: Sales, B.D. and Folkman, S. (eds.). *Ethics in research with human participants*, pp. 195–205. Washington, DC: American Psychological Association.

DuBois, J., Bailey-Burch, B., Bustillos, D., Campbell, J., Cottler, L., Fisher, C., et al. (2011). Ethical issues in mental health: the case for community engagement. *Current Opinion in Psychiatry*, **24**, 208–214.

Gillon, R. (1994). Four principles and attention to scope. *British Medical Journal*, **309**, 185–189.

Hughes, I. (2008). Action research in healthcare. In: Reason, P. and Bradbury, H. (eds.). *The SAGE handbook of action research participative inquiry and practice*, pp. 381–393. London: Sage.

Human, D. and Fluss, S.S. (2001). The World Medical Association's Declaration of Helsinki: Historical and Contemporary Perspectives, 5th draft. World Medical Association, 24 July. http://www.wma.net/en/20activities/10ethics/10helsinki/draft_historical_contemporary_perspectives.pdf

Nowotny, H., Scott, P., and Gibbons, M. (2001). *Re-thinking science: knowledge and the public in an age of uncertainty*. Cambridge: Polity Press.

Pickersgill, M.D. (2011). Research, engagement and public bioethics: promoting socially robust science. *Journal of Medical Ethics*, **37**, 698–701.

Pittaway, E., Bartolomei, L. and Hugman, R. (2010). 'Stop stealing our stories': the ethics of research with vulnerable groups. *Journal of Human Rights Practice*, **2**, 229–251.

Robotham, D., Wykes, T., Rose, D., Doughty, L., Strange, S., Neale, J., and Hotopf M. (2016). Service user and carer priorities in a Biomedical Research Centre for mental health, *Journal of Mental Health*, **25**, 185–188.

Staley, K., Buckland, S.A., Hayes, H., and Tarpey, M. (2014). 'The missing links': understanding how context and mechanism influence the impact of public involvement in research. *Health Expectations*, **17**, 755–764.

Wang, C. and Burris, M.A. (1997). Photovoice concept, methodology and use for participatory needs assessment. *Health Education & Behaviour*, **24**, 369–387.

Wynne, B. (2006). Public engagement as a means of restoring public trust in science–hitting the notes, but missing the music? *Public Health Genomics*, **9**, 211–220.

Chapter 6

Introduction to epidemiological study designs

Tamsin Ford, Jayati Das-Munshi, and Martin Prince

Importance of study design

Epidemiologists must have a sound understanding of the principles of study design. Ethical considerations naturally prevent us from allocating potentially harmful exposures on an experimental basis in human populations, yet observational studies are inherently more vulnerable to the effect of bias and confounding. These problems can be minimized by good study design.

The design (and analysis) of a study aspires to maximize the *precision* and *validity* of its findings. The *precision* of an estimate of the prevalence of depression in a population will be reduced by sampling and measurement error. These errors are generally random, that is, equally likely to deviate from the truth in either direction. Precision can be improved with larger sample sizes and more accurate measures. Confounding and bias lead to non-random error, that is, the effect of the bias or confounder is systematic, tending mainly in one direction, thus reducing the *validity* of a finding. Choices of study design and measurement strategy are key factors in minimizing non-random error and maximizing the validity of the results.

Although the conduct and analysis of epidemiological studies has become increasing sophisticated over time, there are a limited number of basic designs, each with their own advantages and disadvantages. This chapter will provide an overview of study design, illustrated with examples from psychiatric epidemiological studies, while individual types of study will be discussed in greater depth in subsequent chapters.

Classifying study design

Epidemiological studies may be experimental or observational. In observational studies, epidemiologists try to make inferences about diseases through natural observation of groups of people defined by their exposure or disease status. The key difference between experimental and observational studies is that in the latter, the investigator has no control over the events under investigation. In epidemiological contexts, experimental studies are randomised controlled trials (RCTs), which are used to test the effectiveness and cost-effectiveness of interventions, RCT can also be used to investigate the aetiology of a condition or the mechanisms of action of a treatment, the effect of family therapy on expressed emotion and relapse in schizophrenia (Lahey et al., 2009).

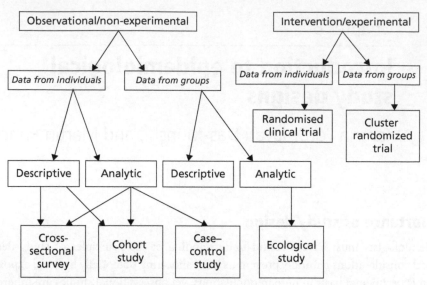

Figure 6.1 Classification of epidemiological studies.

Observational studies can be descriptive or analytic. A descriptive study illustrates an outcome, such as depression, *or* an exposure, for instance, life events, in terms of the characteristics of affected people in a particular place at a particular time. In contrast, analytical studies test for associations between outcomes and exposures. However, this classification is not rigid and as Figure 6.1 suggests, some cross-sectional surveys and cohort studies have both descriptive and analytic elements.

Epidemiological studies may analyse data aggregated across whole populations, for instance, the mean per capita alcohol consumption by region or country, or they report data at the individual level, for example, the number of units consumed by each person on a daily or weekly basis.

The following brief overview of the common study designs should be read in conjunction with Table 6.1, which summarizes the main features of each design.

Descriptive studies

Descriptive studies often use routinely collected statistics, such as mortality data, to investigate the occurrence of a disorder, or an exposure. Accompanying data, for example, on a death certificate, tends to be relatively sparse, limiting the potential for the study of co-determinants to simple variables such as age, gender, occupation, region, and time period. This is a particularly useful approach for rare disorders, and for outcomes that are relatively completely ascertained for official purposes. Suicide is frequently studied in this manner; for example, data from the UK have suggested a reduction in suicide rates from the beginning of the current century to their lowest recorded levels in 2006–2007 (Thomas and Gunnell, 2010) before increasing again (Ibrahim et al., 2019). Descriptive studies can also be used to generate hypotheses, which can then be tested in analytic

Table 6.1 Advantages and disadvantages of different types of epidemiological study

	Cross-sectional	Case–control	Cohort	Ecological	Clinical trial
Subject selection	Defined population	Caseness	Exposure	Aggregated data	Caseness
Source of bias	Selection Non-response Information (recall and observer)	Selection Information (recall and observer)	Information (observer only) Loss to follow-up (selection)	Selection of population Ecological fallacy	Selection Information (reduced by blinding)
Probability of confounding	Medium	Medium	Low	High	Very low if randomized
Resources	Quick and cheap	Relatively quick and cheap	Lengthy and expensive	Relatively quick and cheap	Relatively expensive
Applications	Planning services Mapping secular and geographical trends Identifying correlates	Rare outcomes Single outcomes Multiple exposures	Rare exposure Single exposures Multiple outcomes	Rare outcomes Rare exposures Multiple exposures Population exposures such as air pollution	Efficacy of new interventions Effectiveness of new interventions Hypothesis-testing mechanisms
Measure of effect	Prevalence	Odds ratio	Relative risk	Correlation/regression coefficient	Relative risk/odds ratio/difference between means

studies, for instance, variation in prevalence among subgroups of a population may provide hints about aetiology that warrant further investigation.

The value of routine data may be compromised by incomplete or inaccurate recording. This may complicate secular or regional comparisons, where ascertainment and recording practices differ between geographical areas or over different time periods. For example, the stigma associated with suicide can lead to coroners in some countries tending to return a verdict of misadventure rather than suicide, so that official suicide statistics from these settings are likely to underestimate the true rate in the population. Similarly, the more common use of narrative or accidental verdicts in England over the last decade may have underestimated the incidence rate of suicides by up to 6% in 2009 (Hill and Cook, 2011). Suicide verdicts are not returned for children under 10 years of age and statistics on 10–14-year-olds do not include deaths with an undetermined cause that may relate to neglect or abuse as well as self-inflicted injury in this age group, while self-inflicted injury is assumed for indeterminate deaths in those aged over 15 years (Office for National Statistics, 2014).

Ecological studies

Ecological studies examine the evidence for associations by testing for correlations between the average level of an exposure and the prevalence or incidence of an outcome across different populations. The indices of both exposure and outcome are aggregated at the population level. For example, an ecological study suggested that child well-being is negatively correlated with income inequality in developed countries (Pickett and Wilkinson, 2007).

Ecological studies are useful to study social psychiatric epidemiology, where the aggregate social exposures may take on a meaning distict from that as an individual level exposure. In the example above, while the degree of income-inequality may vary greatly within a region or country, the impact of the aggregate social exposure, in the example above the experience of living within pockets of extreme income inequality, may have an influence on health that is distinct from the individuals socio-economic status.

There are three main problems with ecological studies. Firstly, the association can only be applied to populations not individuals. The incautious application of results obtained from data gathered at population level to individuals can therefore result in an 'ecological fallacy'. A classic example is the assumption made by many that lower levels of cardiovascular disease among countries with high levels of red wine consumption indicated that red wine had cardioprotective properties (Law Malcolm et al., 1999). Red wine consumption, plus morbidity and mortality from cardiovascular disease were both measured at population level, so we cannot be sure that the individuals drinking red wine actually had healthier cardiovascular function; collective wishful thinking perhaps? For a more recent and more psychiatric example, an ecological study mapped areas with high rates of suicide to population level risk factors, citing lower levels of education and higher density of immigrants as risk factors (Rocha et al., 2020). This study should not be intepretated as meaning that individuals with lower levels of education or who were born outside the country in which they live were necessarily at higher risk of suicide; individual level data would be needed to demonstrate this.

Secondly, as ecological studies often use data gathered for reasons other than research, information on potential confounding factors is often lacking and cannot be tested. Finally, as data on the exposure and the outcome are frequently gathered at the same time, we cannot make any inference about the likely direction of causality. It is possible to construct an argument that low levels of child well-being might lead to higher levels of income inequality as well as the other way round.

Cross-sectional surveys

Cross-sectional surveys collect information from a sample from a defined base population about the prevalence of an outcome, and exposure to potential risk factors for that outcome. They are quick and relatively cheap to perform and are often used to demonstrate the extent of the disorder, to plan services, and to identify potential risk factors for further study in hypothesis-driven analytical studies (see later in this chapter). As the disorder and the exposure are recorded simultaneously, a cross-sectional survey can never provide direct evidence of causality.

The population under study may be defined by area, for example, all children in Great Britain under 16 years (Green et al., 2005), or by other characteristics, such as all children looked after by the state because their families cannot care for them at a particular point in time (Ford et al., 2007). The first step is to identify a sampling frame or list to identify all individuals making up the population from which the sample is to be drawn. Administrative lists such as electoral registers are often used, although these can be surprisingly inaccurate. The British Child and Adolescent Mental Health Surveys used the child benefit register, as this benefit was at the time universal and drawn for 99% of children, but inaccurate addresses meant that this method achieved only a 90% coverage of the target base population (Meltzer et al., 2000; Green et al., 2005). An alternative is for the investigators to compile their own sampling frame by a door-knock census of the area to be surveyed. This obviously becomes impractical in large surveys or those covering extensive areas. If the sampling frame is not representative of the base population, the survey may be subject to selection bias; that is, it may either systematically over- or underestimate the true prevalence of the disorder in the base population due to the over- or under-representation of particular subgroups of people. Explicit inclusion and exclusion criteria, formulated in advance, are an essential component for all cross-sectional surveys. For instance, both British Child and Adolescent Mental Health Surveys excluded children who were in foster care, and included children between the ages of 5–15 (Meltzer et al., 2000) or 16 years (Green et al., 2005). These criteria must be carefully justified on the basis of feasibility, logistics, or relevance, and set limits on the generalizability of the survey findings.

A low response rate (<80%) will tend to reduce the validity of the survey's findings, as it is likely that non-responders differ from responders in many ways, some of which may be related to either the exposure and/or the outcome under investigation (Wolke et al., 2009). Non-response bias occurs if the characteristics of those who respond differ systematically from those who do not respond. However, if data is available about those who refused to participate, it may be possible to argue that non-response bias is relatively unlikely. Wolke and colleagues (2009) were able to demonstrate that despite the loss of those more likely to have teacher-reported behavioural difficulties, the associations between a plethora of background characteristics with the presence of behavioural difficulties were strikingly similar regardless of whether the family remained in the Avon Longitudinal Study of Parents and Childhood (ALSPAC) or not. Conversely, one should not assume that a high response rate necessarily eliminates the possibility of biased estimates (Gerrits et al., 2001).

The cross-sectional survey is evidently an inefficient design for investigating rare disorders. For example, the second British Child and Adolescent Mental Health Survey studied 7977 children and reported a prevalence of 0.9% for pervasive developmental disorders (Green et al., 2005). The 67 children with pervasive developmental disorder detected by this survey are too few for anything other than the simplest of analyses of sociodemographic and other characteristics within the group. Chapter 13 describes the use of surveillance and registers, which provide useful methods to gather data on rare conditions and events, or investigators may over-sample small but significant subpopulations in order to obtain sufficiently precise information about the distribution of the outcome among them.

Cohort studies

There are two essential features of a cohort study:

1. Participants are defined by their exposure status rather than by outcome.

2. It is a longitudinal design: exposure status *must* be ascertained before outcome is known.

Cohort studies may be descriptive, only illustrating the rates of disease in one particular group (usually an occupational exposure), but more commonly compare the rates of a disorder in different exposure groups.

Classical cohort studies start with a group of people defined by their exposure status and compare the incidence of a disorder in these groups over time. If the study is prospective, that is, the study commences before the onset of disease and the participants are followed forwards in time, the incidence of the disorder can be directly calculated, information bias is limited, and we can ascertain the direction of causality. However, due to the number of participants required and the length of time required to accumulate sufficient cases, cohort studies can be prohibitively expensive. If one wanted to investigate the impact of obstetric complications on the incidence of schizophrenia in this manner, one would have to follow up the cohort for 25–30 years and would need an enormous number of people in order to generate a sufficient number of cases. For this reason, cohorts are not the design of choice for studying rare disorders.

A variant of the classical cohort study is the *population cohort study*, in which selection of the participants is not based upon exposure to a single putative risk factor. This permits study of multiple exposures as well as multiple outcomes, and findings are broadly generalizable. For instance, the ALSPAC, mentioned earlier, has followed all children born in Avon in the early 1990s (http://www.bristol.ac.uk/alspac/) or the Millennium Cohort Study, which has followed children born in 2000–2001 at regular intervals (https://cls.ucl.ac.uk/cls-studies/millennium-cohort-study/). Both studies are still gathering information and have data available on many disparate issues affecting health and development.

The logistical demands and costs of a cohort study can be minimized by using a *historical cohort study* design. The rate of disorder is still compared across exposure groups, but the disease has already occurred at the time of investigation. The essential element is the availability of information on exposure collected for another purpose before the onset of the disorder. Information bias is excluded since as with a classical prospective cohort study, neither the assessors nor the participants under study knew who would develop the disorder at the time when the exposure was ascertained. Thus Malmberg and colleagues (1998) linked data routinely gathered about the personality of conscripts to the Swedish army to the National Register of Psychiatric Care in order to investigate the role of personality factors in their future risk of developing Schizophrenia. Jones and colleagues (1994) combined data from the UK National Survey of Health and Development, a representative sample of all babies born in one week in 1946 and the Mental Health Enquiry, a central register of all admissions to psychiatric hospitals. They related various indices of child cognitive, behavioural, social, and physical development to the future risk of developing schizophrenia.

Case–control studies

Case–control studies are essentially retrospective designs. The aim is to recruit a random sample of cases and non-cases (controls) from the same defined population, and then to inquire about their history of past exposure to possible risk factors. The odds of being exposed are compared between cases and controls. The resulting measure of effect, the odds ratio, should approximate to the relative risk estimated in a cohort study (see earlier discussion) for rare disorders, although this assumption begins to fail as the population prevalence of the disorder rises above 10%.

Case–control studies are relatively quick and cheap to conduct, and are particularly appropriate for the initial investigation of rare disorders or events. For example, Parker and colleagues (2016) used this approach supplemented with national norms to study the relationship between psychopathology and developmental level with exclusion from school. This design carries the advantage that it can be used to study multiple exposures, but is prone to bias for several reasons. If the chances of being selected as a case or a control are related to your exposure status, the findings of the study will be invalidated due to *selection bias*, which is why it is imperative to define the base population carefully so that cases and controls *only* vary in relation to outcome status. If cases were collected from prospective referrals to a certain clinic, the controls must be selected from the people who would be referred to the same clinic, were they to develop the disorder under study.

As the data on exposure is sought after the onset of disease, there is a real risk that the information obtained is biased according to health status. Over-zealous researchers may look harder for evidence of exposure in cases than controls if they are also aware of the hypothesis under investigation and the participant's disease status, creating *observer bias*. Equally, people suffering from a disorder are likely to have thought about the potential causes in a way that the controls will not, leading to *recall bias*. For example, Kruk and Aboul-Enein (2004) reported an association between breast cancer and life event from a questionnaire-based case–control study, but it is possible that the relationship could be explained women with cancer being more likely to remember negative experiences. This phenomenon is sometimes referred to as 'effort after meaning'. To minimize *information bias* (both recall and observer bias) it is important to apply the same measures of exposure status to cases and controls and to try and use objective methods such as blood tests and medical records in preference to, or to supplement, subjective information. It may also be possible to blind the observer to the outcome status of the participant, and to blind both the observer and the participant to the hypothesis under study.

Intervention studies

In intervention studies, the experimenter allocates the intervention (exposure) either to some individuals or communities and compares the outcome of interest between the treatment groups. By *randomly allocating* participants to the different interventions, the investigator hopes to create groups that are similar in respect to all confounders, both known and unknown. It is also important to ensure, if possible, that both the investigator and the participants do not know which intervention they are receiving, that is to say that trial is *'double blind'*. This prevents *information bias*, which may otherwise arise where perceptions about the interventions influence self-reported or researcher-ascertained outcome. However, blinding is hard to achieve with psychological interventions and drug effects, for example, the parkinsonism associated with conventional neuroleptics can foil blinding. Asking participants and data collectors which group they thought that they were in at the end of the trial can help investigators to assess the extent to which the double blind was maintained, and also to assess the possible impact of information bias upon the findings.

Spontaneous remission is a particular problem with chronic relapsing and remitting conditions such as depression or schizophrenia. People tend to seek help when their symptoms are most intense, and thus by definition, will tend to improve over time even if placebo treatment is allocated. However, random allocation and blinding minimize the possibility that spontaneous improvement accounts for any observed differences between treatments. If a commonly used intervention for the condition under study is available, it should be used in the comparison group, as it would be unethical to use an inert placebo when an evidence-based treatment existed (Hrobjatsson and Gotzche, 2001).

In a rigorously conducted randomized controlled trial, it can be possible to make direct causal and mechanistic inferences from the effects observed. For instance the efficacy of methylphenidate in suppressing the symptoms of hyperkinetic disorder has led to the investigation of the involvement of dopaminergic pathways in inattention and overactivity.

In the mental health field, it is common to find trials of complex psychosocial interventions as well pharmacological treatments, sometimes simultaneously, as in the comparison of the use of cognitive behavioural therapy as an adjunct to selective serotonin inhibitors in young people (Goodyer et al., 2007). Some complex intervention studies involve the application of inventions to groups of people or defined communities such as schools, for example the STARS study (Supporting Teachers and childREn in Schools; Ford et al., 2018), which tested the use of a teacher classroom management course on children's mental health and academic attainment as well as on teachers' mental health, burn out, and self-efficacy. Cluster randomized trials require methodological and analytic approaches that account for the design. For example, the pupils at a particular school are likely to be more similar to each other than to pupils at other schools. Their observations are *clustered* rather than independent and if this is ignored in the analysis, which then assumes that observations are independent, there is an increased likelihood of detecting erroneous associations where none exist. Similarly, the sample size should be based on the number of schools, as well as the number of children, receiving the intervention.

Quasi-experimental designs

Quasi-experimental designs are opportunistic in that they take advantage of unplanned events to assess the impact of an exposure, or an intervention, on a relatively well-defined group of people who happened to be affected by that event. However, the allocation of the exposure is by definition not random, although the study may be controlled by the addition of a group who were not exposed, or did not receive the intervention. The fall of the Ceausescu regime and the need to respond to the plight of children living in profound deprivation allowed Rutter and colleagues (2007) to study the impact of extreme adversity in infancy by following the developmental trajectory of 165 Romanian orphans, most of whom had been placed in institutions, with 52 children from the UK who were adopted before the age of 6 months. This study has provided extremely valuable insights into child development and would have been impossible without this or a similar set of socio-political events.

Qualitative and mixed methods studies

The study designs previously described are all used to gather quantitative data, or information that has numerical qualities (Porta, 2014). Qualitative approaches use systematic approaches to gather non-numeric data about experiences and attitudes (Porta, 2014), and are increasingly used alongside epidemiological studies to enrich the understanding of complex problems and issues. Samples sizes are necessarily smaller, limiting generalizability, yet these data offer a level of detail and description that is not practical on larger scale. A good example of this kind of approach are the process evaluations that often accompany randomized controlled trials of complex interventions, which explore barriers and facilitators that might influence implementation and can provide insights into mechanisms by which moderators and mediators may act. For example, Hansford and colleagues (2015) have published a protocol for the process evaluation accompanying a cluster randomized controlled trial of teacher classroom management that applies descriptive quantitative analysis of attendance, satisfaction, and utility with the qualitative data derived from focus groups and interviews with teachers who attended the course and their colleagues about the application of the strategies learned in their context.

Conduct of studies employing quantitative methods

In the following sections we describe some basic steps in the conduct of studies employing quantitative methodologies, in particular basic methods common to cross-sectional, cohort, and case–control studies. See Chapter 7 for the conduct of qualitative studies,

Chapter 8 for details on conducting ecological studies, and Chapter 12 on randomized controlled trials.

Approaching the participant

The first contact is of vital importance. This will usually be by mail, or by direct contact. The project should be described honestly and comprehensively, but in simple and non-threatening terms. The potential value of the project should be stressed, together with a description of any burden that will be placed on participants in terms of time or discomfort. The layout of printed material should be clear, and should be of a professional appearance. It can sometimes be helpful to include a letter of introduction from some person known to the participant, such as their general practitioner, or some locally prominent person. Participants will need to read, or have read to them, an information sheet describing the research and their role in it. An investigator should be available to answer any questions the potential participant may have. It should be made clear that the choice, whether or not to participate, is for them alone, and that they are free to decline, or to pull out after first agreeing, at any time, without giving reasons and with no adverse consequences. Those who wish to participate should sign a consent form. The investigator and the participant should both keep a copy of the consent form.

The burden imposed on the participant

Potential participants are likely to be put off by lengthy, unwieldy interviews. Special care should be taken if it is proposed to enquire into culturally sensitive areas such as sexual behaviour or marital relationships. Physical examinations and procedures such as taking blood samples may also reduce the response rate. The incorporation of biological measures into epidemiological research poses particular difficulties. However, well-designed studies have demonstrated the feasibility of collecting blood, cheek scrapes for genetic material, saliva for cortisol, and even carrying out carotid artery ultrasonography on large population-based samples (Hofman et al., 1997). Epidemiological studies inevitably involve some element of compromise between the depth and breadth of the data that investigators might ideally wish to gather, and that which can be pragmatically achieved. For example, there is no point in developing a complex survey protocol that achieves a response rate of only 30%. Simpler, less sophisticated measures may be nearly as precise while achieving a much higher response.

The medium for the administration of the research interview

Questionnaire-based measures can be administered in a face-to-face interview, over the telephone, by post, or via the Internet (distributing questionnaires by email or allowing participants to access a web-based survey tool). Postal and Internet-based methods can obviously only be used for self-completion questionnaires. They may seem appealing at first sight because of the apparent savings in personnel time, cost, and efficiency. However, response rates for postal and Internet-based interviews can be very low, typically only

30–40%, although door-knocking surveys may also suffer from low levels of response. Non-responders tend to have lower socioeconomic status, lower educational levels (there is evidently a particular problem with the illiterate), and may be more likely to have mental disorders, than responders; hence this is likely to lead to bias. Postal methods will thus only be acceptable if the questionnaire is exceptionally simple and clearly laid out, and if considerable resources can be allocated to pursuing non-responders by postal reminders, and if need be, with telephone calls or home visits. Internet-based surveys may also exclude individuals who do not have access to the Internet or to the technology to take part in the survey and may lead to people who are less computer literate being unable to take part. A further difficulty is that it may be difficult to monitor who responds to such surveys; individuals may share links to the survey via social media or email, making it difficult to be sure as to the exact sampling frame for the study. Internet-based surveys have the advantage that they can potentially be implemented rapidly; for example, following the 11 September 11 attacks on the World Trade Centre in New York, US, in 2001, investigators used a web-based survey on a pre-existing, nationally representative sample of adults in the US to assess respondents' mental health and the impact of coping strategies, following the attacks (Silver et al., 2002).

Telephone interviews may be an acceptable alternative that still offers economies in terms of time saved taken to travel to a participant's home. Repeated telephone calls can be made to gain access to those who are rarely at home. Response rates can therefore be quite high, and many instruments have been shown to be both feasible and valid when administered in this way. Evidently this method can only be used in settings where a substantial proportion of the population have a telephone in their home, in recent years there has been a trend for individuals to own mobile phones and not telephones in their home; this applies particularly to young people who may be excluded from the sampling frame. In many low- and middle-income countries, people now only own mobile phones, particularly in areas of poor infrastructure where fixed-line technology may not exist. Surveys based on mobile phone calls may potentially be used to good effect in these settings (Hu et al., 2010). Assuming near-complete coverage of a population, the telephone system can even be used to generate representative samples for population surveys, using the technique of random digit dialling (Breslau et al., 1999). Random digit dialling of mobile phones has previously been shown to have equivalent coverage, comparable to traditional sampling methods, especially among younger adults (Gundersen et al., 2014).

Face-to-face interviews offer the participant the convenience of being interviewed in their own home, by an interviewer who should:

- be polite
- be neatly and appropriately dressed
- carry identification
- be sensitive to their position as guests in the participant's home.

Some participants may prefer to be interviewed in a research centre rather than in their own homes, and provision should be made for this eventuality.

The resources committed to following up non-response

Eligible participants who state clearly that they do not wish to participate in a study should not be pressured or otherwise induced into changing their minds. They may however be invited to provide some basic data (e.g. age, gender, social class, and smoking behaviour) that can be used later to check whether their non-response is likely to have led to bias. However, much non-response arises from eligible persons who have not replied at all to the request for an interview, as opposed to having actively refused participation. Many of these may agree to participate if they are approached again. Most researchers would make it their practice to approach such 'passive non-responders' on at least two, and possibly up to four further occasions before accepting that their failure to respond indicates a positive wish not to participate. Initial approaches by letter can be supplemented by telephone calls or even home visits. Home visits may reveal another reason for non-response; the register may be inaccurate and the person has moved away or died. Following up non-response can be time-consuming and costly, so provision needs to be made for this in the survey budget and time schedule.

Interviews/assessments

It is desirable that instruments to be used in the study are valid and reliable, although this may be difficult in the absence of a valid criterion if the question in the study has not been previously asked. The concepts of validity and reliability are dealt with in more detail in Chapter 2 on measurement in psychiatry. Validity refers to the extent to which an instrument measures what it purports to measure. Instruments should be validated *for the population in which they are being used*. Some instruments have been validated for clinical populations, but not for community samples. Others have been validated for one culture (e.g. a high-income anglophone country) but not another (e.g. a low-income country). Establishing validity for an instrument may necessitate pilot work, which may include:

+ translation and back translation
+ checking conceptual validity using ethnographic procedures
+ field trialling for feasibility, and for criterion validity against a local gold standard.

Data collection and processing

Increasingly, data collection for large studies, such as for cross-sectional or cohort studies, proceeds through computer-assisted personal interviewing (CAPI) techniques, whereby the interviewer uses portable electronic devices such as laptops or tablets to collect information on survey participants. These methods have replaced paper-based methods as data can be checked and cleaned on entry (rather than involving a long process later, therefore saving on resources). The equivalent process—computer-assisted self-interviewing (CASI)—can also be used for assessments requiring self-completion, by the participant being handed the device and asked to fill in the questionnaire themselves. Where CAPI or CASI procedures are used, the script of the questionnaire is contained in a computer file. The interviewer reads the question from the screen of the laptop and enters the data directly onto the computer. The data that is entered can then be retrieved in the form of a data spreadsheet. This facility is also available within the EpiData software package (http://www.epidata.dk), although more sophisticated programs are available commercially. Data is stored on the device, and may be uploaded to a cloud server in real time through mobile networks, or transferred to an institutional server on return to base at the end of each day's interviewing, Computer-administered questionnaires offer considerable advantages in terms of flexibility. Complex branching structures can be built into the questionnaire. Thus different sections of the questionnaire can be administered to men and women. Lengthy detailed sections can be omitted unless a particular combination of screening items is endorsed. Data transfer errors are eliminated. The EpiData package is public domain software originally developed by the World Health Organization and Centers for Disease Control, Atlanta, US, and now maintained by the EpiData Association from Denmark; it can be downloaded from http://www.epidata.dk. The package is also available for mobile devices. Validity checks can also be run after all the data has been entered. Frequency distributions can be run for all variables to check that all recorded values are sensible. Cross-tabulations may be used to establish, for instance, that all pregnancies are recorded as occurring in women.

Paper-based methods may still be used, particularly in low-resourced settings. Interviewers may record data on to a paper questionnaire, which should be clearly laid out with variable names and coding boxes for each item of data to be recorded. Data coded on the questionnaires then needs to be entered into a computerized database. Many errors can occur in this process. The data entry clerk may misread the coding on the questionnaire, or their finger may slip on the computer keyboard. Errors are considerably reduced by double entering data. When the data is entered a second time, the computer identifies discrepancies between the first and second entry and requests clarification. Errors can be further reduced by validity checks. These can be incorporated into the data entry program. Thus, the entry field for the variable gender could be set to accept 1 (for male), 2 (for female), and 9 (for missing value), but to reject all other values. Double-data entry and computerized validity checks are available with a variety of data entry software packages. Data management is a crucially important component of any well-conducted study. However, it is often neglected, and few reports give adequate descriptions of the procedures that were followed. Data handling is an important source of random error for many studies.

Practical exercises

Answer the following questions for each of the studies (A–E) described.

1. Is the study descriptive or analytic?
2. Is data aggregated or not?
3. What type of study design was used?

4. What is/are the outcome(s)?

5. What is/are the exposure(s)?

6. What measure(s) of effect might be used?

7. What are the types of bias that the investigators will have to guard against?

A. A study was set up to test the predictive validity of the diagnostic category of depressive conduct disorder. The investigators contacted three groups of adults who had previously attended the same child and adolescent mental health service. As children, the participants had been diagnosed with depressive disorder, conduct disorder, or depressive conduct disorder.

B. A study collected data on symptoms of anxiety and sociodemographic characteristics from children and young people aged between 5 and 18 years sampled via a population register.

C. A study examining the impact of heavy 'ecstasy' use compared regular ecstasy users with ecstasy naïve participants on a psychometric battery, and with structural and functional magnetic resonance imaging scans.

D. In a study designed to examine the effect of a non-steroidal anti-inflammatory drug on the progression of Alzheimer's disease, participants were randomly allocated to receive either the active drug or a placebo.

E. A study was set up to test the predictive validity of the diagnostic category of depressive conduct disorder. The investigators contacted three groups of young adults who had attended a child psychiatric clinic as children. As children, the participants had been diagnosed with depressive disorder, conduct disorder, or depressive conduct disorder.

Further reading

Jenkins, R. and Meltzer, H. (eds.) (2003). A decade of National Surveys of Psychiatric Epidemiology in Great Britain. *International Review of Psychiatry*, **15**, 5–200.

Lee, W., Bindman, J., Ford, T., Glozier, N., Moran, P., Stewart, R., and Hotopf, M. (2007). Bias in case-control studies: a literature survey. *British Journal of Psychiatry*, **190**, 204–209.

Porta, M. (ed.) (2014). *A dictionary of epidemiology*, 6th edn. New York: Oxford University Press.

Wessely, S. and Everitt, B.S. (2004). *Clinical trials in psychiatry*. Oxford: Oxford University Press.

References

Breslau, N., Chilcoat, H.D., Kessler, R.C., Peterson, E.L., and Lucia, V.C. (1999). Vulnerability to assaultive violence: further specification of the sex difference in post-traumatic stress disorder. *Psychological Medicine*, **29**, 813–821.

Ford, T., Vostanis, P., Meltzer, H., and Goodman, R. (2007). Psychiatric disorder among British children looked after by local authorities: a comparison with children living in private households. *British Journal of Psychiatry*, **190**, 319–325.

Ford, T., Edwards, E., Sharkey, S., Okoumunne, O., Byford, S., Norich, B., and Logan, S. (2012). Supporting Teachers And childRen in Schools: the effectiveness and cost-effectiveness of the

Incredible Years Teacher Classroom Management programme in primary school children: a cluster randomised controlled trial, with parallel economic and process evaluations. *BMC Public Health*, **12**, 719.

Ford, T., Hayes, R., Byford, S., Edwards, V., Fletcher, M., Logan, S., Norwich, B., Pritchard, W., Allen, K., Allwood, M., Ganguli, P., Grimes, K., Hansford, L., Longdon, B., Norman, S., Price A., and Ukoumunne O. C. (2018). The effectiveness and cost-effectiveness of the Incredible Years® Teacher Classroom Management programme in primary school children: results of the STARS cluster randomised controlled trial. *Psychological Medicine*, 47(4), 828–842.

Gerrits, M.H., Voogt, R., and van den Oord, E.J.C.G. (2001). An evaluation of non-response bias in peer, self and teacher ratings of children's psychological adjustment. *Journal of Child Psychology and Psychiatry*, **42**, 593–602.

Goodyer, I., Dubicka, B., Wilkinson, P., Kelvin, R., Roberts, C., Byford, S., et al. (2007). Selective serotonin reuptake inhibitors (SSRIs) and routine specialist care with and without cognitive behaviour therapy in adolescents with major depression: randomised controlled trial. *BMJ* 335, 142.

Green, H., McGinnity, A., Meltzer, H., Ford, T., and Goodman, R. (2005). *Mental health of children and young people in Great Britain, 2004*. London: The Stationery Office.

Green, J. (2014). Process to progress? Investigate trials, mechanism and clinical science. *Journal of Child Psychology and Psychiatry*, **56**, 1–3.

Gundersen, D.A., ZuWallack, R.S., Dayton, J., Echeverría, S.E., and Delnevo, C.D. (2014). Assessing the feasibility and sample quality of a national random-digit dialing cellular phone survey of young adults. *American Journal of Epidemiology*, **179**, 39–47.

Hansford, L., Sharkey, S., Edwards, V., Ukoumunne, O., Byford, S., Norwich, B., et al. (2015). Understanding the influences on teachers' uptake and use of behaviour management techniques in the STARS trial: process evaluation for a randomised controlled trial. *BMC Public Health*, **15**, 119.

Hill, C. and Cook, L. (2011). Narrative verdicts and their impact on mortality statistics in England and Wales. *Health Statistics Quarterly*, **49**, 81–100.

Hofman, A., Ott, A., Breteler, M.M.B., Bots, M.L., Slooter, A.J.C., van Harskamp, F., et al. (1997). Atherosclerosis, apolipoprotein E, and prevalence of dementia and Alzheimer's disease in the Rotterdam Study. *Lancet*, **349**, 151–154.

Hróbjartsson, A. and Gøtzsche, P.C. (2001) Is the Placebo Powerless?—An Analysis of Clinical Trials Comparing Placebo with No Treatment. *N Engl J Med*, **344**,1594–1602. DOI: 10.1056/NEJM200105243442106

Hu, S.S., Balluz L., Battaglia M.P., and Frankel M.R. (2010). The impact of cell phones on public health surveillance. *Bulletin of the World Health Organization*, **88**, 799.

Ibrahim, S., Hunt, I., Rahman, M.S., Shaw, J., Appleby, L., and Kapur, N. (2019). Recession, recovery and suicide in mental health patients in England: time trend analysis. *The British Journal of Psychiatry*. https://doi.org/10.1192/bjp.2019.119

Jones, P., Rodgers, B., Murray, R., and Marmot, M. (1994). Child development risk factors for adult schizophrenia in the British 1946 birth cohort. *Lancet*, **344**, 1398–1402.

Kruk, J. and Aboul-Enein, H.Y. (2004). Psychological stress and the risk of breast cancer: a case-control study. *Cancer Detection and Prevention*, **28**, 399–408.

Law Malcolm, Stampfer Meir, Barker D J P, Mackenbach Johan P, Wald Nicholas, Rimm Eric et al. (1999). Why heart disease mortality is low in France: the time lag explanation. Commentary: Alcohol and other dietary factors may be important. Commentary: Intrauterine nutrition may be important. Commentary: Heterogeneity of populations should be taken into account. Authors' response *BMJ*, **318**, 1471.

Layey, B.L. D'Onofrio, B.M., and **Waldman** I.D. (2009). Using epidemiologic methods to test hypotheses regarding causal influences on child and adolescent mental disorders. *Journal of Child Psychology and Psychiatry*, **50**, 53–62

Parker, C., Marlow, R., Kastner, M., May, F., Mitrofan, O., Henley, W., and Ford, T. (2016). The "Supporting Kids, Avoiding Problems"(SKIP) study: relationships between school exclusion, psychopathology, development and attainment - a case control study. *Journal of Children's Services*, **11**(2), 91–110.

Malmberg, A., Lewis, G., David, A., and Allebeck, P. (1998). Premorbid adjustment and personality in people with schizophrenia. *British Journal of Psychiatry*, **172**, 308–313.

Meltzer, H., Gatward, R., Goodman, R., and Ford, T. (2000). *The mental health of children and adolescents in Great Britain*. London: The Stationery Office.

Office for National Statistics (2014). *Suicide statistics in the United Kingdom, 2012 registrations*. London: Office for National Statistics.

Pickett, K. and Wilkinson, R.G. (2007). Child well-being and income inequality in rich societies; an ecological cross sectional survey. *BMJ*, **335**, 1080–1087.

Porta, M. (ed.) (2014). *A dictionary of epidemiology*, 6th edn. New York: Oxford University Press.

Rocha, J.V.M. and Nunes, C. (2019). Community *Ment Health J*. https://doi.org/10.1007/s10597-019-00510-9

Rutter, M., Beckett, C., Castle, J., Colvert, E., Kreppner, J., Mehta, M., et al. (2007). Effects of profound early institutional deprivation: an overview of findings from a UK longitudinal study of Romanian adoptees. *European Journal of Developmental Psychology*, **4**, 332–350.

Silver, R., Holman, E., McIntosh, D.N., Poulin, M., and Gil-Rivas, V. (2002). Nationwide longitudinal study of psychological responses to September 11. *JAMA*, **288**, 1235–1244.

Thomas, K. and Gunnell, D. (2010). Suicide in England and Wales 1861–2007: a time-trends analysis. *International Journal of Epidemiology*, **39**, 1464–1475.

Wolke, D., Waylen, A., Samara, M., Steer, C., Goodman, R., Ford, T., and Lamberts, K. (2009). Does selective drop out lead to biased prediction of behaviour disorders? *British Journal of Psychiatry*, **195**, 249–256.

Chapter 7

Qualitative research

Oana Mitrofan and Rose McCabe

Introduction

Qualitative research is increasingly deployed in health services research, from the development to the evaluation of healthcare processes and interventions. There has also been a rapidly developing field of mixed methods studies, that is, studies combining qualitative and quantitative research methods, in recent years. This chapter offers an overview of the nature and purpose of qualitative research, its methods and processes, quality appraisal, synthesis of qualitative research, and the integration of qualitative and quantitative approaches in mixed methods research.

What is qualitative research?

Qualitative research seeks to answer 'what', 'why', and 'how' questions, rather than 'how many' or 'how often'. It is an interpretative approach concerned with understanding the meanings people attach to phenomena (e.g. beliefs, actions, processes) within their social worlds (Buston et al., 1998). It captures experiences of health, illness, and treatment, thereby contributing towards our understanding of what change is indicated to improve health and healthcare provision (Taylor and Francis, 2013). It is an *inductive* approach as patterns and theories emerge from the data, compared to a *deductive* approach where theories are subsequently empirically verified.

Why use a qualitative approach?

In health research, qualitative methods are used to increase understanding of phenomena, experiences, or processes. Qualitative research is often complementary to quantitative research as it helps to 'look behind the numbers' (Buston et al., 1998) and allows a deeper understanding through the study of 'naturally occurring, ordinary events in natural settings' (Miles and Huberman, 1994). A qualitative investigation may precede quantitative research in the study of new or complex areas to explore unknown variables, generate hypotheses, and inform quantitative research tools (e.g. survey questionnaires). Public involvement (through 'patient and public involvement'), which is an increasingly important aspect of the research process, often adopts a qualitative approach to explore stakeholders' perspectives on research priorities and specific research plans. Qualitative work often also follows quantitative research in order to provide an understanding of unexpected or contradictory findings.

Quantitative and qualitative methods can be combined to examine different phenomena or the same phenomenon from different perspectives in a mixed methods (also known as a multi-method or multi-strategy) study. This involves the planned mixing of qualitative and quantitative methods at a predetermined stage of the research process, which can facilitate the exploration of a complex research topic in both breadth and depth, collecting and integrating quantitative (numbers, frequencies) and qualitative (participants' views and experiences) findings. Although challenging (extensive data collection, the time-consuming nature of analysing both numeric and verbatim text), such studies have grown to become one of the major approaches currently used in health research (Tashakkori and Teddlie, 2003; Dixon-Woods et al., 2004). For example, qualitative methods are often used to study *how* a new treatment or intervention is actually implemented in practice in a randomized controlled trial (RCT).

Before moving on to the next section, we recommend reading the practical exercises at the end of this chapter, which illustrate the basic steps in the design of a qualitative research project.

How do you collect qualitative data?

The most commonly used qualitative methods in health services research are *interviews, focus groups*, and *observational methods*, with the specific method chosen depending on the research question and practical issues such as optimal access to participants. For example, focus groups are often difficult to conduct with healthcare professionals due to the demands on their time and the need to have the group in the same location at the same time. For these reasons, interviews with individual professionals are often more feasible. Table 7.1 presents the most common methods along with their strengths and limitations.

Qualitative interviews

Interviews are the most commonly used qualitative method and can be *semi-structured* or *unstructured*. *Semi-structured* interviews involve the use of an interview (or topic) guide that defines the areas to be explored, in the form of a series of topics and open-ended questions, from which the researcher may further expand or diverge for more detail by using prompts and probes. An *unstructured* interview guide typically includes a few topics only, the line of inquiry depending on how the interviewee responds. The researcher may begin by saying 'Please tell me about your experience of seeing a psychiatrist' and later continue with questions that are not specified ahead of the interview in order to clarify or obtain more detail on the interviewee's initial responses.

The questions in qualitative interviews should be 'open-ended, neutral, sensitive, and clear to the interviewee' (Patton, 1987). The challenge for the qualitative interviewer is to keep a balance between providing an optimum space for the interviewee to describe their experience and uncovering their meanings (i.e. encouraging and allowing

Table 7.1 Common qualitative data collection methods

Data collection method	Subtypes	Raw data	Strengths	Limitations
One-to-one interviews	Semi-structured; in-depth; face-to-face; telephone; online	Verbatim transcripts of audio/video recordings or online discussions, researcher's notes	Allow detailed exploration of individual perspective/experience Interviewee often leads discussion and may reveal issues of particular personal importance Allow exploration of sensitive topics	Little information on behaviour in real-life situations Can be intensive for both interviewee and interviewer Challenges for researcher: avoid being too directive, using leading questions, imposing own assumptions
Focus groups	Face-to-face; online	Verbatim transcripts of audio/video recordings or online discussions, researcher's notes	Allow multiple views to be explored simultaneously, which can further stimulate discussion Can provide rich data through exploration of group interaction	Less useful for exploring sensitive topics or views that go against the majority (some views may not be revealed due to group dynamics) Challenges for researcher: moderate discussion (keep group on topic, encourage everyone's input, monitor/limit domineering individuals, and impact of group hierarchy)
Observational methods	Participant observation; non-participant observation; ethnography; conversation analysis	Verbatim transcripts of audio/video recordings; written narratives; diaries; visual material (e.g. photographs); field notes	Allow access to naturally occurring situations/interactions/behaviours Can reveal what people actually do, not just what they say Allow exploration of topics that may be uncomfortable for participants to discuss	Time consuming Good-quality recordings essential Challenges for researcher: particular skills (e.g. good observational skills and memory, ability to systematically record events in great detail); field access (usually via a 'gatekeeper'); maintaining professional boundaries (avoid becoming too immersed in the field and losing objectivity or becoming emotionally overinvolved); ethical challenges, e.g. ensure fully informed consent (can cause changes in participants' behaviour)

enough time for detailed explanations) and maintaining a focus on the research question. Acknowledging and making efforts to limit imposing the interviewer's own concepts is also key (Britten, 1995).

Focus groups

Focus groups involve convening a group of people to discuss particular issues, with the researcher acting as facilitator (or moderator) and usually assisted by a co-facilitator. Like interviews, focus groups use a topic guide based on the research questions to direct the discussion and allow detailed exploration of particular areas of interest as they arise during the discussion.

This form of data collection makes use of the interaction between individuals and their mutual influence on each other's contribution during the discussion, in order to generate rich insights into the topic of interest. The rationale behind this method is that group processes can facilitate a deep exploration of participants' perspectives and experiences, uncovering 'not only what people think but how they think and why they think that way' through the debate within the group. Focus groups allow the researcher to access various forms of interpersonal communication (e.g. humour, disputes). This can reveal less obvious aspects of people's beliefs and attitudes such as cultural values or group norms, hence the frequent use of focus groups in cross-cultural research and research involving ethnic minorities (Kitzinger, 1995).

One important aspect in the design of a focus group is the composition of the group. Shared characteristics facilitate discussion of common, similar views and experiences, while a more diverse group can highlight different perspectives on a topic. The researcher also needs to monitor the hierarchy within the group for any impact it may have on the discussion and try to ensure that all members are given an equal opportunity to voice their views.

Observational methods

Observational methods involve systematic, detailed observation of people's communication, attitudes, and behaviour: 'watching and recording what people do and say' and then analysing the material (Mays and Pope, 1995). It can involve the researcher becoming immersed in the field, to 'submit oneself in the company of the members to the daily round of petty contingencies to which they are subject' (Goffman, 1961) in order to capture the breadth and depth of their social world. These approaches involve 'naturalistic' research as the activities being observed take place in the normal course of events and have not been created in the course of the research, for example, as interviews or focus groups are. There are different types of observational methods such as participant observation, non-participant observation, ethnographic research, and conversation analysis.

The distinction between participant and non-participant observation depends on the level of interaction between the researcher and those being observed. In participant observation, the researcher has a dual role of participating in the observed social setting while maintaining the necessary professional distance to allow adequate data collection.

Non-participant observation involves limited direct interaction with the individuals observed, and may be useful in situations when such interaction is undesirable or difficult to achieve.

Ethnography is a complex research method derived from the field of anthropology that aims to obtain a holistic picture of the subject of study. It usually involves collecting data through participant observation and in-depth interviews. The researcher needs to observe the everyday lives of the people studied in order to fully capture the ways they describe and structure their world (Fraenkel and Wallen, 1990). One recent study of user involvement in health service development adopted this approach, combining participant observation, semi-structured interviews, and the collection of documentary evidence to explore the ways in which the policy of user involvement is interpreted, and what influences its practical implementation within health services. The approach helped to identify existing challenges, such as differences in the healthcare professionals' and service users' understanding and practice of user involvement, and the need for better evidence of the benefits of user involvement (Fudge et al., 2008).

Conversation analysis has its roots in sociology, and refers to both a method of data collection and data analysis. It focuses on naturally occurring social interaction and is founded on the premise that social interaction is systematic and ordered. In their communication with each other, individuals display their own, and shape one another's, meanings and interpretations of events (Collins and Britten, 2006). Verbal as well as non-verbal aspects of communication (i.e. the words as spoken, pauses, overlapping speech, volume, pace and stress intonation, laughter or crying, eye gaze, gesture, and postural orientation) are transcribed from the audio/visual recording of a naturalistic interaction and micro-analysed (McCabe, 2006). Conversation analysis has contributed to a better understanding of how healthcare is delivered by professionals and received by patients. For example, Heritage and colleagues (2007) have shown the importance of language used by physicians in primary care settings. A single-word intervention consisting of altering the physician's inquiry from 'any other concerns' to 'some other concerns' significantly reduced patients' unmet concerns.

Choosing a data collection method

Choosing a method of data collection is an important decision in the design of a qualitative project, but potentially challenging as there are no straightforward rules. The main factors to consider are the research question, the participants, the research setting, and the researcher's own skills and experience. The underlying rationale is to choose a method that will facilitate an exploration of participants' views and experiences 'as openly as possible in a way that is best suited to them and the aims of the research' (Frith and Gleeson, 2012).

Different methods can be used to explore the same topic in order to uncover different aspects, or to suit the type of participants or research setting. Interviews tend to be seen as more useful in researching sensitive topics, but focus groups can also be appropriate as shyer individuals may be encouraged, and feel supported by other members, in sharing common views. Focus groups can facilitate the exploration of taboo or stigmatized experiences (Kitzinger, 2006). Chapple and colleagues (2013) used in-depth interviews to explore the perspectives of bereaved relatives on newspaper reporting of suicide. The study aimed to recruit a diverse sample including people living in different areas, thus capturing a broad range of experiences of contact with various newspapers across the country, which would have been more difficult to achieve with focus groups.

Schulze and Angermeyer (2003) used focus groups in their study of subjective experiences of stigma among people with schizophrenia. The authors argued that one-to-one interviews would have potentially influenced participants' communication due to similarities to a therapeutic setting (e.g. expectation of expert advice). Other researchers used one-to-one interviews to explore patients' experience of stigma related to mental illness and its consequences for the individual (Dinos et al., 2004). Another example is the exploration of the doctor–patient interaction and the factors involved in clinical decision-making processes: different studies used one-to-one interviews (Seale et al., 2006), focus groups (Pappadopulos et al., 2002), and conversation analysis of doctor–patient encounters (McCabe, 2002).

Electronic media such as the Internet provide novel ways to collect qualitative data and address some of the logistical challenges of face-to-face interviews or focus groups. Online communities/support networks are on the rise, and qualitative methods such as conversation analysis are starting to be employed to explore their use and supportive role along with their challenges (Smithson et al., 2011).

Sampling in qualitative research

An essential aspect of qualitative research, which is markedly different to the quantitative approach, is the sampling procedure. Qualitative research does not seek a representative sample of all people comprising a specific population as it does not aim to generalize findings to a population level. It focuses on relatively small samples, selected *purposefully*, in order to capture information-rich cases for in-depth study. A commonly used *purposive sampling* strategy is 'snowball' or 'chain' sampling, which involves identifying cases of interest from people who can recommend others and know what cases are information rich (Patton, 1990). The sample size depends on several factors such as the research question, type of data, data collection method, and the available time and resources. Sampling until no further analytical insights are identified, that is, until the point of *saturation* (Pope et al., 2006), is often recommended. As a rule of thumb, interview-based studies generally have samples of fewer than 50 participants (Ritchie et al., 2003), and focus group studies commonly involve a few groups only, with a recommended number of four to eight people per group (Kitzinger, 2006).

How do you analyse qualitative data?

In qualitative research, the phases of data collection and analysis do not always represent a linear pathway, rather an iterative one, where creativity, reflexivity, and flexibility are essential (Frith and Gleeson, 2012). The analytical process begins during data collection as data are gathered and analysed and this feeds into the ongoing data collection until *saturation* is reached, when no further analytical themes can be identified. The researcher can move backwards and forwards between the raw data and interpretation, constantly making sense of the data throughout data collection and analysis and regularly revisit and, if necessary, refine the methods used in the pursuit of richer data. Such refinements may consist of adding questions to the topic guide, and conducting additional interviews/focus groups in order to pursue emerging ideas (Pope et al., 2006).

Qualitative research can produce vast amounts of unstructured data. Most forms of qualitative data analysis involve the following generic steps (Creswell, 2003; Spencer et al., 2003).

1. *Data preparation* involves transcribing interviews/focus groups, checking transcripts against original recordings, and typing up notes.

2. *Familiarization* with data involves reading and/or listening/watching the data to become familiar with the data in a general sense and to note general thoughts and ideas.

3. *Coding* (or *labelling*) involves a systematic approach to coding the data with a term (often based in the participants' language), then categorizing all data into 'chunks'. Categories are later refined and reduced, for example, by grouping together. Themes can emerge gradually from the data (a more inductive approach) or can be predefined from the literature, research questions, or topic guide (a more deductive approach).

4. Detailed *descriptions* of the setting, participants, themes/categories, and patterns/typologies.

5. Developing an *explanation/interpretation* of the data, and possibly raising new questions. Researchers' background and experience and existing literature/theories can feed into the interpretation.

The most common form of analysis used in healthcare research is *thematic analysis*. The type of coding depends on the specific methodological approach. The most common approaches are displayed in Table 7.2.

Various computer software packages are available to facilitate qualitative data analysis, especially the more time-consuming aspects of organizing, coding, and retrieving data, such as NVivo, ATLAS, and MAXQDA. It may be challenging to start using any qualitative data collection and analysis methods without some form of training, and there are many training courses available through universities and other research organizations, which are particularly useful before embarking on a qualitative study.

How do you ensure rigour in qualitative research?

There are several ways to ensure scientific rigour in the design, conduct, and reporting of qualitative research. For any qualitative study, a clear and sufficiently detailed description of its theoretical assumptions, methods of data collection and analysis, research procedures, and study findings is essential. This will ensure that the 'journey' from the raw data

Table 7.2 Common forms of qualitative data analysis

Analytic method	Specific features/steps
Quantitative content analysis	Focuses on counts/frequencies of categories that may be statistically analysed
Thematic analysis	Focuses on identifying higher-level themes across data. It involves organizing data into themes and examining all cases to ensure that all manifestations of each theme is accounted for and compared. Findings can be descriptive (reporting of themes) or interpretative (deeper exploration of theme interconnection)
Framework approach	A more deductive approach. Focus on the systematic application of a thematic framework involving main and sub-themes (emerging and predefined) to all data and structuring data in a matrix format (displaying themes/sub-themes across columns and each case as a separate row). The entire analytic process from identifying the thematic framework to explanation/interpretation of themes/sub-themes and their interrelationship is highly transparent
Grounded theory	Inductive approach. Focus on developing theory from the data in a cyclical and iterative approach: analysis feeds into subsequent sampling, further data collection, and testing of emerging theories
Conversation analysis	Focuses on analysing naturally occurring interaction. It involves highly detailed transcription including non-verbal communication and examines the structure of conversation to identify systematic and recurrent patterns of interaction drawing on a large body of conversation analytic studies
Discourse analysis	Focuses on analysing text and language and how knowledge is produced within a particular discourse through the use of distinctive language (e.g. medical discourse)

through each analytical step to the more sophisticated interpretation is 'transparent', allowing an assessment of the evidence for the findings.

A number of ways have been suggested to safeguard validity such as constantly comparing and contrasting examples, examining 'deviant' cases, triangulation, respondent validation, and reflexivity. 'Deviant case analysis' involves searching for and examining elements in the data that appear inconsistent with the emerging explanation (Mays and Pope, 2000). Triangulation refers to using more than one source of information (two or more independent data sources, for example, patients and clinicians, or different data collection methods, such as interviews and observation) to identify patterns of convergence. Respondent validation includes confirming with the study participants that the study findings represent a reasonable account of their views. Reflexivity refers to acknowledging the influence of the researcher's personal characteristics (e.g. age, gender, and professional status), background, knowledge, and experience on the research process and findings.

Reliability in qualitative research can be ensured by keeping sufficiently detailed records of the data collection and analysis methods and research process to allow replication. Often, data are double coded by another researcher/s and inter-rater reliability reported.

A number of guidelines and tools for reporting and appraising qualitative research are available such as the Consolidated Criteria for Reporting Qualitative Research (Tong et al., 2007) and the Critical Appraisal Skills Programme Qualitative Checklist (available at http://www.casp-uk.net).

Combining and appraising evidence from multiple qualitative studies in a systematic review or meta-synthesis is increasingly being undertaken (Thomas et al., 2004). Various methods for synthesizing qualitative research have been developed such as meta-ethnography (Barnett-Page and Thomas, 2009). Such meta-syntheses can provide new insights into an area, for example, a recent systematic review of perceived barriers and facilitators to mental health help-seeking in young people (Gulliver et al., 2010).

What are the key strengths of qualitative research?

Key strengths of qualitative research are the richness of data and the facilitation of a deeper understanding of phenomena. Qualitative research is particularly well suited to exploring lay and professional beliefs and attitudes around mental health and illness, professional and patient experiences of delivering and receiving care, and various aspects of doctor–patient interactions.

The place of qualitative methods in developing and evaluating complex healthcare interventions alongside RCTs has been increasingly recognized, especially following the publication of the Medical Research Council's framework (Craig et al., 2008) and more recent guidance on process evaluations (Evans et al., 2014). Qualitative methods can be used before, during, or after a trial to generate hypotheses and develop outcome measures, assess fidelity and quality of implementation, identify contextual influences, explain variations in effectiveness, and help to refine an intervention. This is particularly the case with complex health and social care interventions involving multiple social and behavioural processes (Lewin et al., 2009).

A recent study provides a useful example of a qualitative study run in parallel with a RCT to explore participant experiences of involvement in a trial to inform future research. Notley and colleagues (2015) conducted a qualitative study alongside a pilot trial of a psychological intervention targeting social disability in young people with emerging psychological difficulties. The data was collected through semi-structured interviews, and analysed using thematic analysis. The researchers identified several important aspects relating to the research process: flexibility in practical arrangements; clear explanation of research processes, particularly randomization, and measures which contributed to participant acceptance and willingness to get involved; researchers' awareness of participant difficulties and having a friendly, individualized approach; and being 'supportive, non-judgemental and empathetic', which was linked to participants' positive experience of disclosure. The study also highlighted the perceived benefits of engagement with the research, in addition to the intervention itself. These findings might benefit future research with vulnerable, hard-to-reach populations where researchers may encounter similar ethical and practical challenges.

What are the key limitations of qualitative research?

Qualitative research generally relies more on the researcher's skills and requires 'a combination of thought and practice and not a little patience' (Dingwall et al., 1998). The influence of the researcher on the process and outcome of the research needs to be acknowledged and assessed during all steps of the research process, and such effects should be discussed when reporting the study findings.

Another limitation refers to generalizability: the ways and the extent to which findings can be shared and applied beyond the study population or setting. Generalizability of qualitative findings should be considered within a particular framework: in relation to the population from which the study sample was drawn, generalizing to other settings which share some common features with the research setting, and as theoretical contributions to new or pre-existing concepts of wider application (Lewis and Ritchie, 2003). Qualitative findings are generally regarded 'not as facts that are applicable to the population at large, but rather as descriptions, notions, or theories applicable within a specified setting' (Malterud, 2001, p. 486).

Practical exercises

For each of the described situations A–D, please answer the following questions:

A. You want to find out about core psychiatry trainees' experience of training, particularly any challenges they are faced with, and factors that prevent or stop young doctors from taking up this specialty. You are particularly interested in getting the views of trainees who left psychiatry for a different specialty/career.

B. You are interested in patients' experience of communication with clinicians around psychiatric assessment and diagnosis, and whether, and to what extent, patients felt engaged in consultation. You would particularly like to find out about the experience of patients referred to secondary mental healthcare for mood difficulties.

C. You want to find out about decision-making processes regarding the start of antipsychotic medication in young people. You wish to explore a range of views including young people, parents, and professionals.

D. You want to find out about the experience of psychiatry trainees in working with young people who engage in self-harm, particularly challenges the trainees may face, and what trainees think about gaps in their training.

1. What would your main research question be?

2. What would be the pros and cons of using a quantitative approach? What would be the pros and cons of using a qualitative approach?

3. What qualitative method could you use to collect your data? What would be the benefits and limitations of using one-to-one interviews? How about focus groups? Can you think of other methods of qualitative data collection that you could use?

4. How would you design your interview/focus group topic guide?

5. How would you analyse your qualitative data?

6. What measures would you take to ensure the scientific rigour of your qualitative study?

Further reading

Denzin, N.K. and Lincoln, Y.S. (2011). *The SAGE handbook of qualitative research*. Thousand Oaks, CA: Sage.

Silverman, D. (2013). *Doing qualitative research: a practical handbook*. London: Sage.

References

Barnett-Page, E. and Thomas, J. (2009). Methods for the synthesis of qualitative research: a critical review. *BMC Medical Research Methodology*, 9, 59–69.

Britten, N. (1995). Qualitative research: qualitative interviews in medical research. *British Medical Journal*, 311, 251–253.

Buston, K., Parry-Jones, W., Livingston, M., Bogan, A., and Wood, S. (1998). Qualitative research. *British Journal of Psychiatry*, 172, 197–199.

Chapple, A., Ziebland, S., Simkin, S., and Hawton, K. (2013). How people bereaved by suicide perceive newspaper reporting: qualitative study. *British Journal of Psychiatry*, 203, 228–232.

Collins, S. and Britten, N. (2006). **Conversation analysis**. In: Pope, C. and Mays, N. (eds.). *Qualitative research in health care*, pp. 43–52. Oxford: Blackwell Publishing.

Craig, P., Dieppe, P., MacIntyre, S., Michie, S., Nazareth, I., and Petticrew, M. (2008). Developing and evaluating complex interventions: the new Medical Research Council guidance. *British Medical Journal*, 337, 979–983.

Creswell, J.W. (2003). *Research design: qualitative, quantitative, and mixed methods approaches*. Thousand Oaks, CA: Sage.

Dingwall, R., Murphy, E., Watson, P., Greatbatch, D., and Parker, S. (1998). Catching goldfish: quality in qualitative research. *Journal of Health Services Research and Policy*, 3, 167–172.

Dinos, S., Stevens, S., Serfaty, M., Weich, S., and King, M. (2004). Stigma: the feelings and experiences of 46 people with mental illness. *British Journal of Psychiatry*, 184, 176–181.

Dixon-Woods, M., Agarwal, S., Young, B., Jones, D., and Sutton, A. (2004). *Integrative approaches to qualitative and quantitative evidence*. London: NHS Health Development Agency.

Evans, R., Scourfield, J., and Murphy, S. (2015). Pragmatic, formative process evaluations of complex interventions and why we need more of them. *Journal of Epidemiology and Community Health*, 69, 925–926.

Fraenkel, J.R. and Warren, N.E. (2009). *How to design and evaluate research in education*. New York: McGraw-Hill.

Frith, H. and Gleeson, K. (2012). Qualitative data collection: asking the right questions. In: Harper, D. and Thompson, A.R. (eds.). *Qualitative research methods in mental health and psychotherapy: a guide for students and practitioners*, pp. 55–68. Oxford: Wiley-Blackwell.

Fudge, N., Wolfe, C.D.A., and McKevitt, C. (2008). Assessing the promise of user involvement in health service development: ethnographic study. *British Medical Journal*, 336, 313–317.

Goffman, E. (1961). *Asylums*. London: Penguin.

Gulliver, A., Griffiths, K.M., and Christensen, H. (2010). Perceived barriers and facilitators to mental health help-seeking in young people: a systematic review. *BMC Psychiatry*, 10, 113–121.

Heritage, J., Robinson, J.D., Elliott, M.N., Beckett, M., and Wilkes M. (2007). Reducing patients' unmet concerns in primary care: the difference one word can make. *Journal of General Internal Medicine*, **22**, 1429–1433.

Kitzinger, J. (1995). Qualitative research: introducing focus groups. *British Medical Journal*, **311**, 299–302.

Kitzinger, J. (2006). Focus groups. In: Pope, C. and Mays, N. (eds.). *Qualitative research in health care*, pp. 21–31. Oxford: Blackwell Publishing.

Lewin, S., Glenton, C., and Oxman, A.D. (2009). Use of qualitative methods alongside randomised controlled trials of complex healthcare interventions: methodological study. *British Medical Journal*, **339**, 732–734.

Lewis, J. and Ritchie, J. (2003). Generalising from qualitative research. In: Ritchie, J. and Lewis, J. (eds.). *Qualitative research practice: a guide for social science students and researchers*, pp. 263–286. London: Sage.

Malterud, K. (2001). Qualitative research: standards, challenges, and guidelines. *Lancet*, **358**, 483–488.

Mays, N. and Pope, C. (1995). Qualitative research: observational methods in health care settings. *British Medical Journal*, **311**, 182–184.

Mays, N. and Pope, C. (2000). Assessing quality in qualitative research. *British Medical Journal*, **320**, 50–52.

McCabe, R. (2006). Conversation analysis. In: Slade, M. and Priebe, S. (eds.). *Choosing methods in mental health research: mental health research from theory to practice*, pp. 24–46. London: Routledge.

McCabe, R., Heath, C., Burns, T., and Priebe, S. (2002). Engagement of patients with psychosis in the consultation: conversation analytic study. *British Medical Journal*, **325**, 1148–1151.

Miles, M.B. and Huberman, A.M. (1994). *Qualitative data analysis: an expanded sourcebook*. Thousand Oaks, CA: Sage.

Notley, C., Christopher, R., Hodgkins, J., Byrne, R., French, P., and Fowler, D. (2015). Participant views on involvement in a trial of social recovery cognitive–behavioural therapy. *British Journal of Psychiatry*, **206**, 122–127.

Pappadopulos, E., Jensen, P.S., Schur, S.B., MacIntyre, J.C., Ketner, S., Van Orden, K., et al. (2002). 'Real world' atypical antipsychotic prescribing practices in public child and adolescent inpatient settings. *Schizophrenia Bulletin*, **28**, 111–121.

Patton, M.Q. (1987). *How to use qualitative methods in evaluation*. London: Sage.

Patton, M.Q. (1990). *Qualitative evaluation and research methods*. London: Sage.

Pope, C., Ziebland, S., and Mays, N. (2006). Analysing qualitative data. In: Pope, C. and Mays, N. (eds.). *Qualitative research in health care*, pp. 63–81. Oxford: Blackwell Publishing.

Ritchie, J., Lewis, J., and Elam, G. (2003). Designing and selecting samples. In: Ritchie, J. and Lewis, J. (eds.). *Qualitative research practice: a guide for social science students and researchers*, pp. 77–108. London: Sage.

Schulze, B. and Angermeyer, M.C. (2003). Subjective experiences of stigma. A focus group study of schizophrenic patients, their relatives and mental health professionals. *Social Science and Medicine*, **56**, 299–312.

Seale, C., Chaplin, R., Lelliott, P., and Quirk, A. (2006). Sharing decisions in consultations involving anti-psychotic medication: a qualitative study of psychiatrists' experiences. *Social Science and Medicine*, **62**, 2861–2873.

Smithson, J., Sharkey, S., Hewis, E., Jones, R.B., Emmens, T., Ford, T., and Owens, C. (2011). Membership and boundary maintenance on an online self-harm forum. *Qualitative Health Research*, **21**, 1567–1575.

Spencer, L., Ritchie, J., and O'Connor, W. (2003). Analysis: practices, principles and processes. In Ritchie, J. and Lewis, J. (eds.). *Qualitative research practice: a guide for social science students and researchers*, pp. 199–218. London: Sage.

Tashakkori, A. and Teddlie, C. (2003). *Handbook of mixed methods in social and behavioural research*. London: Sage.

Taylor, B. and Francis, K. (2013). *Qualitative research in the health sciences: methodologies, methods and processes*. London: Routledge.

Thomas, J., Harden, A., Oakley, A., Oliver, S., Sutcliffe, K., Rees, R., et al. (2004). Integrating qualitative research with trials in systematic reviews. *British Medical Journal*, **328**, 1010–1012.

Tong, A., Sainsbury, P., and Craig, J. (2007). Consolidated criteria for reporting qualitative research (COREQ): a 32-item checklist for interviews and focus groups. *International Journal for Quality in Health Care*, **19**, 349–357.

Chapter 8

Ecological studies

Jayati Das-Munshi

Introduction

Ecological studies assess the association of group-level characteristics (such as income, religion, and ethnic group composition) with group-level outcomes (such as proportions with mental illness at a regional level). Although ecological study designs allow the possibility of assessing associations at a group level, these study designs are limited in not allowing inferences at the individual level to be made. For example, a study which suggests a correlation between country-level per capita consumption of alcohol and liver cirrhosis incidence (Ramstedt, 2001), does not necessarily mean that all individuals who experience liver cirrhosis in countries with high per capita alcohol consumption do so due to the effects of alcohol consumption.

Despite the limitations of ecological studies, studies which take into account features of group-level characteristics are important in psychiatric epidemiology. In particular, there is much interest in understanding the contextual determinants of mental health. This is related to a growing realization that to only concentrate on the individual may lead to a limited view of populations and in particular the contexts in which individuals live. There may also be variables which can only really be assessed at the group level, for example, area-level ethnic density, population density, or income inequality. Understanding the role of an individual's household, neighbourhood, or even country may help to develop interventions or policies which could have beneficial population-level impacts. In addition, temporal trends in disease prevalence/incidence or disease trends following the implementation of a new policy can also be assessed using ecological study designs. There may be circumstances where such study designs are the only possible option, as it may be unethical or not feasible to design a randomized controlled trial to assess the introduction of a population-level intervention or a new policy.

Advances in statistical methods have led to the development of multilevel modelling approaches. These approaches allow the simultaneous analysis of both individual-level and area-level associations. Multilevel modelling approaches may deal with some of the limitations associated with geographical ecological studies and will be briefly introduced in the second part of this chapter.

Historical overview

Perhaps the first ecological study in epidemiology was John Snow's analysis of the cholera epidemic of 1854. Following an outbreak of cholera in the Soho area of London, Snow investigated the occurrence of deaths from the disease in the local area and plotted these on a map. The spatial representation of the outbreak clustered around the water pump on Broad Street and led Snow to conclude that the water supplied by the pump was linked to the incidence of cholera in local residents. Snow convinced local authorities to remove the pump handle. This symbolic gesture ('symbolic' as many, including Snow himself, have suggested that the cholera epidemic was already in decline by that point (McLeod, 2000)) coincided with the end of the cholera epidemic. It was not until almost 30 years later, that Robert Koch was credited for the discovery of the bacterium *Vibrio cholerae*.

A seminal example of an ecological study relevant to psychiatry is Emile Durkheim's study of suicide in the 1890s (Durkheim, 1951). In examining rates of suicide, Durkheim assessed the association of religion (Protestant versus Catholics) with suicide rates across European countries. His analysis suggested higher rates of suicide in countries with a higher proportion of Protestants. Durkheim maintained that higher levels of individualism and lower levels of traditional constraints and social cohesion in Protestant countries led to higher suicide rates which he characterized as 'egoistic' suicides. For Durkheim, suicide was the end product of an individual's lack of social integration or bond with their community. His study has received intense criticism over the years. In particular, commentators have shown through later work that the Protestant–Catholic differences highlighted in Durkheim's study could have been due to the under-counting of suicide in Catholic areas, where suicide was considered more taboo than in Protestant areas. Moreover, differences in Protestant and Catholic communities may be through a number of factors not just restricted to levels of social cohesion typified in each community ('confounding'), which he did not consider. It has also been suggested that Durkheim's analysis may have hid differences at the individual level (Morgenstern, 1982). For example, it is possible that all of the suicides reflected in states with greater proportions of Protestants were committed by Catholics (Morgenstern, 1982), perhaps due to Catholics in these areas holding a minority status and being socially isolated. Mistakenly assuming that group-level correlations equate to individual-level differences is to commit the 'ecological fallacy', described in further detail in Box 8.1.

Types of ecological studies

Broadly, there are two types of ecological study (Box 8.2):

1. Ecological studies with a focus on geography. These types of study designs have a special place in research focused on the interrelationships of place and health, but may also provide important information on population-level variations in health as well as clustering of disease. For example, investigators may assess how disadvantage correlates with levels of mental health problems, with both of these measured at the neighbourhood-level. Ecological studies may also be exploratory, simply relating to the spatial variation of disease.

Box 8.1 Fallacies: some definitions

- *Ecological fallacy*: falsely attributing findings from analyses conducted on group-level data to individuals.
- *Individualistic fallacy*: falsely attributing findings from analyses based on individual-level data to the group.
- *Cross-level inference*: inferences about individuals are based on group-level data or inferences about groups are based on individual-level data. Where these inferences are incorrect, ecological or individual fallacies, respectively, may be said to have occurred.

2. Ecological studies which assess disease trends over time. These studies can also be used to assess the impact of an exposure, such as a population-level policy or intervention, on disease trends. These studies can also be exploratory, simply assessing disease trends over time.

In both types of ecological study design, the unit of investigation is the group and not the individual. Therefore the power of the study should be based on the number of groups (and not on the number of individuals within each group or on the size of group).

Ecological studies with a focus on geography

In their classic study, Faris and Dunham (1939) identified that admission rates for schizophrenia were more than nine times greater in the centre of Chicago (Illinois, US) compared to the outskirts. Building on a theoretical model of 'social disorganization' where they postulated that the innermost zones of the city were more socially disorganized compared to the outskirts, Faris and Dunham suggested that levels of social disorganization within the city were implicated in the aetiology of schizophrenia (Figure 8.1). Although there have been many developments since this study in understanding the role of the environment in contributing to the aetiology of schizophrenia, their work made an important contribution in considering the role of place in mental health (March et al., 2008).

Ecological studies which assess disease trends over time

Ecological studies may also be useful for assessing secular trends or changes in population health following the introduction of policies or interventions. Like ecological studies of geographical areas, ecological studies assessing time trends may give important clues as to the aetiological origins of a disorder. Although these studies may be relatively quick to perform and cost-effective as investigators conducting these types of studies can take advantage of routinely collected data, in practice it can be difficult to deduce whether observed changes in disease trends are as a result of an intervention, particularly if the trend was already falling prior to the introduction of the intervention (Figure 8.2).

Box 8.2 Some types and examples of ecological studies

Ecological studies with a geographical focus

♦ Studies which identify geographical 'clusters' of disease.

Example: John Snow and the Broad Street pump (cholera epidemic of 1854).

♦ Studies which identify differences in health outcomes between populations.

Example: the age-standardized prevalence of dementia varies fourfold from western Sub-Saharan Africa (2.07%) to Latin America (8.5%) (Prince et al., 2013).

♦ Studies which identify correlations between group-level exposures and group-level outcomes.

Example: studies which have shown a positive correlation between country-level inequality and country-level mental health outcomes (Pickett and Wilkinson, 2010).

Ecological studies with a temporal focus

♦ Studies which identify temporal trends in disease over time.

Example: an ecological study which suggested that reduced exposure to sunshine in the perinatal period is associated with increased rate of schizophrenia in men (McGrath et al., 2002). The authors speculated that perinatal environmental risks (such as perinatal vitamin D levels and altered host response to infection) could be important in the pathogenesis of schizophrenia (McGrath et al., 2002).

♦ Studies which identify changes to disease trends over time, following the introduction of policies or changes in practice.

Example: a study which suggested a reduction in paracetamol overdose deaths as well as a reduction in registrations for liver transplant due to paracetamol hepatotoxicity, following the introduction of legislation in the UK to reduce pack sizes of paracetamol (Hawton et al., 2013).

In order to take into account underlying trends, analytic methods such as 'interrupted time series' analyses permit the possibility of examining changes to underlying trends in disease following the introduction of an intervention or policy (Ramsay et al., 2003). These methods have the advantage of taking into account underlying trends (i.e. the observed trend in disease following the introduction of the intervention compared to what the trend would have otherwise been had the intervention not been introduced) (Ramsay et al., 2003). For example, in a study assessing the impact of legislation on sales of paracetamol (Hawton et al., 2013), the authors showed that the introduction of a law which led to a reduction in pack sizes of paracetamol available to consumers, was associated

(a) The concentric zone model of urban organization.

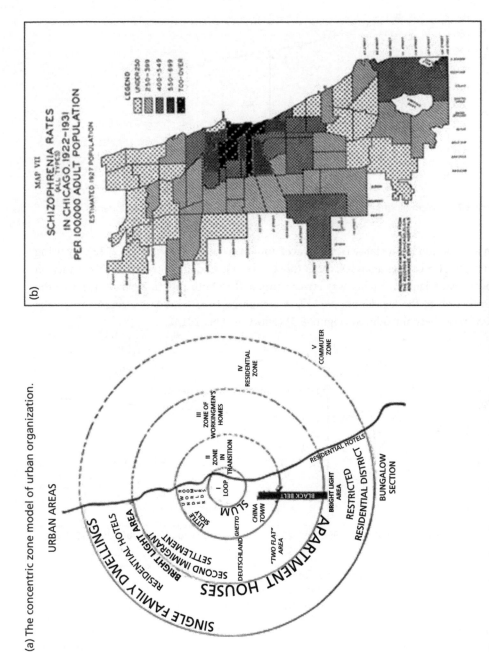

Figure 8.1 Faris and Dunham's 1939 ecological study of Chicago neighbourhoods.
Reproduced with permission from *Mental Disorders in Urban Areas* by R. Faris and H. Dunham, University of Chicago Press, Chicago, Illinois, 1939.

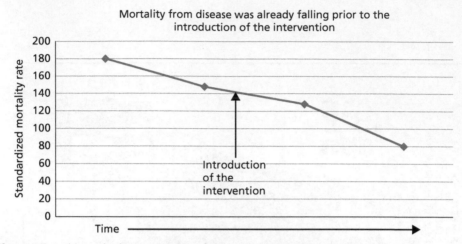

Figure 8.2 Problem of inferring causation from ecological studies assessing time trends.

with a reduction in mortality from paracetamol overdose (Hawton et al., 2013). By using interrupted time series analyses, the authors were able to demonstrate that this reduction in overdose-related mortality was lower compared to both the time period prior to the introduction of the legislation, as well as compared to an alternative scenario had the policy never been introduced (Figure 8.3) (Hawton et al., 2013).

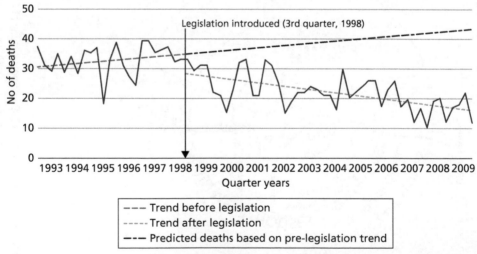

Figure 8.3 Suicide and open verdict deaths involving paracetamol in people aged 10 years or over in England and Wales and best-fit line relating to 1998 legislation which restricted pack sizes of paracetamol sold.

Ecological studies which assess trends following the introduction of an intervention can provide valuable insights, especially where a randomized controlled trial may not be feasible (e.g. in instances where policies at a national level are introduced affecting the whole population, or in instances where to randomize may not be ethically acceptable). A limitation of ecological studies assessing time trends following the introduction of a policy is that as they do not include a randomized control group, they cannot be used to rule out that other events (outside of the factors studied) impacted disease trends. In addition, the time frame over which exposure and disease outcomes should be measured is not always clear cut—especially if a time lag for the intervention on disease outcome is anticipated.

Advantages and disadvantages of ecological studies

See Figure 8.4 and Box 8.3.

A brief diversion: ecological studies versus ecological variables

Ecological studies should not be confused with ecological *variables*. Ecological variables are group-level variables and can be used in other types of study designs aside from ecological studies. Ecological variables may be derived from the individuals who make up

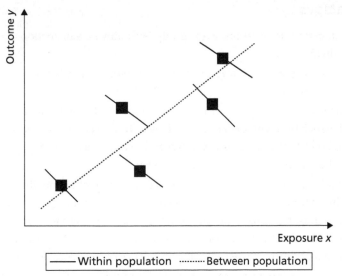

Figure 8.4 Ecological bias. Ecological bias is said to have occurred when what is seen at the group level does not correspond to the individual level. In this figure, over the five population groups (represented as boxes) as exposure *x* increases, so too does outcome *y*. However, for individuals *within* each of the population groups, exposure *x* is inversely associated with outcome *y*.

Adapted with permission from *Epidemiologic Methods: Studying the Occurrence of Illness* by Thomas Koepsell & Noel Weiss. Oxford University Press (2014). Reproduced with permission of the Licensor through PLSclear.

Box 8.3 Advantages and disadvantages of ecological studies

Advantages

1. Cheap and quick to conduct. Aggregated sources of data are readily available in publicly accessible archives and registries (e.g. at the country level, county level, and state level). For this reason, ecological studies may be a good starting point for generating hypotheses.

2. We may be interested in group-level phenomena: measures of disease occurrence (e.g. prevalence) can be obtained at the group level and measures of exposure effect (correlation coefficients or regression coefficients) can be derived.

3. The focus of study is the group. This minimizes the potential for *individual fallacies* (Box 8.2).

4. Some exposures can only be studied at the group or population level (e.g. policies affecting health at country, state, or regional level).

5. Improvements in precision as dichotomous outcomes (e.g. prevalence) become continuous.

6. Information bias less likely as exposure and outcome are usually ascertained separately.

7. Data are aggregate: fewer ethical issues surrounding confidentiality.

Disadvantages

1. *Ecological biases*: observations at the group level may be a distortion of differences at the individual level.

2. Cannot assume that group-level characteristics represent individuals; to do so is to commit an *ecological fallacy* (Figure 8.3) (Box 8.2).

3. There may not be enough variation in the group-level variable to allow an assessment of association with dependent variables. To detect an association there need to be different levels of exposure; however, in studies using group-level variables this may be less evident at the aggregated level.

4. There may be differences in ascertainment of exposure or outcome either according to geography (in the case of ecological studies of place) or over time (for ecological studies assessing trends over time). This may lead to misleading estimates which suggest differences in disease by place or over time, which are due to differences in methods as opposed to true difference in underlying prevalence or incidence of disease.

5. Ecological studies are prone to confounding and it is especially difficult to be certain about causal associations. It may not be possible to collect information on aggregate data on key confounders.

6. Many ecological studies rely upon routine data. This makes them best suited to data which is readily available and reliable (e.g. mortality). Variations in data which depend upon service utilization (e.g. number of admissions) may be due to factors other than prevalence of a disorder (e.g. due to the availability of services).

the groups in a study (e.g. proportion of ethnic minorities in a neighbourhood, mean household income for a borough, etc.) or alternatively, ecological variables may have no individual-level equivalent. An example of an ecological variable without an individual-level equivalent may be 'relative country-level income inequality' (e.g. assessed through the Gini coefficient), or policy and legislative procedures impacting regions or countries.

Including individuals in studies of groups: multilevel modelling

Ecological studies tell us something about the group but should not be used to make inferences about individuals. It has been suggested that twentieth century trends in epidemiology shifted the focus of disease on to individuals and prioritized individualized 'risk' over environmental and social determinants of health. This focus on 'risk factor' epidemiology obfuscated the role of the wider environment or context in patterning adverse health outcomes. Health behaviours became conceptualized as located within individuals, yet wider social determinants (such as neighbourhood, region, or country) may also play a role in patterning health behaviours and outcomes (Diez-Roux, 1998). Indeed, experiences located within the context (which could be a neighbourhood or a country) in which a person resides may have effects on health which are independent to individual-level experiences (Diez Roux, 2001). Some of the most successful policy interventions to address health behaviours have been at the population level, for example, taxation on alcohol to curb levels of alcohol consumed (Wagenaar et al., 2009).

To draw inferences about the group solely from individual-level studies may be to commit an 'individualistic fallacy' (Susser, 1994; Diez Roux, 2002) (Box 8.1). This is in contrast to the ecological fallacy (Box 8.1). The properties of the 'group' may not just be the sum of the individuals who make up the group and so may need to be studied in their own right (Diez-Roux, 1998; Susser, 1994; Diez Roux, 2001). For example, using results from mostly ecological study designs (Wilkinson, 1992; Wilkinson and Pickett, 2010), Wilkinson and Pickett (2010) have suggested that there is a positive correlation between more unequal societies and adverse health outcomes. This has been observed across a range of health indicators, from life expectancy to mental health and substance misuse (Wilkinson, 1992; Wilkinson and Pickett, 2010). Although hotly contested, the central facet of this debate is that greater relative deprivation and inequality (as opposed to absolute levels of material deprivation (Wilkinson, 1992)) is important for national health outcomes such as mortality (Wilkinson and Pickett, 2010). These interactions between individuals can only be social, thus arguably can only be studied at the group level. Moreover, as these health differences relate to poverty relative to wider society, they may not be observed at lower levels of geographical area (Pickett and Wilkinson, 2010). Thus group-level experiences may impact individual-level experiences and may be more than the sum of the individuals which make up that group. These are described as 'contextual' effects (Diez Roux, 2002). Conversely, if the composition of the group fully accounts for group-level phenomenon, these are referred to as 'compositional' effects (Diez Roux, 2002). Ecological studies can characterize the variation in disease prevalence by geographical area, but they cannot be used to tell us if observed differences are due to the areas themselves, or due to the individuals which make up those areas; that is, this type of study design cannot be used to distinguish between contextual versus compositional effects (Diez Roux, 2001).

Developments in statistical techniques have meant that it is now possible to analyse both group-level and individual-level attributes in statistical models, which are able to assess the role of individual variables in accounting for group-level phenomenon and vice versa. These models are known as multilevel models and are also referred to as 'mixed effects' models, 'random effects' models, and 'random intercepts' models in the literature. The application of multilevel techniques to the analysis of epidemiological studies (e.g. in the analysis of repeated measures or in the analysis of clustered data) is discussed in detail later in this book (see Chapter 18). The following section will briefly consider the way in which the application of multilevel modelling techniques have enhanced studies of context on mental health; whereas previously these types of study were mainly reliant on ecological study designs.

Multilevel models and studies of place/context on mental health

Whereas ecological studies only have information on groups of individuals, within a multilevel analytic framework there is information on groups (such as neighbourhoods, countries, and counties), as well as information on the composition of the groups (e.g. individuals or households). In this way, the data is said to have a 'hierarchical' structure. Individuals may be 'nested' within households; households may be 'nested' within neighbourhoods; and so on (Figure 8.5).

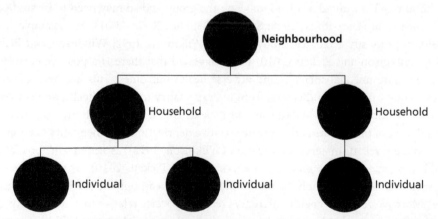

Figure 8.5 Multilevel data: example of a hierarchical structure. There are three 'levels' (individual level, household level, and neighbourhood level) with observations 'clustered' or 'nested' within each level (individuals nested within households, households nested within neighbourhoods).

It is useful to think of each of the groups within the dataset as a 'cluster' in which observations which make up each cluster (e.g. individuals) share common characteristics. The way in which individuals nested within a larger group (whether it is a household or neighbourhood or county) share the attributes of the group is referred to as 'within-cluster correlation'. Individuals within a neighbourhood (or 'cluster') may also be different to individuals living in other neighbourhoods; this is referred to as 'between-cluster variation'. Standard regression procedures (see Chapter 18 for details) assume that observations are independent of each other. Since people living within the same neighbourhood are likely to be similar to each other, and therefore non-independent, it is likely that assumptions of standard regression procedures will be violated. If we were to proceed with standard regression procedures which did not take into account the way in which individuals living within neighbourhoods shared common attributes, this would lead to biased estimates in the form of small standard errors and therefore small p-values and narrow 95% confidence intervals. There are a number of statistical techniques which can be used to deal with the clustering or non-independence of observations within a group[1] but most of these techniques tend to deal with clustering as if it were a 'nuisance'.

In social epidemiology, this statistical nuisance of clustering may actually be of interest, since it may tell us something about the neighbourhood or geographical context in which people live (Merlo et al., 2005). The more alike people in neighbourhoods are, or in statistical terms appear to 'cluster', the more likely it will be that individual health will be related to the contextual or neighbourhood environment (Merlo et al., 2005). Multilevel models explicitly model the variance between neighbourhoods, and allow the possibility of partitioning the variance between neighbourhoods and the individuals which make up those neighbourhoods and allow investigators to assess how far the neighbourhood context accounts for individual-level health differences. Further details on multilevel modelling approaches are described in chapter 18.

It should be emphasized that multilevel models are an analytic technique and not a study design. For studies assessing geographical context, these statistical methods tend to be used with data which are collected as a result of observational study designs, for example, collected during cross-sectional surveys. Therefore, although ecological bias may be avoided by using these analytic methods, these types of studies will still be prone to confounding, problems with identifying temporal associations (for cross-sectional studies), as well as potential observation and selection biases.

---

1 It is beyond the scope of the present chapter to detail statistical methods which deal with clustering in data. Interested readers are encouraged to consult statistical textbooks (e.g. see Kirkwood, B. and Sterne, J. (2003). *Medical statistics*, 2nd edn. Malden, MA: Blackwell Publishing).

Conclusion: is there a place for ecological study designs and studies which consider place or context in psychiatric epidemiology?

Ecological study designs have a long history in psychiatric epidemiology. Prior to the rise of 'methodological individualism' they were used by investigators to make inferences about individuals, especially where individual-level data were unavailable (Susser, 1994). However, to make incorrect inferences about individuals based on group-level attributes leads to ecological fallacy as attributes of the individual do not necessarily correlate with that of the group. With the rise of (individualized) risk factor epidemiology, ecological study designs fell out of favour (Susser, 1994). Yet these study designs are a valuable asset in psychiatric epidemiology as they can be used to generate hypotheses and are useful in assessing geographical and temporal trends in disease. They can also be used to assess trends following the implementation of policies or interventions. In some cases, ecological studies may be the only way to assess the impact of population-level interventions or policies, as it may be unethical or impractical to use randomized controlled trials. To forego any study of the group in favour of the individual is also to have a blinkered view of the causal web of disease, leading to a focus solely on individual risk factors, to the detriment of wider contextual determinants.

The advent of multilevel modelling strategies in psychiatric epidemiology have meant that analyses of 'place', as well as of the individuals who live in them, allow an understanding of the contextual determinants of mental health. Despite the advantage of multilevel models in being able to simultaneously model individual-level and neighbourhood-level variance, these analytic techniques still need to be used cautiously as they deal with observational data (usually from a cross-sectional study) and therefore still remain prone to the limitations of observational study designs.

Practical exercises

1. There are concerns that suicide mortality in some countries is greater than in others. Consider the types of information available at country level which you could use in an ecological study examining country-level factors associated with suicide. What are the advantages and disadvantages of this type of study? What other types of study could you design to deal with these limitations?

2. Investigators of a study unexpectedly find that the prevalence of common mental disorders is reduced in neighbourhoods which are more deprived, relative to less deprived neighbourhoods. The study has utilized information at the neighbourhood level only (area/neighbourhood-level indices for deprivation). Estimates for common mental disorders were obtained from a national survey of mental health—the investigators took a measure for proportion of individuals with common mental disorders at the neighbourhood level and used this as an outcome measure. What are the limitations of this study design? Can you think of a way to deal with these limitations, bearing in mind that additional information at the individual level might also be available?

References

Diez-Roux, A.V. (1998). Bringing context back into epidemiology: variables and fallacies in multilevel analysis. *American Journal of Public Health*, **88**, 216–222.

Diez Roux, A.V. (2001). Investigating neighborhood and area effects on health. *American Journal of Public Health*, **91**, 1783–1789.

Diez Roux, A.V. (2002). A glossary for multilevel analysis. *Journal of Epidemiology and Community Health*, **56**, 588–594.

Durkheim, E. (1951). *Suicide: a study in sociology*. New York: The Free Press.

Faris, R.E.L. and Dunham, W. (1939). *Mental disorders in urban areas*. Chicago, IL: University of Chicago Press.

Hawton, K., Bergen, H., Simkin, S., Dodd, S., Pocock, P., Bernal, W., et al. (2013). Long term effect of reduced pack sizes of paracetamol on poisoning deaths and liver transplant activity in England and Wales: interrupted time series analyses. *BMJ* **346**, f403.

March, D., Hatch, S.L., Morgan, C., Kirkbride, J.B., Bresnahan, M., Fearon, P., and Susser, E. (2008). Psychosis and place. *Epidemiologic Reviews*, **30**, 84–100.

McGrath, J., Selten, J.-P., and Chant, D. (2002). Long-term trends in sunshine duration and its association with schizophrenia birth rates and age at first registration—data from Australia and the Netherlands. *Schizophrenia Research*, **54**, 199–212.

McLeod, K.S. (2000). Our sense of Snow: the myth of John Snow in medical geography. *Social Science & Medicine*, **50**, 923–935.

Merlo, J., Chaix, B., Yang, M., Lynch, J., and Råstam, L. (2005). A brief conceptual tutorial of multilevel analysis in social epidemiology: linking the statistical concept of clustering to the idea of contextual phenomenon. *Journal of Epidemiology and Community Health*, **59**, 443–449.

Morgenstern, H. (1982). Uses of ecologic analysis in epidemiologic research. *American Journal of Public Health*, **72**, 1336–1344.

Pickett, K.E. and Wilkinson, R.G. (2010). Inequality: an underacknowledged source of mental illness and distress. *British Journal of Psychiatry*, **197**, 426–428.

Prince, M., Bryce, R., Albanese, E., Wimo, A., Ribeiro, W., and Ferri, C.P. (2013). The global prevalence of dementia: a systematic review and metaanalysis. *Alzheimer's & Dementia*, **9**, 63–75.e2.

Ramsay, C.R., Matowe, L., Grilli, R., Grimshaw, J.M., and Thomas, R.E. (2003). Interrupted time series designs in health technology assessment: lessons from two systematic reviews of behavior change strategies. *International Journal of Technology Assessment in Health Care*, **19**, 613–623.

Ramstedt, M. (2001). Per capita alcohol consumption and liver cirrhosis mortality in 14 European countries. *Addiction*, **96**, 19–33.

Susser, M. (1994). The logic in ecological: I. The logic of analysis. *American Journal of Public Health*, **84**, 825–829.

Wagenaar, A.C., Salois, M.J., and Komro, K.A. (2009). Effects of beverage alcohol price and tax levels on drinking: a meta-analysis of 1003 estimates from 112 studies. *Addiction*, **104**, 179–190.

Wilkinson, R. and Pickett, K. (2010). *The spirit level: why equality is better for everyone*. London: Penguin.

Wilkinson, R.G. (1992). Income distribution and life expectancy. *British Medical Journal*, **304**, 165–168.

Chapter 9

Cross-sectional surveys

Martin Prince and Jayati Das-Munshi

Introduction

This chapter considers the strengths and limitations, and the uses and abuses of cross-sectional surveys in psychiatric epidemiology. Certain basic aspects of research methodology, the concept of the base population, sampling strategies, representativeness, the problem of non-response, and the practical logistics of population-based research are introduced here, although they are in practice equally relevant to other study designs. The chapter also introduces the problem of bias, arising both from non-response and misclassification. In conclusion, major surveys of psychiatric morbidity are reviewed in a historical context, highlighting methodological developments and discussing the yield of information to be gleaned from them.

Uses and applications of cross-sectional surveys

Cross-sectional surveys can be used to measure the prevalence of a disorder within a population. This may be useful for:

- drawing public and political attention to the extent of a problem within a community
- planning services—identifying need, both met and unmet
- describing the burden of a condition within a population—its prevalence, the level of associated disability, the demands on services, and the economic costs.

Such surveys may seek to make comparisons with other populations or regions (in a series of comparable surveys conducted in different populations), or to chart trends over time (in a series of comparable surveys of the same population).

They can also be used to compare the characteristics of those in the population with and without the disorder, thus

- identifying cross-sectional associations with potential risk factors for the disorder
- identifying suitable (representative) cases and controls for population-based case–control studies.

Findings from population-based cross-sectional surveys can be generalized to the base population for that survey and, to some extent, to other populations with similar characteristics.

Box 9.1 Examples of base populations taken from the psychiatric literature

Cross-sectional surveys should have a defined base population such as:

- all children in one or more schools (Stansfeld et al., 2004)
- all prisoners in a given country (Brinded et al., 2001)
- all residents in two South London boroughs (Hatch et al., 2012)
- all residents of several catchment areas taken to be broadly representative of national diversity (Regier et al., 1984)
- all adult residents of a country (Slade et al., 2009; MacManus et al., 2016).

The results can be generalized to the base population and also, possibly, to other populations with similar characteristics.

The main drawback of cross-sectional surveys for analytical as opposed to descriptive epidemiology is that they can only give clues about aetiology. Because exposure (potential risk factor) and outcome (disorder or health condition) are measured simultaneously one can never be sure, in the presence of an association, which is the cause and which the consequence. The technical term is 'direction of causality'. Thus, in the 10/66 Dementia Research Group surveys in Latin America, China, and India (Albanese et al., 2013), dementia was associated with lower systolic blood pressure—did low blood pressure lead to dementia, or dementia to low blood pressure?

The design of cross-sectional surveys

Conduct of surveys

The basic procedures which should be followed in the conduct of cross-sectional and other types of study design have been covered previously, in Chapter 6. In the following sections, some of the specific issues which need to be considered when conducting cross-sectional surveys are further highlighted.

The base population

Cross-sectional surveys survey a defined base population, from which the sample for the survey is drawn. The random element of the sampling selection procedure should ensure that the sample is *representative* of this wider population. The findings of the survey should then be *generalizable* to this group.

From the examples given in Box 9.1 it should be clear that the base population might be a special subpopulation (prisoners, homeless people, hospital inpatients) or the general population. Whichever, the first step is to identify a sampling frame defining eligibility. Criteria need to be thought through carefully. For population surveys they usually include an age criterion, a place of residence criterion, and a period criterion; thus all residents of a defined area, resident on a particular day or month. Participants may occasionally need to be excluded from the survey because of health or other circumstances that render their participation difficult or impossible. Exclusion criteria should be specified in advance. Every effort should be made to be as inclusive as possible, in order to maximize the potential for generalizing from the survey findings.

Sampling frames require an accurate register of all eligible participants in the base population. In most countries, such registers are drawn up and updated regularly for general population censuses, taxation, and other administrative purposes, and for establishing voting entitlement in local and national elections. However, there are problems associated with using such registers. Some may not contain all of the information (e.g. age, sex, and address) that is needed to identify and contact a sample with a specified age range. Many governments will either not allow researchers to have access to these registers, set limits on the information that can be gleaned from them, or will limit the way in which the data is used. Also many administrative registers are surprisingly inaccurate, particularly in the case of highly mobile urban populations. Thus people move address without informing the relevant agency, or move or die in the interval between regular updates of the register. For government censuses this problem is referred to as undercounting. If a sociodemographic group (ethnic minorities or older people), or people with a health condition under study (depression) are particularly likely to be underrepresented this can lead to significant biases. Because of these deficiencies, some population-based surveys draw up their own register by carrying out a door-knock census of the area to be surveyed. While this is practical for a small catchment area survey, a survey of a larger base population such as the population of a whole country would need a different strategy. Often investigators draw a random sample of households, which are then visited by researchers who interview either all eligible residents, or individuals selected at random from among the eligible residents in the household.

Sampling strategies

It is clearly not necessary to interview every resident of a country to estimate the prevalence of major depression with reasonable precision. Sample size calculations may be carried out to determine the minimum sample size required to measure a given prevalence with a given precision (e.g. ± 1%). Sampling is guided by two overriding aims:

- to achieve the maximum precision for a given outlay of resources
- to avoid bias.

Bias in sampling arises when

- the sampling is non-random
- the sampling frame (list, register, or other population record) does not cover the population adequately, completely, or accurately
- some sections of the intended population are difficult to find or are likely to refuse to cooperate.

Table 9.1 Overview of sampling strategies

Simple random samples	For example, 1 in 5 residents of an area
Stratified random samples—with a fixed sampling fraction	For example, 1 in 5 selected at random from each age group, or both genders, or each housing district. This eliminates between strata sampling error
Stratified random samples—with a variable sampling fraction	For example, 1 in 10 of those aged 65–74, 1 in 5 of those aged 75–84, and 1 in 2 of those aged 85 years and over. The aim is to over-sample strata with low numbers or high standard errors in order to ensure adequate precision in each subgroup. When the final prevalence estimate for the whole population is calculated, the over-sampling of the subgroups will have to be taken into account. Estimates for subgroups are *weighted back* to their distribution within the whole population by using *weights* that are calculated according to the different *sampling fractions* applied
Cluster random sample	For example, a random sample of schools in the UK, a random sample of classes within the selected schools, and a random sample of children within the selected classes. A simple random sample of all UK schoolchildren would necessitate negotiating access to and visiting a much larger number of schools. As long as the cluster sampling is truly random and the analysis is appropriately weighted, unbiased and generalizable estimates should result

Definitions: simple random samples—members of a population all have an equal chance of being selected for a study; stratified random samples—the population is split into subpopulations which are relatively homogeneous; cluster random samples—'clusters' (e.g. schools, villages) are randomly selected, from which participants are randomly selected.

There are several different possible sampling strategies. Note, however, that each of these involves random selection. Table 9.1 provides some examples of base populations, which could form the basis for representative cross-sectional surveys.

Response rates/representativeness

The size of the achieved sample (those who have been interviewed and contributed data) will differ from that of the target sample because of non-response. Some participants will refuse to be interviewed, others will have died or moved away since the register or sample was established. In establishing the sample or register, some data (usually at least age and gender) is available on all potential participants. It is therefore possible, at least to some extent, to check the representativeness of the achieved sample. Systematic differences between the characteristics of those who were interviewed and those who were not can lead to biased estimates of prevalence, and bias in investigations of aetiological associations. The best way to limit non-response bias is to ensure the highest response rate possible. See Box 9.2 for factors that can influence the response rate.

Box 9.2 Factors that can influence the response rate

Certain characteristics of the study may affect the response rate and should be considered in the survey design:

♦ The manner of the initial approach to the participant.

♦ The burden imposed on the participant by the survey.

♦ The medium for the administration of the research interview.

Interviews/assessments

In cross-sectional surveys of psychiatric morbidity it may be necessary to assess large numbers of participants. For this reason, assessments tend to be made by lay interviewers rather than by trained clinicians. Great reliance is placed on highly structured diagnostic instruments that are validated for lay administration. Reliability is achieved partly through the highly structured nature of the assessments, and by rigorous training of lay interviewers, with continuing monitoring during the course of the survey for quality control. The most widely used instruments for the assessment of psychiatric disorder in adults are the Composite International Diagnostic Interview (CIDI), the Mini-International Neuropsychiatric Review (MINI), and the Clinical Interview Schedule—Revised (CIS-R) (Jenkins et al. 1997; Sheehan et al. 1998; see also Chapter 2). These have been demonstrated to be capable of identifying a range of psychiatric disorders in the community with reasonable sensitivity and specificity. However, concerns have been raised regarding the validity of these diagnoses against the gold standard of semi-structured assessments administered by experienced clinicians. These have revealed generally poor concordance for common mental disorders (Brugha et al. 1999a, 1999b). There have also been particular problems in the rating of symptoms of psychosis that requires some degree of interviewer judgement as to the pathological significance of the behaviour or experience described (Cooper et al., 1998).

Common standardized diagnostic measures used with children and young people include the Development and Well-Being Assessment (Goodman et al., 2000), the Schedule for Schizophrenia and Affective Disorder for children (K-SADS), the Child and Adolescent Psychiatric Assessment (CAPA), and the Diagnostic Interview Schedule for Children (DISC). The Development and Well-Being Assessment (DAWBA) is novel in that it is a structured measure based on the fifth edition of the *Diagnostic and Statistical Manual of Mental Disorders* (*DSM-5*) and tenth edition of the International Classification of Diseases and Related Health Problems (ICD-10) (World Health Organization (WHO), 1992; American Psychiatric Association, 2013), that combines information from parents, children aged 11 years or more, and teachers if the family consents; multiple informants increase validity in standardized diagnostic assessments (Garb, 2005). The DAWBA is also the only standardized diagnostic assessment to combine these structured (thus highly reliable) questions with semi-structured probes (which increase validity) when the structured questions identify problem areas. The structured and semi-structured data from all informants can then be reviewed by suitably trained clinicians to assign diagnoses, which reduces misclassification due to respondent misunderstanding and allows the detection of disorders that are asymptomatic due to active treatment.

Much more work is required to validate lay-administered structured assessments in general population samples, and to identify the source and significance of discrepancies with clinician semi-structured diagnoses. Whatever approach is used, there will be some misclassification. This may either be random (not related to actual caseness or exposure) or systematic. Systematic misclassification may bias the estimate of prevalence, and may also bias investigations of aetiological associations.

Two-phase surveys

For rare conditions, such as schizophrenia, a two-phase diagnostic procedure may be indicated. Here the investigator deploys a short measure which can be cheaply used on large populations to identify likely cases. Those with a high probability of being a case are then given a more extensive and definitive second-stage clinical assessment, often carried out by a psychiatrist. A similar two-phase approach is often used in the diagnosis of dementia, in which a cognitive test is used as a screening instrument; those performing badly receive a more detailed neuropsychological assessment, a clinical interview, a physical examination, and an informant interview to establish a definitive diagnosis. These designs are superficially attractive, providing diagnostic precision, but with considerable economies of research effort. The rarer the condition, the greater the economy. However, they should be used with extreme caution given several significant caveats and disadvantages (Dunn et al., 1999):

1. The screening measure should have high sensitivity and specificity.

2. For a rare condition, the positive predictive value of the screening instrument will tend to be low, even when specificity is high. Most of the screen-positive participants will be false positives, and significant resources may need to be allocated to the second phase.

3. Unless (and this is most unusual) one can be confident that the screening measure has 100% specificity, that is, there are no false negatives, one must interview a sufficient number of randomly selected false negatives to assess the false-negative rate with reasonable precision.

4. The analysis of the data is complicated, particularly with respect to estimates of standard errors (and confidence intervals) and in testing for statistical significance of differences between prevalences observed in subgroups (see 'Analysis of data from cross-sectional surveys' for further details).

5. Further more serious complications arise where, as is usual, there is non-response in the more burdensome second phase, and this non-response, whether it arises from deaths, refusals, or moving away is non-random with respect to the exposure and the outcome had it been measured (informative censoring).

Although most of these problems have been recognized for some time (Deming, 1978), two-phase surveys are enduringly popular but often incorrectly designed, analysed, and inferenced. For example, in a recent systematic review of population-based studies of the prevalence of dementia, 77% of studies had use a multiphase design, but only 17% of these had correctly applied the design and appropriately analysed the results (Prince et al., 2016).

Analysis of data from cross-sectional surveys

The frequency of the mental health condition in the population is generally expressed in terms of prevalence. Prevalence refers to the proportion of persons in a defined population that has the condition at the instant of the survey. Some mental health conditions (e.g. depression) are relapsing and remitting disorders, and for that reason period prevalence rates are sometimes quoted. A period prevalence (e.g. 12-month prevalence) is the proportion of those in a defined population, who *either* have the condition at the instant of the survey *or* have had it at any time over the previous 12 months. Several standard assessments (e.g. the CIDI and the Schedules for Clinical Assessment in Neuropsychiatry (SCAN)) enquire after lifetime experience of mental disorders, and generate lifetime prevalence estimates. The validity of this approach is understandably controversial, relying as it does upon accurate recall of symptoms experienced many years previously (Parker, 1987; Wittchen et al., 1989).

Cross-sectional surveys tend by their very nature to be descriptive and exploratory rather than being driven by specific hypotheses. The strategy for analysing cross-sectional surveys should nevertheless be closely linked to prior research objectives. The following are some basic principles:

♦ Start with simple description, univariate comparison between groups and classical stratified analysis. Proceed to more complex analyses, for example, multivariable modelling with caution, and only when strictly indicated.

♦ Prevalence estimates should be weighted back to the composition of the base population, taking account of the sampling fractions applied in a two-phase survey. This is not a straightforward matter. Although point estimates can be calculated accurately by simple algebra (the Horvitz–Thompson estimator), standard errors will be underestimated and require the application of special techniques. Dunn and colleagues (1999) provide an excellent overview. It is also not appropriate to test for the statistical significance of observed differences between proportions in subgroups (e.g. the prevalence of depression in men and women) using standard chi-squared tests. More recent versions of SPSS provide some features to support design-based analysis, but only certain more specialized statistical software packages (e.g. STATA (StataCorp, 2015)) provide a full range of appropriate techniques. From all of these factors it should be evident that the economies of two-phase designs are to a considerable extent offset by the complications implicit in the correct analysis of these complex data sets. Expert statistical advice *must* be sought in the planning of such studies, and will almost certainly be required to assist in their analysis.

- Prevalence estimates should be accompanied by 95% confidence intervals, giving an indication of the precision of the estimate given the sample size (see earlier section for the special circumstances of the two-phase survey). Theoretically, this may not be appropriate or necessary in catchment area surveys where the whole population has been surveyed, since sampling error cannot occur when there has been no sampling. Nevertheless, conventionally, confidence intervals are still provided.

- Potential risk factors for the main outcome can be investigated by comparing the characteristics of cases and non-cases. In the first instance these comparisons should be univariate, for example, the t-test for differences in the mean age of cases and non-cases, or the chi-squared test for differences in the proportions of people who smoke.

- Bear in mind that the risk of making one or more type 1 errors increases with the number of statistical comparisons being made. It is important to be judicious in the way in which you explore the data, and honest in the way in which you report the conduct of your analysis. Thus if you make 60 statistical comparisons it would be wrong to report the 2 'statistically significant' differences without referring to the 58 'non-significant' tests.

- As in analytical epidemiology, multivariable modelling can be used to control for confounding and to test for interaction (effect modification). See Chapters 10 and 11 for more details.

Major psychiatric morbidity surveys: a historical review of methodological developments, scope, and achievements

The US NIMH Epidemiologic Catchment Area (ECA) programme

The ECA programme was the first large-scale attempt to estimate the prevalence of psychiatric morbidity in a nationwide survey (Regier et al., 1984). This was a governmental initiative developed during the presidency of Jimmy Carter (1976–1980) to inform future mental health policy in the US. Five catchment area communities were selected for study, to represent broadly the ethnic, socioeconomic, and geographic diversity of the nation. A probability sample of over 18,000 adults was drawn from these sites. The survey interview was the comprehensive, lay administered, fully-structured Diagnostic Interview Schedule (DIS) (Robins et al., 1981). The principal focus of the ECA was upon 1-year and lifetime prevalences of diagnoses according to the then current *DSM-III* criteria (Weissman et al. 1988). Aspects of the ECA have been criticized, particularly the validity of the DIS lifetime diagnoses (Burvill, 1987; Parker, 1987), the appropriateness of lay interviews, the applicability of the diagnostic ascertainment for older people, and its failure to assess the findings of the survey in the context of the existing epidemiological data (Burvill, 1987).

The US National Comorbidity Survey (NCS)

The NCS was the second major national survey conducted in the US. It differed from the ECA in its sampling methodology; a truly representative national sample was drawn of 8098 persons 15–54 years of age (Blazer et al., 1994). On this occasion, the survey interview was a modified version of the WHO's CIDI, a fully structured, lay-administered interview generating diagnoses according to *DSM-IV* criteria. The focus of the survey was to measure prevalence and to identify the extent of comorbidity between major and minor mental disorder and alcohol and substance use disorders (Blazer et al., 1994; Kendler et al., 1996; Kessler et al., 1997). Extensive analyses were conducted of lifetime experience of mental disorders using reported ages of onset, and sequence of onset of comorbid disorders to identify windows of opportunity for preventive interventions in younger adults (Kessler et al., 1998). A further feature of the NCS was the investigation of possible aetiological factors for mental disorders. Certain of these investigations were limited by the problem of attributing direction of causality to the observed associations, for example, between social support and depression (Zlotnick et al., 2000) and smoking and mental disorder (Lasser et al., 2000). Other reported associations, for example, that between child sexual abuse and adult mental disorder (Molnar et al., 2001), are more likely to reflect causal processes because of the latency between the reported exposure and the outcome, although recall bias may still be a problem.

Since the original NCS survey in 1992, there has been one follow-up survey of the original respondents, conducted in 2001–2002 (NCS-2). There has also been a replication survey (National Comorbidity Survey Replication (NCS-R)) which was conducted on another sample of nationally representative respondents. In addition, there has also been the National Comorbidity Survey of Adolescents (NCS-A), which was a survey of 10,000 adolescents sampled through representative schools or NCS-R households.

The remarkably prolific published output from the NCS may be explained in part by the decision to archive the data set in the public domain, making it available to the whole scientific community. This is now a standard procedure for surveys funded by the US National Institutes of Health.

The UK National Psychiatric Morbidity Surveys (NPMS) and Adult Psychiatric Morbidity Surveys (APMS) (England)

The UK APMS (previously referred to as the NPMS) was first commissioned by the UK Department of Health's Office of Population Censuses and Surveys in 1993 to conduct a survey of psychiatric morbidity in a nationally representative household sample of 10,108 adults aged 16–65, living in England, Scotland, and Wales (Jenkins et al., 1997). Since this time, there have been surveys every 7 years, with subsequent cross-sectional surveys in 2000 in England, Scotland, and Wales (Singleton et al., 2001), and in 2007 and 2014 in England only (McManus et al., 2009, 2016). In addition, surveys conducted in 2007 and 2014 included people over the age of 65 years. Core methodologies and questionnaires have stayed the same over waves of survey, in order to allow an assessment of changes to the prevalence of mental disorders over time. The survey interview was the CIS-R (Lewis et al., 1992). This generated diagnoses of common mental disorders (i.e. excluding psychoses) according to ICD-10 criteria, and a scalable score allowing exploration of the impact of psychiatric morbidity as a continuum in the general population. Psychoses were assessed using a two-phase method in which participants reporting psychotic disorders or symptoms suggestive of psychotic disorders or responding positively to items from the Psychosis Screening Questionnaire were subsequently interviewed with the comprehensive semi-structured clinical assessment SCAN. Each of the surveys has also included questions enquiring after suicidality as well as an assessment of alcohol and substance use. Earlier surveys included an assessment of personality disorders, later surveys (from 2007) focused on antisocial and borderline personality disorders (McManus et al., 2009). Following a realization that there were gaps in epidemiological knowledge, later surveys (2007) have also included assessments of attention deficit hyperactivity disorder, autism spectrum disorders, post-traumatic stress disorder, and eating disorders (McManus et al., 2009, 2016).

The UK national surveys were part of a wider UK policy-driven initiative to estimate the extent and impact of mental disorders with particular reference to implications for service delivery. This acknowledged the limitations of household surveys, which might miss vulnerable and dependent persons with mental disorders. To complete the picture, several complementary surveys of special settings, using comparable methods, were therefore conducted by the Office for National Statistics:

1. A sample of residents of institutions caring for the mentally ill ($N = 1191$); hospitals, nursing homes, residential care homes, hostels, group homes, and supported accommodation (Meltzer et al., 2003a).

2. A sample of homeless people ($N = 1166$) accessed through hostels, night-shelters, private sector leased accommodation, and day centres (Gill et al., 2003), with an analysis specifically focused on homeless people in Glasgow (Kershaw et al., 2003).

3. A supplementary sample of people with psychosis, known to services and living in private households (Foster et al., 1996; O'Brien et al., 2002)

4. A survey of prisoners and young offenders conducted in England and Wales (Singleton et al., 1998; O'Brien et al., 2001; Lader et al., 2003).

5. A survey of children looked after by local authorities (2001–2002) (Meltzer et al., 2003b).

6. There have also been two surveys of children and young people, one in 1999 and one in 2004 (Green et al., 2005), both of which were followed up 3 years later (Ford et al., 2017). A follow-up survey on children and young people has also been published (Sadler et al., 2018).

The Australian National Survey of Mental Health and Wellbeing

There have been two Australian National Surveys of Mental Health and Wellbeing, the first one in 1997 and the most recent one in 2007 (Slade et al., 2009). The 2007 survey drew a nationally representative probability sample of private households, leading to a representative sample of 8841 adults aged 18–85 years (Slade et al., 2009). The survey interview was the CIDI version 3.0 and was used to derive 12-month prevalence of mental disorders, modified to the Australian context (Slade et al., 2009). The findings from the first survey played an important role in informing the delivery of mental healthcare in Australia (Slade et al., 2009). The second survey was designed with the intention to assess the severity and impairment of mental disorders as well as impact on healthcare service use (Slade et al., 2009). The second survey revealed a high prevalence of lifetime common mental disorders and substance misuse, with just under half (45.5%) meeting criteria (Slade et al., 2009). The second survey also revealed high levels of comorbidity associated with disability and greater service use; the patterns reported were similar to those reported in the 1997 survey (Teesson et al., 2009). Investigators for the second survey also found that overall levels of service use had not changed substantially in the 10 years from the first survey (although they proposed a number of potential reasons for this, including differences in methodology across the two surveys) (Burgess et al., 2009) but that by the second survey, there had been an increase in reported use of psychologists (Burgess et al., 2009).

The World Mental Health (WMH) surveys

The World Mental Health (WMH) initiative, coordinated by the WHO's International Consortium in Psychiatric Epidemiology (ICPE), is the most ambitious attempt yet to generate data on the prevalence and impact of mental disorders, which has permitted valid comparisons between countries and regions worldwide (Kessler, 1999). The initiative includes representative surveys from 28 countries worldwide with just under 160,000 interviews (http://www.hcp.med.harvard.edu/wmh/index.php). Most of the surveys have been nationally representative, with the exception of a few regional surveys conducted in Brazil and Japan.

The core instrument for the surveys is the WHO World Mental Health Composite International Diagnostic Interview (WMH-CIDI). Diagnoses according to the WMH-CIDI have been validated against the Structured Clinical Interview for *DSM-IV* (SCID) using WMH samples across three countries in Europe and in the US (Haro et al., 2006). Impact has also been assessed in terms of associated impairment and disability, using the WHO's Disability Assessment Scale (WHODAS II) and the Sheehan Disability Scale (SDS). A further aspect of the CIDI has been in its incorporation of assessment of mental disorder severity (as opposed to a simple assessment of mental disorder prevalence), which was noted by the original investigators as crucial in the planning and delivery of healthcare services (Kessler et al., 2009).

Dissemination of findings from cross-sectional surveys

In addition to publication in peer-reviewed scientific journals, investigators should always consider alternative methods to reach the target audience, the consumers, for their research. Findings from cross-sectional surveys may be of relevance to:

+ politicians
+ health policymakers
+ non-governmental organizations and mental health advocacy groups
+ public health physicians
+ health practitioners
+ community leaders
+ the wider community
+ participants taking part in the survey.

Action research will be firmly orientated towards the public health and policy priorities for the population under study. It should gauge its success by the impact that it achieves in terms of raising awareness, altering priorities, and informing better preventive and treatment interventions. Achievement of these goals will certainly depend upon well-designed and focused research, but equally upon an effective and balanced dissemination strategy (Box 9.3). This should certainly extend beyond publications in high-quality peer-reviewed publications, and presentations at research conferences (which will influence the academic community, but may be relatively ineffective in other respects).

Final conclusions

In conclusion, cross-sectional surveys are a powerful study design which have been used across international settings to determine the prevalence of mental disorders, as well as associated demographic, clinical, and social 'risk factors' for disorders. Cross-sectional surveys may be nationally representative and therefore have the advantage of potentially

---

Box 9.3 A balanced dissemination strategy for action research

+ High-impact publications in peer-reviewed scientific journals.
+ Research presentations at national and international conferences.
+ Feedback to participants (e.g. plain English summaries via social media/websites).
+ Special local and national workshops including policymakers, clinicians, and community leaders.
+ Community meetings.
+ Fact sheets.
+ Press releases.
+ Media interviews.
+ Via institutional and study websites.

being generalizable to the base population of the country and therefore can be used to determine the prevalence of psychiatric morbidity in a population, thus assisting with the planning and delivery of services. They do, however, need to be conducted appropriately, with adequate levels of response, in order to ensure that bias is minimized.

Advantages of cross-sectional surveys include the following:

1. If well designed can give an assessment of morbidity and associated risk factors in a population and may generalize well to the base population.

2. Good for assessing common conditions at a population level.

3. Can be conducted with lay interviewers using appropriately validated instruments (e.g. CIDI or CIS-R) thus are associated with lower costs.

4. If well designed are potentially informative to policymakers, politicians, community leaders, public health, and others outside of academic community, and therefore are potentially impactful.

Disadvantages of cross-sectional surveys include the following:

1. Certain groups of people may be less likely to take part in the survey despite measures to minimize this. For example, people with mental disorders or who are socially disadvantaged may be less likely to take part, or conversely, people who are in full-time employment may be underrepresented if the conduct of the survey occurs only during working hours.

2. Even though cross-sectional surveys may be used to infer 'risk factors' for disease, they only capture data at one point in time, and therefore cannot be used to make inferences around direction of association of potential exposures with outcomes.

3. As cross-sectional surveys only occur at one point in time, participants may be asked to recall previous events during the survey, with survey instruments designed to assess lifetime recall of mental disorder diagnoses. This may be prone to recall bias.

4. One-stage cross-sectional surveys are well suited to common or prevalent conditions (e.g. for the assessment of the common mental disorders) but are less well suited to rare conditions such as schizophrenia. In these circumstances, two-stage surveys may be considered but are fraught with difficulties (see earlier section on this).

Practical exercises

1. How might you set about drawing a representative sample for a cross-sectional survey measuring the prevalence of *DSM-5* major depression in each of the following four settings (think of the example of your own country)?

    a. All inpatients in a general hospital.

    b. All general hospital inpatients in the whole country.

    c. All residents of a particular city borough aged 65 and over.

    d. All residents of the whole country (aged 18–65).

2. Consider the following questions:

   a. How did these two surveys establish their register/sampling frame?

   b. What efforts were made in the two surveys to deal with non-response?

   c. How might misclassification bias have caused problems in the two surveys?

   d. What do you think is the practical usefulness of SELCoH?

References

Albanese, E., Lombardo, F.L., Prince, M.J., and Stewart, R. (2013). Dementia and lower blood pressure in Latin America, India, and China: a 10/66 cross-cohort study. *Neurology*, **81**, 228–235.

American Psychiatric Association (2013). *Diagnostic and statistical manual of mental disorders*, 5th edn. Washington, DC: American Psychiatric Association.

Blazer, D.G., Kessler, R.C., McGonagle, K.A., and Swartz, M.S. (1994). The prevalence and distribution of major depression in a national community sample: the National Comorbidity Survey. *American Journal of Psychiatry*, **151**, 979–986.

Brinded, P.M., Simpson, A.I., Laidlaw, T.M., Fairley, N., and Malcolm, F. (2001). Prevalence of psychiatric disorders in New Zealand prisons: a national study. *Australian and New Zealand Journal of Psychiatry*, **35**, 166–173.

Brugha, T.S., Bebbington, P.E., and Jenkins, R. (1999a). A difference that matters: comparisons of structured and semi-structured psychiatric diagnostic interviews in the general population. *Psychological Medicine*, **29**, 1013–1020.

Brugha, T.S., Bebbington, P.E., Jenkins, R., Meltzer, H., Taub, N.A., Janas, M., and Vernon, J. (1999b). Cross validation of a general population survey diagnostic interview: a comparison of CIS-R with SCAN ICD-10 diagnostic categories. *Psychological Medicine*, **29**, 1029–1042.

Burgess, P.M., Pirkis, J.E., Slade, T.N., Johnston, A.K., Meadows, G.N., and Gunn, J.M. (2009). Service use for mental health problems: findings from the 2007 National Survey of Mental Health and Wellbeing. *Australian and New Zealand Journal Psychiatry*, **43**, 615–623.

Burvill, P.W. (1987). An appraisal of the NIMH Epidemiologic Catchment Area Program. *Australian and New Zealand Journal of Psychiatry*, **21**, 175–184.

Cooper, L., Peters, L., and Andrews, G. (1998). Validity of the Composite International Diagnostic Interview (CIDI) psychosis module in a psychiatric setting. *Journal of Psychiatric Research*, **32**, 361–368.

Deming, W.E. (1978). An essay on screening, or two-phase sampling, applied to surveys of a community. *International Statistical Review*, **45**, 28–37.

Dunn, G., Pickles, A., Tansella, M., and Vazquez-Barquero, J.L. (1999). Two-phase epidemiological surveys in psychiatric research. *British Journal of Psychiatry*, **174**, 95–100.

Ford, T., MacDiarmid, F., Russell, A.E., Racey, D., and Goodman, R. (2017). The predictors of persistent DSM-IV disorders in 3-year follow-ups of the British Child and Adolescent Mental Health Surveys 1999 and 2004. *Psychological Medicine*, **47**, 1126–1137.

Foster, K., Meltzer, H., Gill, B., and Hinds, K. (1996). *OPCS surveys of psychiatric morbidity in Great Britain, report 8: adults with a psychotic disorder living in the community*. London: HMSO.

Garb, H.N. (2005). Clinical judgement and decision making. *Aunnual Review of Clinical Psychology*, **1**, 67–89.

Goodman, R., Ford, T., Richards, H., Meltzer, H., and Gatward, R. (2000). The Development and Well-being Assessment: description and initial validation of an integrated assessment of child and adolescent psychopathology. *Journal of Child Psychology and Psychiatry* **41**, 645–657.

Gill, B., Meltzer, H., and Hinds, K. (2003). The prevalence of psychiatric morbidity among homeless adults. *International Review of Psychiatry*, 15, 134–140.

Green, H., McGinnity A., Meltzer H., Ford T., Goodman R. (2005). *Mental health of children and young people in Great Britain, 2004*. London: HMSO.

Haro, J.M., Arbabzadeh-Bouchez, S., Brugha, T.S., de Girolamo, G., Guyer, M.E., et al (2006). Concordance of the Composite International Diagnostic Interview Version 3.0 (CIDI 3.0) with standardized clinical assessments in the WHO World Mental Health surveys. *International Journal of Methods in Psychiatric Research*, 15, 167–180.

Hatch, S.L., Woodhead, C., Frissa, S., Fear, N.T., Verdecchia, M., Stewart, R., et al. (2012). Importance of thinking locally for mental health: data from cross-sectional surveys representing South East London and England. *PLoS One* 7, e48012.

Jenkins, R., Bebbington, P., Brugha, T., Farrell, M., Gill, B., Lewis, G., et al. (1997). The National Psychiatric Morbidity surveys of Great Britain—strategy and methods. *Psychological Medicine*, 27, 765–774.

Kendler, K.S., Gallagher, T.J., Abelson, J.M., and Kessler, R.C. (1996). Lifetime prevalence, demographic risk factors, and diagnostic validity of nonaffective psychosis as assessed in a US community sample. The National Comorbidity Survey. *Archives of General Psychiatry*, 53, 1022–1031.

Kershaw, A., Singleton, N., and Meltzer, H. (2003). Survey of the health and wellbeing of homeless people in Glasgow. *International Review of Psychiatry*, 15, 141–143.

Kessler, R.C., Aguilar-Gaxiola, S., Alonso, J., Chatterji, S., Lee, S., Ormel, J., et al. (2009). The global burden of mental disorders: an update from the WHO World Mental Health (WMH) Surveys. *Epidemiologia E Psichiatria Sociale*, 18, 23–33.

Kessler, R.C. (1999). The World Health Organization International Consortium in Psychiatric Epidemiology (ICPE): initial work and future directions—the NAPE Lecture 1998. Nordic Association for Psychiatric Epidemiology. *Acta Psychiatrica Scandinavica*, 99, 2–9.

Kessler, R.C., Olfson, M., and Berglund, P.A. (1998). Patterns and predictors of treatment contact after first onset of psychiatric disorders. *American Journal of Psychiatry*, 155, 62–69.

Kessler, R.C., Zhao, S., Blazer, D.G., and Swartz, M. (1997). Prevalence, correlates, and course of minor depression and major depression in the National Comorbidity Survey. *Journal of Affective Disorders*, 45, 19–30.

Kessler, R.C., Aguilar-Gaxiola, S., Alonso, J., Chatterji, S., Lee, S., Ormel, J., et al. (2009). The global burden of mental disorders: An update from the WHO World Mental Health (WMH) Surveys. *Epidemiologia E Psichiatria Sociale*, 18, 23–33.

Lader, D., Singleton, N., and Meltzer, H. (2003). Psychiatric morbidity among young offenders in England and Wales. *International Review of Psychiatry*, 15, 144–147.

Lasser, K., Boyd, J.W., Woolhandler, S., Himmelstein, D.U., McCormick, D., and Bor, D.H. (2000). Smoking and mental illness: a population-based prevalence study. *JAMA*, 284, 2606–2610.

Lewis, G., Pelosi, A.J., Araya, R., and Dunn, G. (1992). Measuring psychiatric disorder in the community: a standardized assessment for use by lay interviewers. *Psychological Medicine*, 22, 465–486.

McManus, S., Bebbington, P., Jenkins, R., and Brugha, T. (eds.) (2016) *Mental health and wellbeing in England: Adult Psychiatric Morbidity Survey 2014*. Leeds: NHS Digital.

McManus S., Meltzer H., Brugha T., Bebbington P., and Jenkins R. (2009). *Adult psychiatric morbidity in England 2007: results of a household survey*. Leeds: The Health & Social Care Information Centre, Leeds.

Meltzer, H., Gill, B., Hinds, K., and Petticrew, M. (2003a). The prevalence of psychiatric morbidity among adults living in institutions. *International Review of Psychiatry*, 15, 129–133.

Meltzer, H., Gatward, R., Corbin, T., Goodman, R., and Ford, T. (2003b). *The mental health of young people looked after by local authorities in England*. London: The Stationery Office.

Molnar, B.E., Buka, S.L., and Kessler, R.C. (2001). Child sexual abuse and subsequent psychopathology: results from the National Comorbidity Survey. *American Journal of Public Health*, 91, 753–760.

O'Brien, M., Mortimer, L., Singleton, N., and Meltzer, H. (2001). *Psychiatric morbidity among women prisoners in England and Wales*. London: The Stationery Office.

Parker, G. (1987). Are the lifetime prevalence estimates in the ECA study accurate? *Psychological Medicine*, 17, 275–282.

Prince, M., Comas-Herrera, A., Knapp, M., Guerchet, M., and Karagiannidou, M. (2016). *World Alzheimer report 2016: improving healthcare for people living with dementia*. London: **Alzheimer's Disease International**. https://www.alz.co.uk/research/WorldAlzheimerReport2016.pdf

Regier, D.A., Myers, J.K., Kramer, M., Robins, L.N., Blazer, D.G., Hough, R.L., et al. (1984). The NIMH Epidemiologic Catchment Area program. Historical context, major objectives, and study population characteristics. *Archives of General Psychiatry*, 41, 934–941.

Robins, L., Helzer, J.E., Croughan, J., and Radcliff, K.S. (1981). National Institute of Mental Health Diagnostic Interview Schedule: its history, characteristics and validity. *Archives of General Psychiatry*, 38, 381–389.

Sadler, K., Vizard, T., Ford, T., Goodman, A., Goodman, R., and McManus, S. (2018). *The mental health of children and young people in England 2017: trends and characteristics*. London: Health and Social Care Information Centre.

Sheehan, D.V., Lecrubier, Y., Sheehan, K.H., Amorim, P., Janavs, J., Weiller, E., et al. (1998). The Mini-International Neuropsychiatric Interview (M.I.N.I.): the development and validation of a structured diagnostic psychiatric interview for DSM-IV and ICD-10. *Journal of Clinical Psychiatry*, 59, 22–33.

Singleton, N., Meltzer, H., Gatward, R., Coid, J., and Deasy, D. (1998). *Psychiatric morbidity among prisoners in England and Wales*. London: The Stationary Office.

Singleton N., Bumpstead R., O'Brien M., Lee A., and Meltzer H. (2001). *Psychiatric morbidity among adults living in private households, 2000*. London: The Stationary Office.

Slade, T., Johnston, A., Browne, M.A.O., Andrews, G., and Whiteford, H. (2009). 2007 National Survey of Mental Health and Well-being: methods and key findings. *Australian and New Zealand Journal of Psychiatry*, 43, 594–605.

Stansfeld, S.A., Haines, M.M., Head, J.A., Bhui, K., Viner, R., Taylor, S.J.C., et al. (2004). Ethnicity, social deprivation and psychological distress in adolescents. *British Journal of Psychiatry*, 185, 233–238.

StataCorp (2015). *Stata statistical software: release 14*. College Station, TX: StataCorp LP.

Teesson, M., Slade, T., and Mills, K. (2009). Comorbidity in Australia: findings of the 2007 National Survey of Mental Health and Wellbeing. *Australian and New Zealand Journal of Psychiatry*, 43, 606–614.

Weissman, M.M., Leaf, P.J., Tischler, G.L., Blazer, D.G., Karno, M., Bruce, M.L., and Florio, L.P. (1988). Affective disorders in five United States communities. *Psychological Medicine*, 18, 141–153. [Erratum in Psychological Medicine 1988;18(3):following 792.]

Wittchen, H.U., Burke, J.D., Semler, G., Pfister, H., Von Cranach, M., and Zaudig, M. (1989). Recall and dating of psychiatric symptoms. Test-retest reliability of time-related symptom questions in a standardized psychiatric interview. *Archives of General Psychiatry*, 46, 437–443.

World Health Organization (1992). *International classification of diseases and related health problems, 10th revision (ICD-10).* Geneva: World Health Organization.

Zlotnick, C., Kohn, R., Keitner, G., and **Della Grotta, S.A.** (2000). The relationship between quality of interpersonal relationships and major depressive disorder: findings from the National Comorbidity Survey. *Journal of Affective Disorders,* **59,** 205–215.

Chapter 10

The case–control study

Lisa Aschan and Matthew Hotopf

Introduction

Imagine an investigator wants to test the hypothesis that obstetric complications are more common in schizophrenia than in the general population. There are two main approaches to this problem. The first involves identifying babies who have had a complicated birth and following them up to see whether they have a higher risk of schizophrenia in later life than babies with an uncomplicated births. This would be a cohort study—the 'ticket of entry' into the study is the exposure status of the individual. Under these circumstances, a well-designed prospective cohort study would undoubtedly give the answer, but it would be a very long time in coming, require a huge sample, and be extremely expensive. This is because schizophrenia is a rare disorder, which develops in early adulthood. Therefore, large numbers of individuals would have to be followed over many years in order to find each case of schizophrenia.

The alternative approach is to use the case–control design. This involves identifying cases with schizophrenia and comparing them with controls who are unaffected. The investigator would then use some method to *look back* and determine the exposure status of cases and controls.

The rationale for the case–control study

The decision about whether to use a case–control or cohort study depends on a number of considerations, which this example illustrates. Case–control studies are most appropriate when (1) the disorder under study is rare, (2) it takes a long time to develop after the exposure (sometimes referred to as the latent period), and (3) the exposure is common. Cohort studies are more appropriate when (1) the disorder is common, (2) it does not take long to develop, and (3) the exposure is rare.

This may be illustrated using a series of hypothetical sample size calculations. Table 10.1 shows the sample sizes required for cohort studies where equal-sized cohorts (exposed and unexposed) are compared over a 10-year period. The investigator sets the power at 80% and the confidence at 95% and looks for a twofold increase in risk in the exposed group. For a condition with an incidence rate of 10/100,000/year, the investigator will require 52,000 participants. Important psychiatric outcomes such as suicide

Table 10.1 Sample sizes required to detect a twofold risk in a cohort study run over 10 years with 80% power and 95% confidence

Incidence rate of disorder	Sample size
10/100,000/year	52,000
100/100,000/year	5,300
1000/100,000/year	650

and schizophrenia have incidences of approximately this order. Therefore, cohort studies would have to be very large and expensive to cope with such conditions.

Table 10.2 shows the same power calculation for a case–control study. Instead of varying the incidence of the disorder, the frequency of the exposure has been changed. This illustrates that when the prevalence of the exposure is very low, case–control studies have to be very large.

Table 10.2 Sample sizes required to detect a twofold risk in a case–control study with 80% power and 95% confidence

Frequency of the exposure	Sample size case–control study
0.1%	52,000
1%	5200
10%	620

Some additional points are worth making in relation to these tables. Firstly, note that for the cohort study, the frequency of the exposure was not mentioned. This is because in cohort studies the investigator typically manipulates exposure status by selecting individuals into the study on the basis of their exposure status. This means that rare exposures can be studied, so long as populations with those exposures can be identified (as classically would happen in occupational cohorts where the exposure is a toxin one particular occupational group has considerable exposure to). In Table 10.2, the prevalence of the illness under study was not mentioned, because in case–control studies this is what the investigator manipulates. Thus in each study design the investigator has control over either the frequency of the exposure (cohort) or the outcome (case–control).[1]

Secondly, although the sample sizes for the examples in Tables 10.1 and 10.2 may *look* similar, Table 10.1 relies upon a 10-year follow-up, while for Table 10.2, the results are—at least theoretically—available immediately. Cohort studies, by virtue of their longitudinal

1 These remarks apply to classical cohort study designs, however, as discussed in Chapter 11, many cohort studies assessing psychiatric outcomes have used *panel designs*, where a detailed baseline study assesses multiple exposures and potential outcomes, and the entire population is followed up, often over several time points. Given that several potential exposures are studied, the sample is not selected based on a particular exposure, as in a classical cohort design.

Table 10.3 Derivation of risks and odds in a cohort study

	Disorder		Total	Risk of disorder	Odds of disorder
	Yes	No			
Exposure					
Yes	a	b	a + b	a/(a + b)	a/b
No	c	d	c + d	c/(c + d)	c/d
Total	a + c	a + d			
Odds of exposure	a/c	b/d			

component are time-consuming. The exception to this is the retrospective or historical cohort study, where participants are still identified according to exposure status, but the exposure is ascertained using historical records (see Chapter 11).

Case–control studies may assess the role of *multiple* exposures on a *single* disorder. In contrast, cohort studies assess the role of a *single* exposure on *multiple* disorders. In the example of obstetric complications, a cohort study would not just be able to look at its impact on schizophrenia, but could also investigate other psychiatric disorders or physical diseases. A case–control study would not be able to do that, but would be able to investigate a wide range of risk factors.

Risk, odds, and the relationship between cohort and case–control studies

In both cohort and case–control studies the main purpose is to determine the relationship between an exposure and an outcome. This is expressed as the risk or rate ratio in cohort studies and the odds ratio in case–control studies. The relationship between these parameters is important to understand, and in describing this relationship one can gain a better grasp of the assumptions underlying case–control studies.

Cohort studies and risk

Cohort studies follow individuals who are free from a disorder to determine their risk of developing that disorder over a particular period of time. The *risk* is a proportion, namely the number of individuals who develop the disorder divided by the number studied. In cohort studies, risks are calculated separately for those exposed and those who are unexposed to the factor under study. The relative risk is derived from this.

Table 10.3 describes the situation in a cohort study when two groups (exposed and not exposed) are followed to determine the number who develop a disorder over a fixed length of time. The risk of the disorder in those exposed is:

$$p_1 = a / (a + b)$$

and in the unexposed is:

$$p_2 = c/(c+d)$$

The risk ratio (RR) is simply calculated as the proportion of these two fractions:

$$RR = \frac{p_1}{p_2} = RR \frac{a/(a=b)}{c/(c=d)}$$

The odds and odds ratio

The odds ratio may be calculated in a cohort study in a similar fashion. The odds is simply the proportion calculated by dividing the number of the times the event happens by the number of times it does not happen, so from Table 10.3, the odds in the two groups are:

Odds of disorder in exposed $= a/b$

Odds of disorder in unexposed $= c/d$

The odds is an intuitively difficult concept to grasp, but has some mathematical advantages over risk. Risk is, by definition, a fraction with a value from between zero and one. The odds can take any value from zero to infinity, and this property makes it an easier parameter to manipulate. Another important feature of the odds is its relation to the risk. Provided the disorder under study is rare, the odds will closely approximate to the risk. In other words, if a is small in relation to b (i.e. many more people do not develop the disorder than do develop it), the odds will approximate to the risk. This is the basis of the so-called *rare disease assumption* which states that if a disease or disorder is sufficiently rare, the odds will approximate to the risk.

The next step is to calculate the odds ratio (OR), which is simply:

$$OR = (a/b)/(c/d)$$

which can be simplified algebraically to the 'cross products' of Table 10.3:

$$OR = ad/bc$$

A worked example

The following example is taken from a cohort study on the effects of unemployment on depression (Weich and Lewis, 1998). This was a prospective cohort study of 7726 individuals who were interviewed at baseline and 1 year later. Depression was measured on the General Health Questionnaire. The main analysis used individuals who were not depressed at baseline, and recorded depression at follow-up according to employment status at baseline (Table 10.4).

$$RR = 0.206/0.181 = 1.14$$

$$OR = 53 \times 3102/686 \times 204 = 1.17$$

Note that as the disorder (depression) is quite common, the risks and odds are slightly different, and the odds ratio is bigger than the risk ratio.

Odds ratios in the case–control study

So far, we have worked from the perspective of the cohort study, in defining the risks and odds of developing the disorder according to exposure status. However, if we were to turn the problem on its head, it would be possible to calculate the odds of *having the exposure according to disorder status*. Returning to Table 10.3 we see that:

Odds of exposure if a participant develops the disorder = a/c

Odds of exposure if a participant does not develop the disorder = b/d

Once again we can determine the odds ratio, which will be

$$OR = (a/c)/(b/d) = ad/bc$$

This value is identical to the odds ratio calculated previously for depression according to exposure status. In other words, the odds ratio is symmetrical—it is the same whichever way it is calculated, this mathematical property makes the odds ratio easier to manipulate than the risk ratio.

We can now consider the same example from the perspective of a case–control study, where individuals were identified not on the basis of their exposure status, but on the basis of whether or not they developed the disorder under study. In the unemployment and depression example, we would need to define cases as individuals with a recent onset of depression, and controls as individuals who were not depressed. Returning the data presented in Table 10.4, let us assume that we identified *all* the cases of depression, and selected an equal number of controls. The table would look something like Table 10.5.

Table 10.4 Risk and odds of depression according to employment status

	Depression		Total	Risk of depression	Odds of depression
	Yes	No			
Exposure					
Unemployed	53	204	257	0.206	0.260
Employed	686	3102	3788	0.181	0.221
Total	739	3306			
Odds of exposure to unemployment	0.077	0.066			

Table 10.5 Case–control study of depression and unemployment

Exposure	Depression Yes (cases)	Depression No (controls)	Total	Risk of depression	Odds of depression
Unemployed	53	46	99	NA	NA
Employed	686	693	1379	NA	NA
Total	739	739			
Odds of exposure to unemployment	0.077	0.066			

The cells for the cases are identical to those in Table 10.4, but for the controls we have attempted to keep the odds of exposure to unemployment as close to the value in Table 10.4 as possible (in order to get it identical we would have had to give fractions of people). Note now that we are unable to calculate the risk of depression in the two exposure groups. Because of the case–control design, we have no denominator data with which to calculate the risk or odds of depression according to exposure status. However, what we are still able to do is calculate the odds of exposure according to disorder status, and we are therefore able to calculate the odds ratio:

Odds ratio = odds of exposure in cases/odds of exposure in controls = 0.077/ 0.066 = 1.17

We can see that this is identical to the odds ratio calculated from the cohort study data. Any differences here would arise from the approximation used to avoid having fractions of people in the table.

Steps to take in conducting a case–control study

Define a problem

Unlike cohort studies, which can give estimates of the incidence of a disorder, and cross-sectional studies, which can give estimates of the prevalence of a disorder, the sole purpose of case–control studies is to explore relationships between exposures and outcomes. Schlesselman (1982) distinguished the exploratory from the analytic case–control studies. In an *exploratory* study, the starting point is often a new problem—for example, a clustering of new cases of a disease—and the investigators seek to identify the cause from a wide range of candidate exposures. Because the disorder may be new (or described in a novel group), too little may be known to narrow the search for exposures, so a wide range of possibilities is explored. The problem with this unfocused approach is that if a high number of possible associations are explored, there is a strong chance that some will turn out 'positive' by chance (so-called type 1 error). A probability of 0.05 indicates a chance of 1 in 20 of obtaining that finding by chance. Therefore, exploratory studies should usually be followed by analytic studies, where the list of candidate exposures is reduced to allow fewer hypotheses to be tested.

Identifying cases

1. Definition of cases

As full a definition of cases as possible should be included in the protocol. In psychiatry, this will usually be based on operational criteria using International Statistical Classification of Diseases and Related Health Problems (ICD), or *Diagnostic and Statistical Manual of Mental Disorders (DSM)* systems. However, such systems are not necessarily the most appropriate means of defining cases: for example, if one was studying common mental disorders in their broadest sense, it would be valid to use a predetermined level of severity on a psychiatric questionnaire or interview, and compare those who fell above and below the cut-off. Similarly, one might want to describe risk factors across entire groups of disorders such as psychotic illness or somatoform disorders. If psychiatric symptom screens are used, it is important that the screening method has been validated for the population of interest.

2. Source of cases

The source of cases should be defined. The key decision is usually whether cases are to be recruited from known clinical samples, or whether they should come from the community. For example, cases of schizophrenia could be identified from mental health services. A clinical service would be used, and all individuals with schizophrenia within that service would be identified. This is usually a much easier and cheaper approach than defining a community or catchment area, and trying to identify all cases of schizophrenia within that area.

An important consideration is whether cases identified from healthcare settings are *representative* of the broader population of individuals with the disorder, or whether they are a selected group. How much this matters depends on the disorder under study and the nature of the healthcare system: when dealing with psychosis in a high-income country, a high proportion of those with psychosis in the population will have been admitted to hospital or been under the care of a community mental health team at some time in their illness. Thus, identifying service users from specialist mental health services will probably lead to a reasonably representative sample of the population of people with psychosis being identified (Boeing et al., 2007). In contrast, the vast majority of those with depression or anxiety never reach mental healthcare services, and therefore samples from these services are likely to be highly unusual and not very representative. People who reach specialized mental healthcare are likely to have more severe illness, greater comorbidity, more treatment failures, and so on.

In low- and middle-income countries, where psychiatric services are scarce, many individuals with psychosis may never be treated in specialist mental health services, and those who are may be an unusual group. For example, they may have wealthy relatives who can afford psychiatric care, or they may have displayed more severely disturbed behaviours which have led them to come to the attention of services. If there are specific risk factors which predict whether an individual with the disorder under study is referred to the setting where recruitment takes place, this can cause selection bias. In this case, we would not necessarily be testing whether the exposures are associated with the disorder, but whether they are associated with psychiatric admission.

A further consideration is the ease of recruiting from a wider community. It is difficult to screen communities to identify patients with psychosis—unless one is prepared to administer lengthy and costly psychiatric interviews to very large numbers of individuals. In close-knit communities, for example, in rural areas, it may be possible to use key informants to identify individuals with psychotic illness, but this approach is likely to be much less feasible in big cities.

3. Prevalent or incident cases?

Most illnesses have a number of potential outcomes: patients may get better, they may have fluctuating symptoms, they may remain chronically ill, or they may die. For example, many patients with depression recover, at least in the short term. Some go on with a chronic illness, some die from suicide or other causes, and some many have a relapsing and remitting course. It is usually most convenient to select cases from a population who are *currently* unwell. However, the problem with this is that those who are currently unwell are also more likely to have chronic illness, as opposed to those who recover or those who fluctuate. The sample of selected cases may therefore no longer be representative of the wider population of individuals with the disorder. The study may thus end up finding risk factors for *chronicity* of the condition, instead of its cause. This is sometimes referred to as prevalence bias. A way around this problem is to use only new or *incident* cases of the disorder.

This approach may not always be practical, especially in psychiatric epidemiology. Many psychiatric disorders have an insidious onset, and run a relapsing and remitting course. Depression may have gone unrecognized for some months or even years before it is detected. 'Incident' cases of depression identified from a general practice or psychiatric outpatient clinic may therefore be no such thing, but instead represent individuals who have had several previous episodes of depression which went undetected. Nonetheless, it is useful to consider how prevalence bias may affect the results reported.

Defining the controls

Defining the controls is one of the most difficult problems in designing case–control studies. The best way to define the control group is to ask: 'If this individual (whom I have called a control) were to get the condition under study, would he/she been included as a case?' If the answer to this question is 'No' then the control group is invalid. Thus if a list of exclusion criteria is used for the cases, the same list should be applied to the controls.

Box 10.1 Some sources of controls in case–control studies

Hospital (or clinic) controls: individuals with other disorders presenting to the same hospital or community mental health service as the cases.

Primary care: in UK and some other health services, a high proportion of the population are enrolled with a general practitioner. It is often possible to identify controls who attend the same general practitioner as the case, even if the case is identified from specialized mental health services.

Electoral or other population registers: electoral registers provide a sampling frame of adults. This method may underestimate certain groups (e.g. young, mobile individuals, or those who are disaffected and disinclined to vote).

Dead controls: for suicide research it may be reasonable to select controls who have died by other means.

Random digit dialling: if cases all have telephones in their homes, another method is to contact controls by random dialling of telephone numbers with the same area codes.

---

1. Source of controls

This depends largely on how the cases were defined. If they are a population-based sample of all new cases with the disease over a 1-year period, then it would make sense to draw controls directly from the same population. If cases came from clinical samples gathered from a general hospital serving a defined area, it would be reasonable to pick controls living in the same area who would also be likely to be treated in the same hospital were they to get ill. However, if cases were gathered from a highly specialized hospital, which attracts referrals from all over the country, the population of controls is much less easy to define. There may also be all sorts of factors independent of the disease which lead to patients being referred to a specialist units, including socioeconomic status. This introduces the possibility of *selection bias* (see 'Selection bias'). Some approaches to the selection of controls are shown in Box 10.1.

2. Matching

Matching is a method of avoiding confounding (see later in this section for a definition of confounding, which is dealt with in Chapters 15 and 16 on inference and covered later in this chapter). In a case–control study, it is desirable to have cases and controls who differ only in terms of disease status, therefore matching is one way to ensure that cases and controls are of similar age, gender, ethnic group, and so on. Although matching is intuitively appealing, it may cause a number of problems including:

Logistical difficulties
Potential controls may be lost in order to find one which matches the cases. If cases and controls are to be matched on several variables (age, gender, social class, ethnic group),

Box 10.2 Mechanisms for avoiding confounding in case–control studies

Design

Restriction: individuals with the confounder are excluded from the study. For example, a case–control study of anorexia nervosa might exclude male patients, as this is an unusual subgroup, and gender could be an important potential confounder.

Matching: controls are matched to cases on several key potential confounding variables—for example, gender, age group, or setting from which they are recruited.

Sampling: rather than individually match, controls may be selected such that they are broadly similar to cases as a group. If 30% of cases are male, the controls can be selected to ensure that 30% of controls are male.

Analysis

Stratification: the analysis is effectively done separately according to the presence or absence of the confounder, and a summary odds ratio taking this into account may be calculated.

Logistic regression analysis: the odds of being a case or control are modelled according to the presence of a number of exposure variables simultaneously. This allows for independent effects of the exposure to be estimated, corrected for the presence of confounders.

one may have to exclude many potential controls because they do not exactly match the case.

Problems in the analysis of data

Matched designs require matched analyses, which are somewhat more complex and less easy to follow than unmatched analyses.

Modern statistical techniques or alternative methods of controlling confounding in the design of studies may be more suitable methods to avoid confounding. Box 10.2 describes some approaches to manage confounding in the design and analysis stages of case–control studies. One approach in the design is to sample the controls in such a way that they are broadly similar to the cases on certain key variables such as gender and age.

3. How many control groups should be used?

An investigator may want to test the hypothesis that childhood sexual abuse is a risk factor for bulimia nervosa. He or she could either use healthy controls, or controls with different psychiatric diagnoses. The choice of control group changes the question being asked. If cases with bulimia nervosa had much more reported sexual abuse than healthy controls, the conclusion might be that sexual abuse causes bulimia. However, if an

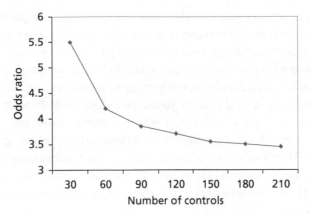

Figure 10.1 The relationship between the number of controls and the odds ratio which may be detected at 80% power and 95% confidence for an exposure with 20% prevalence.

additional control group with depression was included, and they were found to have the *same* frequency of childhood sexual abuse, it could be argued that abuse was a general risk factor for psychiatric morbidity, and was not *specifically* associated with either.

4. How many controls per case?

Imagine that a disorder was so rare it was only possible to recruit 30 patients. One way to increase statistical power in this situation would be to have more controls than cases. Figure 10.1 demonstrates that by having more than one control per case, it is possible to increase statistical power. With one control per case (i.e. 30 in each group), and assuming that the exposure was present in 20% of the control population, the study would only have sufficient power to detect a very big odds ratio of 5.5. In designing studies, one wants to have sufficient power to detect a much smaller effect. By doubling the number of controls to 60 the odds ratio falls to 4.2 and by having four controls per case it falls to 3.7. However, after this there is a law of diminishing returns and having 210 controls (i.e. 7:1) allows an odds ratio of 3.45 to be detected.

Selection bias

The main point of much of the previous discussion on the definition of cases and controls is to avoid selection bias. This is the most challenging aspect of designing a case–control study. Selection bias occurs when the exposure status of cases or controls influences the likelihood that they are entered into a study. In addressing selection bias it is worth considering all the factors which lead to a case or control being enrolled into the study.

An example of the importance of selecting cases can be illustrated by socioeconomic patterns of autism spectrum disorder (ASD) observed in the US. Initial observations by Kanner (1943) indicated that children of families of higher socioeconomic status were more likely to have ASD. Subsequent case–control studies and other types of studies consistently supported such patterns. However the cases were typically identified from healthcare records, while controls were often sampled from the community. Since healthcare access requires insurance in the US, critics argued that children with ASD from higher socioeconomic groups were more likely recruited into the study, creating a bias in case ascertainment. That is, the exposure—high socioeconomic status—influenced the chances of becoming a case in the study. A recent study put this hypothesis to the test using a nested case–control study within a population cohort of children in Stockholm, Sweden, where healthcare coverage is universal (Rai et al., 2012). In contrast to the US findings, a reverse socioeconomic gradient was observed where children from lower socioeconomic status families were at greater risk of ASD diagnoses, suggesting that case ascertainment bias played a role in the US studies. This illustrates the importance of considering the healthcare context and its potential impact on findings.

Another example arises when new syndromes are identified by enthusiastic clinicians. In the 1980s, there was growing interest in fatigue syndromes which were considered to have been caused by viruses (Wessely et al., 1998). A number of papers suggested that individuals with such fatigue syndromes had more antibodies to certain viruses in their blood than healthy controls. However, many of the studies were performed by physicians or virologists who recruited patients referred to their clinics. But these patients were often referred because general practitioners had noticed they had raised viral antibodies, and wanted a virological opinion. Thus the exposure (prior viral infection) and the outcome (chronic fatigue) were not independent in the way cases were selected. These problems could have been resolved by identifying cases of chronic fatigue syndrome from primary care and comparing with controls from within the same setting—the process of referral often involves subtle processes which can lead to selection bias.

Selection biases are important no matter what exposure is being measured. It is often assumed in psychiatric genetics, for example, that genes are unlikely to impact one's likelihood of participating in a study. However, the polygenic risk score of schizophrenia has a powerful impact on likelihood of participation (Martin et al., 2016). This might imply, for example, that in case–control studies of psychosis, controls with a strong genetic predisposition to the disorder are selected out, whereas cases, in touch with services, are included, the implication being that genetic risk for the disorder may be overestimated.

Estimating exposure status

Once cases and controls have been defined, the task is to estimate their exposure to the risk factor under study. This may be done by giving the participants (or their relatives) questionnaires, using historical records, taking blood, or measuring other biological markers. The main aim is to avoid *information bias*.

The procedure by which cases and controls are approached and interviewed should be as similar as possible. They should receive the same interview schedule and the same questions. If an informant, such as a relative, is used to elicit information about cases, an informant should also be used for controls.

Recall bias

There are two important forms of information bias which are pertinent to case–control studies. The first is *recall bias*. This occurs when the experience of having a disease in itself affects the process of recalling prior exposures. An obvious example is in dementia: patients with dementia have global cognitive deficits, including memory problems, therefore they are unlikely to be able to recall prior events. If the question under study was whether prior head injury causes dementia, asking sufferers from dementia would clearly cause problems, as they may well have forgotten past events. One would instead have to use contemporaneous records (e.g. hospital notes) or ask an informant who knew the individual well.

A more common problem is that the illness being studied *increases* the recall of prior exposure. Most individuals when they get ill may want to make sense of their suffering and think of many different prior events which could be implicated. This *effort after meaning* may mean that when asked about prior events they put more effort into recall than someone without the illness. For example, the parent of a patient with schizophrenia may spend considerably more effort recalling past exposures such as obstetric complications than the parent of a healthy individual. This also is a potential problem for life events research, where individuals with existing depression are asked to recall life events over the previous 6 or 12 months, and events are contextualized in order to determine the severity of their impact. Individuals with depression often have distortions in their thought processes which may lead them to preferentially recall negative events.

Recall bias may be reduced by:

- using alternative sources of information which do not depend upon the memory of participants (e.g. previous hospital records)
- disguising the hypothesis from the subject by nesting questions related to the exposure of interest in an interview which covers other aspects of lifestyle
- using controls who have another disorder. This may change the nature of the question being asked, because many risk factors in psychiatry are not specifically related to individual diagnoses, but increase the risk of a wide variety of psychiatric disorder.

Observer bias

The second form of information bias is observer bias. This occurs when the interviewer's knowledge of the participant's disease status affects the way he or she asks them questions. This could either be conscious cheating on the part of the interviewer, but more commonly a subtle process by which the interviewer is more diligent when asking cases than controls.

Observer bias may be overcome by the following techniques:

- 'Blinding' the interviewer to the hypothesis under study, by nesting key questions about the exposure in a more extensive interview about other aspects of lifestyle.
- 'Blinding' the interviewer to the disease status of participants. This may be very difficult to achieve in psychiatric epidemiology.

- Using highly structured interviews which force the interviewer to ask each participant the same question in an identical manner.

- Using questionnaires or computerized interviews which the participants complete themselves.

Examples of case–control designs in psychiatric epidemiology

The following section describes a number of recent, well-conducted case–control studies in psychiatry.

Case–control studies nested in cross-sectional studies

We have already seen that selection bias is a major problem for case–control studies. One way around this is to perform a case–control study within an existing cross-sectional study. Cross-sectional studies aim to identify all cases of a disorder within a study sample representative of a given population—they therefore provide a ready-made sampling frame for the case–control study. While cross-sectional studies are often able to assess risk factors, when a detailed ascertainment of risk factors is required, it is usually unnecessary to apply this to all participants in the cross-sectional study. Instead, a nested case–control study can be performed. An example of this is a study of life events in elderly individuals with depression (Brilman and Ormel, 2001). Cases of depression were identified in a cross-sectional study. Controls were selected randomly from non-depressed participants in the same study. Cases and controls were then given a detailed interview (the Life Events and Difficulties Schedule (LEDS; Brown and Harris, 1978)). The main rationale for this approach is that the LEDS is a long interview, and it would have been wasteful to have administered it to the entire population studied in the cross-sectional study. The use of a population-based sampling frame radically reduced the possibility of selection bias in the case–control study.

Case–control studies nested within cohort studies

Nested case–control studies are usually considered to be sub-studies of larger cohort studies, where information on specific exposures may be expensive to obtain. For example, one might be interested in the relationship between conjugal loss and depression, and perform a cohort study to compare rates of depression in individuals who recently lost a spouse, compared to those who were still married. After describing the key associations in the cohort study, there might be data which were thought relevant and important, but expensive to collect for the entire cohort. For example, one might decide that a key risk factor for bereavement outcome was the quality of the relationship, and devise an interview for participants to complete. This approach might be prohibitively expensive to do on the entire cohort, and one might instead select all those who develop depression (the cases) and compare them with a proportion of randomly selected individuals who did not develop depression (the controls). This would change the design to a *nested* case–control study, as the selection of participants now would depend on their mental health status.

In the section on risk and odds, the relationship between cohort studies and case–control studies was explored. Rothman (2012) has argued that all case–control studies can be thought of as being 'nested' within either real or theoretical cohort studies. A good example is a case–control study that assessed the school performance cases with schizophrenia and controls without schizophrenia (Cannon et al., 1999). The authors set out to test the hypothesis that individuals with schizophrenia have difficulties in childhood (which might reflect problems in neurodevelopment) which manifest as poorer school performance. The study was 'nested' within a birth cohort—namely all individuals born in Helsinki, Finland, between 1951 and 1960. This was in effect a 'virtual' cohort—it existed as a theoretical entity, but no one had previously collected data from all its members. This nesting, however, allowed the researchers to define a population base to recruit into the case–control study. Cases were identified from national databases which allowed all known cases of schizophrenia to be identified. The researchers linked these records with child health cards in Helsinki, which determined whether they had been educated in that city. Controls were identified as the next individual to appear on the child health cards, who was also born in Helsinki between 1951 and 1960 and who did not grow up to develop schizophrenia. Cases and controls were then compared according to school performance by going back to school records. The main result was that while academic performance and behaviour at school were no different in the children who developed schizophrenia and those who did not, individuals who developed schizophrenia had poorer performance on other non-academic activities.

The psychological autopsy study

Suicide is an especially difficult area to study. It is a rare outcome, whose definition may vary over time, and between countries, according to legal and cultural factors. Obviously, once suicide has happened the 'participant' is by definition dead. Case–control studies of suicide have therefore tended to use the 'psychological autopsy' approach, where a detailed interview is administered to a relative of the suicide victim. This presents difficulties for ascertaining the same information in the controls—if living controls are used, it is necessary to use the same technique. Information bias would result from any approach where the information was being gathered differently on controls as opposed to cases—hence there is a need to ensure that information on controls is gathered by asking an informant rather than directly asking the living control. An example is a study from New Zealand (Milner et al., 2014) which used this method to compare the impact of involuntary job loss on suicide and suicide attempts with a control population drawn from the general population. Suicides were defined from routine death registrations. Suicide attempt cases were identified from local hospitals. Relatives and friends of the two groups of cases and controls were asked to provide information on job dismissal or redundancy of the participants in the previous 12 months. This approach is probably the closest one can get to an unbiased estimate of risk factors in suicide; however, there are still major problems with potential recall bias. Suicide is frequently associated with powerful feelings of guilt in the relatives of the victim, and such feelings may act to emphasize or de-emphasize risk factors.

Genome-wide association studies (GWASs)

In psychiatric genomics, case–control designs are widely used for GWASs. Psychiatric genomics involves characterizing the genetic architecture that is associated with the risk of psychiatric disorders. This had been an area of emerging importance as results from such studies could not only uncover clues to the aetiology of disorders, but also drive advances in treatments, and accurately identify persons at risk. Adopting this genome-wide approach by searching wide sets of genetic variants has revealed that a large number of contributing genetic loci contribute to the heritability of psychiatric disorders. This is an advance from previous genetic research using a 'candidate gene' approach, which produced unreliable and inconsistent findings (Gratten et al., 2014).

A typical case–control GWAS involves measuring genetic variations in single nucleotide polymorphisms (SNPs) in large samples of cases with the psychiatric disorder and in many thousands of healthy controls. The aim is to identify individual genetic loci associated with the disorder by comparing SNPs present in individuals with and without the disorder.

In a case–control study, a GWAS identified 108 genetic loci associated with schizophrenia (Schizophrenia Working Group of the Psychiatric Genomics Consortium et al., 2014). By combining data from multiple study sites, the investigators overcame previous sample size limitations due to the rarity of the disorder, to produce the largest GWAS of schizophrenia to date comprising 36,989 cases and 113,075 healthy controls. In addition to identifying specific SNPs associated with schizophrenia, the investigators produced polygenic risk scores—weighted summary scores of associated SNP alleles. These scores were then tested as exposure variables in independent samples hypothesizing that the higher scores would be associated with cases. The results indicated that the polygenic risk scores could distinguish cases from controls with accuracy levels above chance, although not sufficiently well to be used as predictive tools yet. As such, this multistage study performed both the *exploratory* and *analytic* case–control analyses identified by Schlesselman (1982), illustrating the utility of this study approach.

The case-crossover design

Case-crossover studies are a particular type of case–control design used to investigate exposures with relatively short-latency effects and outcomes with a clearly defined time of onset. Instead of characterizing a group of people as cases, and comparing them to another group of individuals defined as controls, the case-crossover study takes a single group of individuals who have experienced an outcome and compares their exposure status between 'case' and 'control' time periods. If an exposure has a short-term effect on an outcome then it should be present at a higher frequency in the time period just before the outcome occurs than in a time period further back.

It is perhaps easiest to illustrate this with an example. In a study by Wu and colleagues (2015), the authors wanted to investigate possible short-term effects of antipsychotic exposure on risk of acute myocardial infarction. Clearly the potential longer-term adverse effects of these agents (e.g. obesity, insulin resistance, and diabetes risk) are well recognized and can be investigated using a traditional cohort study design or as a secondary outcome in a randomized controlled trial. However, there are also potentially important 'acute' effects such as QT interval prolongation and ventricular arrhythmias (change in heart rhythm) which might occur in certain people shortly after starting an antipsychotic and are less easily investigated in a cohort study (because of the logistical challenges of recruiting people at the point of medication initiation in sufficient numbers to detect this rare outcome). The approach taken by Wu and colleagues was to use a large national healthcare database to ascertain all people with a diagnosis of schizophrenia or bipolar disorder who had experienced an acute myocardial infarction (heart attack). The date of this event was classified as the 'index date'. In primary analyses, antipsychotic use was ascertained in two time periods: (1) the 'case' period of 1–60 days prior to the index date, and (2) the 'control' period of 61–120 days prior to the index date. If antipsychotic agents have a short-term risk effect on acute myocardial infarction then this exposure should be present more often in the case than the control period, and this hypothesized association was indeed demonstrated in the analysis reported.

A key feature of the case-crossover design is that each person acts as their own control (with the individual being the matching variable and the time periods being the cases and controls). This means that differences between individuals cannot act as confounding factors and can therefore be ignored as alternative explanations for an observed association—a very important feature not dissimilar to the advantage conferred by randomization in a trial. The important confounding factors that *do* need consideration are other features which might vary between time periods. For example, Wu and colleagues adjusted analyses for changes in healthcare contacts and other medications, although were still left with some uncertainty as to whether it was the initiation of an antipsychotic which was the risk factor for acute myocardial infarction or a deterioration in the mental disorder being treated. Nonetheless, the design is potentially powerful in terms of inferring causality and is widely used in other fields of health research. The drawback for psychiatric epidemiology is that it does depend on being able to define discrete events and short-term risk effects, whereas many of our outcomes of interest involve gradually developing (and/or fluctuating) conditions with risk factors that accumulate over a life course. As well as adverse effects of medication, short-term precipitants of suicide attempt/completion are an obvious potential area for applying a case–control approach, and exposures recently investigated have included selective serotonin reuptake inhibitor initiation, acute air pollution, bereavement, and substance use (Björkenstam et al., 2013; Bakian et al., 2015; Morgensen et al., 2016; Bagge and Borges, 2017). The analysis is essentially the same as that of a traditional matched case–control study.

Analysis and reporting of case–control studies

The Strengthening the Reporting of Observational Studies in Epidemiology (STROBE) recommendations are a useful set of guidelines for researchers to use when reporting the results from observational studies such as case–control studies (von Elm et al., 2014). These are summarized in checklists that specify standard methods of reporting results, and are particularly helpful in critical appraisals of observational research. The steps outlined as follows include key features of the STROBE checklist for case–control studies.

Once the data have been collected on cases and controls, they are entered into a statistical software package and analysed. The first step should be a description of the population from which cases and controls came, how many potential cases and controls were excluded, and how many refused to participate. In practice, these simple but important data are rarely presented (Lee et al., 2007). This gives the reader a view of the representativeness of the sample. Key features of the cases should be described: for example, how long had they been ill? How many were in-patients? What was the severity of their illness?

The next step should be a comparison of the main sociodemographic characteristics of cases and controls. The reader should be able to see any major differences in terms of their age, gender, social class, occupational group, and so on. There are two main reasons for this. It may be that these sociodemographic variables are to be studied as risk factors in their own right. Alternatively, the study may aim to examine other risk factors, and it is important to know whether any relationships could be due to confounding by these sociodemographic variables.

Statistical tests are frequently reported to demonstrate that differences between cases and controls are 'non-significant'. However, it should be emphasized that when statistically non-significant differences are found between cases and controls, the variables involved can still act as a confounder. It is more important to look for the *size of the difference* between the two groups.

The relationship between exposure and outcome: the odds ratio and 95% confidence interval

Subsequent tables should show how the exposures of interest may be distributed throughout cases and controls. The odds ratio is the basic measure of relative risk in the case–control study, and has been described in detail earlier in this chapter. Ideally, odds ratios should be presented with their 95% confidence intervals. This gives an indication of the precision of any effect size determined. Returning to Table 10.5, we can calculate the confidence interval for the odds ratio as follows. First the standard error (SE) is calculated:

$$SE = \sqrt{\left(\frac{1}{a} + \frac{1}{b} + \frac{1}{c} + \frac{1}{d}\right)}$$

This is then multiplied by 1.96 (to get 95% confidence).

And then exponentiate this term to get an error term (ET):

$$ET = e^{1.96SE}$$

The 95% confidence intervals are derived by multiplying and dividing the odds ratio by the error term. From the example shown in Table 10.5 the standard error is:

$$SE = \sqrt{\frac{1}{53} + \frac{1}{46} + \frac{1}{686} + \frac{1}{693}} = 0.209$$

$$ET = e^{1.96 \times 0.209} = 1.51$$

The odds ratio was 1.17 so the upper boundary of the 95% confidence intervals is:

$$1.17 \times 1.51 = 1.77$$

and the lower boundary of the 95% confidence interval is:

$$1.17/1.51 = 0.77$$

This gives us an odds ratio of 1.17 with a 95% confidence interval of 0.77–1.77. This indicates that we can be 95% confident that the true odds ratio lies somewhere between 0.77 and 1.77. As the null value for the odds ratio is 1 (i.e. an odds ratio of 1 indicates no difference) and these 95% confidence intervals include 1, we can infer that the relationship is not statistically significant at $p < 0.05$. More importantly, these confidence intervals would indicate the degree of precision of this estimate. Note that the standard error is heavily influenced by the cell sizes of the study; with one or two very small cell sizes, the standard error will be large, and the 95% confidence will be wide, even if the case–control study has been huge.

More than one level of exposure

Many exposures have more than one level of severity. For example, individuals may have experienced no life events, one life event, two events, or more than three events. This may be handled by making a table like Table 10.6.

Table 10.6 More than one level of exposure

Sample	Cases	Controls
No life events	a	b
One event	c	d
Two events	e	f
Three or more events	g	h

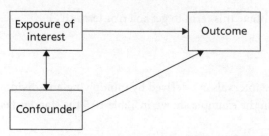

Figure 10.2 Illustration of the mechanism of confounding. The confounder causes the outcome under study, and is also associated with the exposure of interest. Thus the confounder can confuse the investigator into believing that the exposure is causal.

The odds ratio for each level of exposure may be calculated on its own *using 'no life events' as the reference*:

- for those with three or more events it would be: *ah/bg*
- for those with one event it would be a*d/bc*.

The 95% confidence intervals are calculated by pretending that there are a series of 2×2 tables for each exposure compared with the no life event group.

Controlling for confounding

The main issue in the analysis of case–control studies is to control for potential confounders. Confounders are defined as variables which are causally related to the *outcome*, and are associated with the exposure of interest, but are not simply on a causal pathway between exposure and outcome (Figure 10.2).

Stratification

Here the 2×2 table shown earlier is broken down (or *stratified*) according to the presence or absence of the confounder. If controlling for gender, there would be a 2×2 table for men and another for women. The odds ratios for each could then be compared, and using classic Mantel–Haenszel techniques a combined odds ratio controlled for gender may be derived.

Modelling

Logistic regression techniques model the odds of being a case according the presence of one or more additional variables simultaneously. The computer derives an odds ratio for each of these variables. Logistic regression may be used to control for multiple confounders simultaneously.

The analysis of the matched case–control study

These comments on the analysis of case–control studies have focused on unmatched designs. When cases and controls have been matched, different statistical methods are required. A detailed discussion of such techniques is outside the scope of this chapter. The main difference is that all statistical tests should take into account the matching, so instead of performing independent *t*-tests, paired *t*-tests should be used, and instead of using the chi-squared test, the McNemar test is used. For modelling in matched case–control studies, conditional logistic regression, which takes into account the clustered nature of each matched pair, should be used.

Interpretation of case–control studies

Once the analysis has been performed, the results are interpreted. As always in epidemiological studies, five possible explanations for an association exist:

- reverse causality
- bias
- confounding
- chance
- causality.

The roles of bias and confounding have been explored in this chapter and elsewhere in some detail. However, it is worth considering how reverse causality and chance may be especially relevant in case–control studies.

Reverse causation

Case–control studies are usually unable to rule out this possibility, since by definition the illness has already occurred when the cases are recruited. Thus it is always possible that the illness led to the exposure and not vice versa. This is especially true in social psychiatry, where exposures such as unemployment and life events may arise directly from the effects of the illness on behaviour. This is less of a concern if previous records can be used in order to ascertain the exposure. In the literature on schizophrenia and obstetric complications, for example, it has been possible to determine the presence of obstetric complications from hospital records, which were recorded long before the individual developed the illness.

Chance

Statistical testing and the use of confidence intervals are the techniques most widely used to deal with chance in studies. One advantage of case–control studies is that they can assess the role of *multiple* exposures simultaneously. If the level of significance is set at 95%, this means that a *p*-value of 0.05 or less may be detected 1 time in 20 *just by chance*. If the investigators have assessed the role of 40 exposures, one would expect that 2 of these would come up as having an association *by chance alone*. This is one reason why it is important for findings in exploratory case–control studies to be replicated in subsequent more rigorous analytic studies.

Conclusion

The case–control study, if well conducted, is able to give unbiased estimates of effect sizes between exposures and outcomes. They are a particularly efficient design—and this efficiency makes them a more viable approach in the study of rare disorders than cohort studies.

Practical exercises

This practical involves using two examples of case–control studies, and discussing some of the advantages and disadvantages of the approaches used in these papers.

Questions

Paper 1: Yousef et al. (1988)

This paper describes a case–control study assessing the relationship between chronic enterovirus infection and a fatigue syndrome. Consider the following questions:

1. How were the cases identified and selected? Is there adequate information?

2. How were the controls selected? Are there any possible problems with this method?

3. Was this a matched case–control study? If so, was a matched analysis performed?

4. Were confounding variables considered?

5. What alternative explanations might there be for the reported association?

6. What improvements could be made to the design which would address these concerns?

Paper 2: Dalman et al. (2001)

This is a population based case–control study assessing the relationship between obstetric complications and schizophrenia.

1. Describe the main advantages of the design chosen. What particular features of the design make this a good study?

2. What was the main problem with their use of obstetric records?

3. How could observer bias be minimized in this study?

Answers

Paper 1

1. There is no information on the selection of cases for this study. The authors worked in a general hospital, and it is possible that some of the patients had been referred to see a virologist. This leads to selection bias, because the exposure under study is a virus—it is likely that individuals suffering from fatigue were preferentially selected into the study because of their history of viral illness.

2. Controls were nominated by cases. This is an unsatisfactory approach to selection of controls because it is likely that exposure status (viral illness) also plays a role in determining whether the control is selected. If the cases were aware of the question under

study, it is possible that they were *less likely* to select controls who had a recent history of viral illnesses.

3. It was a matched design, but the analysis appears to have been unmatched. Note that there was a major imbalance between the numbers of cases and controls, which is curious in a matched case–control study—usually one would expect the same number of controls as cases, or that the number of controls would be a multiple of the number of cases.

4. No confounding variables were considered.

5. The most likely explanation for the association is selection bias, caused by the method of selection of cases.

6. The use of a population-based case–control design would have been preferable, in which cases could have been identified from general practice, or cross-sectional surveys. Alternatively, this question may be better addressed using a cohort design.

Paper 2

1. This paper had a number of strengths: the investigators used a population-based design, which minimized the chances of selection bias. They used obstetric records, which removes the possibility of recall bias. The study was large, so it had adequate statistical power to address the main questions under study, and the authors used both matching and conditional logistic regression in order to control for confounders.

2. The main problem with the use of obstetric records was that many of the records did not contain an Apgar score (which is a method of recording asphyxia at birth). They therefore had to rely on entries into the notes about the various items of the Apgar score (heart rate, breathing, colour, tone, and the excitability of the infant). This introduces the possibility of misclassification (i.e. some of the infants who might have had a low Apgar score, might have been categorized as healthy, and vice versa). Another possibility is observer bias—as the information gathering depended to some extent on the researcher's judgement, the researcher may have been more thorough when assessing the notes of the cases (who later developed schizophrenia) compared with the controls.

3. Observer bias could be avoided (and in this paper was avoided) by asking midwives to rate the notes without any knowledge of the case–control status of individuals in the study.

Further reading

Lee, W., Bindman, J., Ford, T., Glozier, N., Moran, P., Stewart, R., and Hotopf, M. (2007). Bias in psychiatric case-control studies. *British Journal of Psychiatry*, 190, 204–209.

Lewis, G. and Pelosi, A.J. (1990). The case-control study in psychiatry. *British Journal of Psychiatry*, 157, 197–207.

Rothman, K.J. (2012). *Epidemiology: an introduction*, 2nd edn. New York: Oxford University Press.

Schlesselman, J.J. (1982). *Case-control studies*. New York: Oxford University Press.

References

Bagge, C.L. and Borges, G. (2017). Acute substance use as a warning sign for suicide attempts: a case-crossover examination of the 48 hours prior to a recent suicide attempt. *Journal of Clinical Psychiatry*, **78**, 691–696.

Bakian, A.V., Huber, R.S., Coon, H., Gray, D., Wilson, P., McMahon, W.M., and Renshaw, P.F. (2015). Acute air pollution exposure and risk of suicide completion. *American Journal of Epidemiology*, **181**, 295–303.

Björkenstam, C., Möller, J., Ringbäck, G., Salmi, P., Hallqvist, J., and Ljung, R. (2013). An association between initiation of selective serotonin reuptake inhibitors and suicide—a nationwide register-based case-crossover study. *PLoS One*, **8**, e73973.

Boeing, L., Murray, V., Pelosi, A., McCabe, R., Blackwood, D., and Wrate, R. (2007). Adolescent-onset psychosis: prevalence needs and service provision. *British Journal of Psychiatry*, **190**, 18–26.

Brilman, E.I. and Ormel, J. (2001). Life events, difficulties and onset of depressive episodes in later life. *Psychological Medicine*, **31**, 859–869.

Brown, G.W. and Harris, T.O. (1978). *Social origins of depression: a study of psychiatric disorder in women*. London: Tavistock Publications.

Cannon, M., Jones, P., Huttunen, M.O., Tanskanen, A., Huttumen, T., Rabe-Hesketh, S., and Murray, R.M. (1999). School performance in Finnish children and later development of schizophrenia: a population-based longitudinal study. *Archives of General Psychiatry*, **56**, 457–463.

Dalman, C., Thomas, H.V., David, A.S., Gentz, J., Lewis, G., and Allebeck, P. (2001). Signs of asphyxia at birth and risk of schizophrenia. Population based case-control study. *British Journal of Psychiatry*, **179**, 403–408.

Gratten, J., Wray, N.R., Keller, M.C., and Visscher, P.M. (2010). Large-scale genomics unveils the genetic architecture of psychiatric disorders. *Nature Neuroscience*, **17**, 782–790.

Kanner, L. (1943). Autistic disturbances of affective contact. *Nervous Child*, **2**, 217–250.

Lee, W., Bindman, J., Ford, T., Glozier, N., Moran, P., Stewart, R., and Hotopf, M. (2007). Bias in psychiatric case-control studies. *British Journal of Psychiatry*, **190**, 204–209.

Martin, J., Tilling, K., Hubbard, L., Stergiakouli, E., Thapar, A., Davey Smith, G., et al. (2016). Association of genetic risk for schizophrenia with nonparticipation over time in a population-based cohort study. *American Journal of Epidemiology*, **183**, 1149–1158.

Milner, A., Page, A., Morrell, S., Hobbs, C., Carter, G., Dudley, M., et al. (2014). The effects of involuntary job loss on suicide and suicide attempts among young adults: evidence from a matched case-control study. *Australian and New Zealand Journal of Psychiatry*, **48**, 333–340.

Morgensen, H., Möller, J., Hultin, H., and Mittendorfer-Rutz, E. (2016). Death of a close relative and the risk of suicide in Sweden: a large scale register-based case-crossover study. *PLoS One*, **11**, e0164274.

Rai, D., Lewi, G., Lundberg, M., Araya, R., Svensson, A., Dalman, C., et al. (2012). Parental socioeconomic status and risk of offspring autism spectrum disorders in a Swedish population-based study. *Journal of the American Academy of Child and Adolescent Psychiatry*, **51**, 467–476.

Rothman, K.J. (2012). *Epidemiology: an introduction*, 2nd edn. New York: Oxford University Press.

Schizophrenia Working Group of the Psychiatric Genomics Consortium, Ripke, S., Neale, B.M., Corvin, A., Walters, J.T.R., Farh, K.-H., et al. (2014). Biological insights from 108 schizophrenia-associated genetic loci. *Nature*, **511**, 421–427.

Schlesselman, J.J. (1982). *Case-control studies*. New York: Oxford University Press.

von Elm, E., Altman, D.G., Egger, M., Pocock, S.J., Gøtzsche, P.C., and Vandenbroucke, J.P. (2014). The strengthening the reporting of observational studies in epidemiology (STROBE). *International Journal of Surgery*, **12**, 1495–1459.

Weich, S. and Lewis, G. (1998). Poverty, unemployment, and common mental disorders: population based cohort study. *British Medical Journal*, 317, 115–119.

Wessely, S., Hotopf, M., and Sharpe, M. (1998). *Chronic fatigue and its syndromes*. Oxford: Oxford University Press.

Wu, S.-I., Chen, S.-C., Kao, K.-L., Juang, J.J.M., Lin, C.-J., Fang, C.-K., et al. (2015). Antipsychotic exposure prior to acute myocardial infarction in patients with serious mental illness. *Acta Psychiatrica Scandinavica*, 131, 213–222.

Yousef, G., Bell, E., Mann, G., Murgesan, V., Smith, D., McCartney, R., and Mowbray, J. (1988). Chronic enterovirus infection in patients with postviral fatigue syndrome. *Lancet*, 1, 146–150.

Chapter 11

Cohort studies

Laura Goodwin and Nicola Fear

Introduction

A cohort is defined as 'a group of people banded together or treated as a group'. A cohort study follows over time a group of participants who share a particular 'exposure' but are free of the outcome of interest at the time of 'exposure'. This 'exposed' cohort is compared with another group of participants who are deemed to be 'unexposed'. The exposed and unexposed cohorts are followed up over time to determine the presence or absence of the outcome(s) of interest. Data are often collected through questionnaires and interviews but can also be collected through medical assessments or the use of routinely collected data (e.g. hospital events and death certificates). Cohort studies require large numbers of participants and are best suited to common outcomes. Boxes 11.1 and 11.2 summarize the differences between cohort studies and case–control studies and randomized controlled trials (RCTs).

Historically, cohort studies were set up to look at chronic diseases (e.g. the Framingham Heart Study (https://www.framinghamheartstudy.org/)) but now include cohort studies which were primarily set up to explore mental health outcomes (e.g. the King's Military Cohort Study (Hotopf et al., 2006; Fear et al., 2010)).

The essential features of a cohort study are:

◆ participants are defined by their exposure (rather than outcome)

◆ exposure is ascertained before the outcome is known.

Types of cohort

There are different types of cohorts:

Birth cohort: this includes individuals born in a certain area and during a specific time period. An example is the National Survey of Health and Development (NSHD) which is the oldest of the British birth cohort studies (http://www.nshd.mrc.ac.uk/). It has collected data from birth on the health and social circumstances of a social class stratified sample ($N = 5362$) of all babies born in England, Scotland, and Wales between 3 and 9 March 1946. Birth cohorts can be highly informative about developmental trajectories and patterns of onset of psychiatric disorders—for example, the Dunedin Multidisciplinary

Box 11.1 How does a cohort study differ from a case–control study?

Case–control studies recruit participants based upon whether they have a particular illness, which means that they can ensure that the sample size of 'cases' is large enough. Even in extremely large cohort studies, there may not be the statistical power to study rare outcomes, or illnesses with long latency periods. In a case–control study, the data will normally be collected retrospectively, whereas many cohort studies can study the prospective effects of different exposures or risk factors from childhood or even conception. Cohort studies are widely used as a tool in social sciences (e.g. looking at education or occupational attainment), whereas case–control studies typically have a more limited focus.

Health and Development Study (New Zealand) has provided some of the best evidence available on peak onset of and risk factors for various disorders (Newman et al., 1996).

'Exposure' cohort: this includes individuals who have been exposed to the factor of interest, but does not necessarily include a comparison group. An example is the Nuclear Industry Family Study (UK) which was set up to investigate possible links between reproductive and child health and parents' exposure to ionizing radiation at work (Maconochie et al., 1999).

Other types of cohort studies include following individuals who have a shared factor, for example, geographical region or work place. An example is the Whitehall study which was established to investigate the social determinants of health, specifically the

Box 11.2 How does a cohort study differ from a randomized controlled trial?

A cohort study is much like an RCT except that the intervention in an RCT is investigator controlled, while the intervention in a cohort study is a naturally occurring phenomenon. There is more likely to be self-selection to an exposure in a cohort study, for example, smokers will generally have chosen to smoke. This means that the exposed and unexposed groups may not be comparable. However, it would not be ethical to randomize people to particular exposures, such as smoking or heavy drinking in pregnancy, which is why these associations cannot be studied in a RCT. It is normally possible to adjust for many of the potential confounders in a cohort study, if they are known confounders and if they have been measured. RCTs are more likely to be shorter term than a cohort study and are less likely to track individuals across the life course. It would also be difficult in a RCT to ensure that a particular treatment or exposure had occurred over a maintained period.

cardiovascular disease prevalence and mortality rates among British male civil servants between the ages of 20 and 64 years (http://www.ucl.ac.uk/whitehallII/). The initial study, the Whitehall I Study, examined over 18,000 male civil servants, and was conducted over a period of 10 years, beginning in 1967. A second study, the Whitehall II Study, examined the health of 10,308 civil servants aged 35 to 55 years, of whom two-thirds were men and one-third women, who were recruited from the British Civil Service in 1985.

Retrospective versus prospective cohort study

Retrospective (or historical) cohort studies

Retrospective cohort studies rely on records of exposure of individuals from the past. These records then allow individuals to be categorized as exposed or unexposed. The ability to do this depends on the quality of the records available. This may give rise to bias in the classification of exposure as these data were collected for other purposes and often the data can be incomplete or inaccurate. So why do these studies? The main advantage is reducing the time required between exposure and outcome, particularly if the outcome can take a long time to develop/emerge (e.g. cancer). These types of study are more commonly used to examine physical health rather than mental health outcomes. A recent example of a retrospective cohort is the study of British participants in the chemical tests at Porton Down (Carpenter et al., 2009; Venables et al., 2009) (see Example 11.1).

Example 11.1 Historical cohort study of UK military participants in the chemical tests at Porton Down

The Porton Down cohort was set up using historical records to study the long-term effects on mortality and cancer incidence among UK military participants in experimental research related to chemical warfare agents from 1941 to 1989. Archive data from Porton Down and UK military personnel records were linked with national death and cancer records, and 18,276 male members of the UK military personnel who had spent time at Porton Down and a comparison group of 17,600 non-Porton Down veterans were followed up to 31 December 2004. The mortality rate ratio of Porton Down compared with non-Porton Down veterans and the standardized mortality ratio of each veteran group were compared with the general population. Ratios were adjusted for age group and calendar period. All-cause mortality was slightly greater in Porton Down veterans. There was no clear relation between type of chemical exposure and cause-specific mortality. The mortality in both groups of veterans was lower than that in the general population. With a lack of information on factors, such as smoking or deployment, it is not possible to attribute the small excess in mortality to chemical exposures at Porton Down.

Example 11.2 The King's Centre for Military Health Research cohort study

The KCMHR cohort study was set up in 2003 to study the mental health effects of deployment to Iraq (the exposure). Cohort members were followed up in 2007–2009 and at this time many had been deployed again to either Iraq or Afghanistan. At the second wave, 68% of the wave 1 sample participated, and two new subsamples were also added to the sample to ensure that it was representative of the composition of the Armed Forces. Data from wave 2 did not show that individuals who had been deployed to either Iraq or Afghanistan were more likely to meet the criteria for post-traumatic stress disorder (PTSD). However, further analysis of the 'exposed' (deployed) sample showed that those who had been deployed in a combat role were more likely to report PTSD.

Prospective cohort studies

A prospective cohort study allows data on the exposure to be collected now, which ensures that the most up-to-date measurement techniques are used, thus minimizing bias in exposure classification. These studies can take time to conduct if the outcome has a long latency period. If the outcome has a short latency period, then a prospective cohort study is appropriate. An example of a prospective cohort study is the King's Centre for Military Health Research (KCMHR) military cohort study which follows up those who were deployed to Iraq in 2003 and Afghanistan in 2006 (Hotopf et al., 2006; Fear et al., 2010) (see Example 11.2).

Design and methodological considerations

Exposed group

Exposure is the factor which is being considered as a possible cause of 'disease'. This might be a lifestyle factor (e.g. smoking), an occupation (e.g. the Armed Forces), an occupational exposure (e.g. radiation), a treatment (e.g. chemotherapy), or some inherent trait (e.g. neuroticism). These exposures may be present or absent and, for those with the exposure, the level of this exposure may be considered (e.g. by duration of exposure, intensity, or severity of exposure).

It is unlikely that the exposure of interest can be measured perfectly. But misclassification must always be minimized. Misclassification of the exposure can either be random or non-random. Random misclassification occurs when the exposure is misclassified to the same degree in all groups, thus making the groups more alike and biasing any observed associations towards the null. This is the most likely type of misclassification in cohort studies. Non-random misclassification occurs when the exposure is either over- or underreported and that this does not happen to the same extent within all study groups.

This can either result in an over- or underestimation of the association. This is unlikely to occur in prospective cohort studies.

Unexposed group

An important aspect in the design of a cohort study is the ascertainment of the unexposed group and this must be carefully considered to minimize bias. Ideally, one selects an unexposed group which is similar to the exposed group with the exception of the exposure. This is not always easy and, therefore, the selection of an appropriate comparison group is one of the most difficult aspects of designing a cohort study. For example, a problem which commonly arises is whether the comparison group can be considered as completely unexposed. Thus the potential for exposure should be considered and measured within the comparison group. However, the use of multivariable data analysis methods means that multiple and varying levels of exposure can be taken into account in the analysis.

Researchers often select more than one comparison group but this can be costly and introduce challenges in the interpretation of the results if differences are observed depending on the comparison group used.

In general, there are three types of comparison commonly used in cohort studies:

1. General population
2. Selected non-exposed group
3. Internal comparison.

One of the disadvantages of using the general population as a comparison group is that they may not be comparable to the exposed cohort, especially if this is an occupational cohort. Why is this important? Those in employment are, on average, more likely to be well compared to those in the general population which includes those unable to work due to illness. This means that disease rates are often higher in the general population group, implying that the exposure is thus 'protective'. This is known as the 'healthy worker effect' (Li and Sung, 1999).

Outcome(s)

A major advantage of a cohort study is the ability to look at a range of outcomes. These outcomes can be short term (e.g. well-being) or long term (e.g. cancer and mortality). Whatever the method, the same approach must be used in the exposed and unexposed cohort. A particularly important aspect of outcome measurement is the completeness of follow-up. It is essential that a high proportion of participants are followed up, otherwise bias may be introduced (see 'Non-response and attrition').

Outcome data can be ascertained from a range of sources—depending on what is being studied:

◆ Routine data (e.g. death certificates, cancer registrations).
◆ Self-reported data from the study participants (e.g. questionnaire or interviews).
◆ Clinical assessment or examination (e.g. height, weight, blood tests, cognitive tests).

Like exposure data, outcome data can be prone to misclassification, random and non-random. In psychiatric epidemiology, self-reported data may be subject to bias caused by high-profile media coverage.

It is worth stating that classic epidemiological studies often focus on binary outcomes taking place at one point in time (disease incidence), while in psychiatric epidemiology the outcome may be multidimensional and it may be more difficult to determine the time of onset.

Confounding factors

A confounder is a factor that is associated with both the exposure and outcome under study (also see Chapter 15 for further discussion of this). It is important to measure and consider the role of confounders in a cohort study, as if the exposure is not allocated at random it may lead to differences in experiences of the groups other than the exposure of interest. This is important when considering if the exposure under study is the cause of the outcome. As long as information on these other factors is collected, confounding can be taken into account in the analysis. Thus any data collected must of good quality and be of sufficient detail. This can often be a problem with retrospective (historical) cohort studies as the required level of detail may not be available.

Non-response and attrition

One of the main challenges for researchers working with cohort study data relates to attrition of participants and missing data. If attrition is random then the implications of this are much less than when particular individuals are more likely to leave a study. Plewis (2007) outlined three reasons why participants may be lost from a longitudinal study: (1) if they can't be located or traced, (2) if their address is known but they can't be contacted at this address, and (3) if they choose to leave a study. Participants can temporarily drop out of a particular wave of a cohort study (wave non-response), but attrition refers to the permanent loss of participants from the cohort. Unit non-response refers to the loss of individuals, who were identified in the target sample, from the outset of the study (Hawkes and Plewis, 2006).

A number of studies have examined which factors are associated with attrition and non-response in the British birth cohorts. Work on the Millennium Cohort Study examined predictors of both unit non-response and attrition from waves 1 to 2. Hawkes and Plewis used data from Child Benefit records to examine associations with unit non-response. A number of factors were found to explain non-participation, including families in minority ethnic wards and younger age of the mother (Hawkes and Plewis, 2006). There is evidence from some studies that mental health status may be associated with attrition (de Graff et al., 2000), which can be problematic if this is also the outcome of interest.

There are statistical methods which can be used to counteract the effects of attrition. These include applying non-response weights or using multiple imputation.

Techniques to reduce attrition in cohort studies

There are a number of strategies which can be used to try and retain cohort members. Booker and colleagues (2011) conducted a systematic review of different retention strategies used in population-based cohort studies. They found that there were 45 different strategies which could be categorized into (1) incentives (monetary and non-monetary); (2) reminder methods, repeat visits or repeat questionnaires, or alternative modes of data collection; or (3) other methods. Incentives were found to increase retention, with one study randomizing participants to different monetary incentives, finding that retention was highest in the groups that received the most money. Offering a different mode of data collection, particularly a different location for face-to-face interviews, was found to be most successful in increasing retention. This may also be helpful for retaining particular groups in a study, for example, older participants for whom travelling to an interview could be more difficult.

The British birth cohorts are unique in that they recruit individuals based upon the fact that they are all born in the same week. Many of the birth cohorts send out birthday cards to all participants with the aim to keep participants engaged and make them feel valued. It is less logistically challenging to do this in a birth cohort, than in a study which includes participants whose birthdays are spread around the year.

Advantages and disadvantages of a cohort study

Cohort studies have a number of advantages over other study designs, the key advantage being that this type of study can allow the determination of causality due to the longitudinal nature of the assessment of exposure(s) and outcome(s). However, this means that they can be logistically challenging to conduct; they require engagement from participants over time meaning that they can be vulnerable to bias (Table 11.1).

Table 11.1 Advantages and disadvantages of a cohort study

Advantages	Disadvantages
Can assess prevalence and incidence	Not suitable for studying rare outcomes
Can infer causality as allows assessment of timing and direction of effect	Requires large sample size
Allows several outcomes to be assessed	Expensive
Ideal for studying rare or opportunistic exposures	Time-consuming
Can often include multiple exposures	Recruitment can be difficult (potentially leading to participation bias)
	Vulnerable to attrition (and hence bias)

Analytical approaches and interpretation

Data from a cohort study are used to estimate risks or rates of the outcome(s) in both the exposed and unexposed groups. Risks and rates are both measures of outcome frequency. These measures of outcome frequency can then be used to determine the association between outcome frequency and exposure. The most commonly used measure of effect is a ratio, that is, a risk ratio or rate ratio. The ratio estimates the size of the effect of the exposure on the outcome.

Risks and risk ratios

Risk is defined as the probability of the outcome among individuals in an outcome-free population during a specified time period. Risk is calculated using the number of outcome onsets observed divided by the number of persons in the cohort at risk at the beginning of the study.

A risk ratio is defined by calculating the ratio of the risks in the exposed to the unexposed.

Rates and rate ratios

A rate relates to the number of outcome onsets that occur among the overall person years at risk, which take into account the changes in the size of the at-risk population over the time period of interest. It is calculated using the number of outcome onsets observed divided by the person-years at risk. The person-years at risk is the sum of total number of years each individual included in the study was at risk of developing the disease of interest. This means that participants who develop the outcome or leave the study for other reasons (i.e. death) only contribute the 'time' they were at risk. The ability to determine person-years at risk allows the estimate of effect to be more precisely determined.

A rate ratio is defined by calculating the ratio of the rates in the exposed to the unexposed.

Example of risks, rates, and ratios

Tables 11.2 and 11.3 present data for 20 participants included in a study of exposure X and outcome Y. Follow-up was for a 10-year period. During the follow-up period some individuals developed the outcome of interest, others died, and others remained free from the outcome. Table 11.2 presents the follow-up data for those exposed to X and Table 11.3 presents the data for the unexposed comparison group.

Population attributable fraction

The population attributable fraction (PAF) gives an index of the maximum potential for prevention at the population level as it provides the proportion of cases in the population which would be prevented if the exposure was removed.

PAF = prevalence of exposure in the general population (RR − 1/RR)

where RR can be the risk or rate ratio.

Table 11.2 Exposed study subjects

Study ID	Follow-up (in years)										Person-years at risk
	1	2	3	4	5	6	7	8	9	10	
1										+	10
2							X				7
3											10
4	X										1
5		+									2
6				X							4
7											10
8									+		9
9			+								3
10					X						5
										Total person-years at risk:	61

+ = death; X = outcome.
Risk in the exposed = number of cases/number of study subjects = 4/10 per 10 years.
Rate in the exposed = number of cases/person years at risk = 4/61 = 66 per 1000 person years.

What this equation shows is that if an exposure is common in the general population, and the rate ratio is high showing a strong association, then there will be a major impact on population health by eradicating the exposure. An example would be smoking and lung cancer.

Multiple comparisons

While a traditional cohort is set up to test the consequences of a specific exposure, the birth cohorts typically collect data on a range of exposures and outcomes. This offers the benefit of providing scope for research from a wealth of disciplines, but there is the potential for these data to be misused. It is important that work using the birth cohort data has clear research hypotheses and that the exposures of interest are clearly defined a priori. If multiple risk factors are tested in the same study, then corrections can be made for multiple testing.

Age, period, and cohort effects

One of the advantages of studying multiple cohorts is that it is possible to investigate whether the effects that are shown are likely to apply across all situations and cohorts, or if they may be specific to the group being studied at that time. For example, certain research areas may be more likely to be studied at a time when these issues are most

Table 11.3 Unexposed study subjects

Study ID	Follow-up (in years)										Person years at risk
	1	2	3	4	5	6	7	8	9	10	
1			X								3
2	+										1
3											10
4											10
5											10
6											10
7								+			8
8										X	10
9											10
10					+						5
										Total person years at risk:	77

+ = death; X = outcome.
Risk in the unexposed = number of cases/number of study subjects = 2/10 per 10 years.
Rate in the unexposed = number of cases/person years at risk = 2/77 = 26 per 1000 person years.
Risk ratio = risk in the exposed/risk in the unexposed = 4/2 = 2.0.
Rate ratio = rate in the exposed/rate in the unexposed = 66/26 = 2.54.

salient or relevant to society, and investigation at another point in time could show different results. These effects have been labelled as age, period, or cohort effects. They can be examined across all types of cohort studies and are not restricted to investigation of the exposure in a traditional cohort study. In the field of mental health there are many risk factors which are more likely to have a greater consequence for particular age groups, such as adolescents.

An age effect is a common effect that is associated with a particular age or stage in the life course. It generally refers to the accumulated exposure of physiological changes associated with the process of ageing and examples include the incidence of coronary heart disease and cognitive decline. Age effects should not differ if you look at different cohorts across different time periods, even if the prevalence of a disorder changes across different generations.

A period effect can be defined as the result of widespread environmental changes, which are not specific to a particular age group. It is a population-wide exposure which occurs at a particular point in time, such as the Dutch famine that occurred at the end of World War II in an area of the Netherlands that was occupied by Germany. This was also referred to as 'hunger winter' and over 20,000 individuals died during this famine and all survivors may have had poorer health outcomes, regardless of their age (Lumey et al., 2007).

A cohort effect, sometimes also referred to as a generation effect, can be thought of as a period that is experienced through an age-specific exposure to an event or cause. For example, if there is variation in the risk of a health outcome through year of birth, as a result of the age-specific effect of an environmental effect at that time. In the earlier example of the Dutch famine, a cohort study was set up to study the effects of maternal nutrition in pregnancy, following up survivors who had become pregnant during the famine. This is because the health consequences of famine may be more likely to seen for children who were in the gestation period at this time (Lumey et al., 2007). A further example relates to the social consequences of the 2008 financial recession, as while the effects of employment and job insecurity may have a widespread impact on mental health, it was greater in particular groups. There is evidence from a number of countries that suicide increases most in young people during a recession as the impact of the recession on their future career may be greater than for those more established in a job (Gunnell et al., 1999; Ostamo et al., 2001).

Mediation analyses

Mediation analysis examines the effect of one variable (the mediator) in explaining the association between two other variables. Order in this relationship is assumed, in that the exposure predicts the mediator and then the mediator predicts the outcome. For this reason, mediation analysis is intended for longitudinal research, when the exposure, predictor, and mediator are ordered in time. An example is in considering the association between mental health and cardiovascular disease, which may be explained by the fact that individuals with a mental disorder are more likely to perform unhealthy behaviours such as smoking and risky alcohol use. Unhealthy behaviours which occur after the onset of the mental disorder could therefore be mediators of this association. The pathway from the exposure to the outcome, via the mediator, can also be referred to as an indirect effect.

Trajectory analyses

Cohort studies (and panel studies) which follow the same individuals up over time, and which tend to use the same measurement across phases, offer the opportunity for trajectory analyses. This can include latent curve modelling which examines how a particular outcome changes within a sample over time, for example, looking at the pattern of change in depression symptoms. There are also methods which can be used to examine different trajectories (or patterns) within a sample. These approaches look at how individuals are clustered based upon their longitudinal patterns. An example of latent class growth analysis was in the 1946 British birth cohort, which identified six distinct longitudinal trajectories of depression and anxiety symptoms. Examples of these trajectories include the most common group with the 'absence of symptoms' and a group with 'adult-onset moderate symptoms' (Colman et al., 2007).

Conclusion

A cohort study determines the size and strength of the association between an exposure and an outcome. As cohort studies are longitudinal in nature, they can be used to determine the sequence of events. There are many types of cohort, each being appropriate depending on the exposure and outcome under study. Advantages of these types of study include their ability to examine rare exposures and multiple outcomes; and, if designed (and conducted) appropriately they can minimize misclassification. However, they can be expensive, time-consuming, and vulnerable to attrition and hence non-response bias.

Practical exercises

Questions

1. Three different research studies are described (a–c). Match each of these descriptions with the following study designs: (i) case–control design, (ii) prospective cohort study, and (iii) retrospective cohort study. For each study you should also state what is the exposure of interest and what is the outcome.

   a. A UK study recruited a representative sample of pregnant women between 2000 and 2001 and after the birth of the child, the mother–child pairs were followed up. When the child was 9 months old, the mothers were interviewed on whether they had breastfed their child and if they did, for what duration. When the child was 5 years old, behavioural problems in the child were assessed using the Strengths and Difficulties Questionnaire. Results suggested that after adjustment for confounders, the odds of the child having behavioural problems were reduced in children who had been breastfed for 4 months or longer.

   b. A Scottish study examined the association between receipt of multidisciplinary care and survival in breast cancer patients. The Scottish Cancer Registry was used to identify all residents who had breast cancer between 1990 and 2000 and this was linked to death records from the General Register for Scotland. It was already known that multidisciplinary team care was introduced to particular health board areas in Scotland in 1995, but not in others. Results showed that the introduction of multidisciplinary care for the treatment of breast cancer was associated with an 18% lower breast cancer mortality rate compared to the health boards who did not implement this change in practice.

   c. A study tested whether there was an association between the use of high-potency cannabis and psychosis. They recruited 410 patients with first-episode psychosis for an inpatient psychiatric unit and 370 controls recruited using volunteer sampling. All participants completed a questionnaire on cannabis use, duration, frequency, and age of first use. Results showed that patients with psychosis were more likely to report using cannabis every day and use of high-potency cannabis compared to controls.

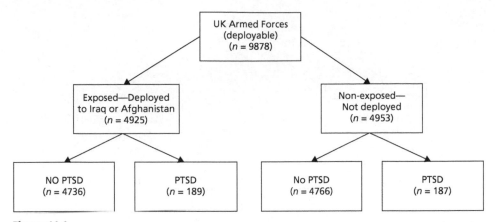

Figure 11.1

2. Read the following paragraph and try and identify what are the (a) age, (b) period, and (c) cohort effects.

A study using US and Canadian data examined the distribution of depressive and anxiety symptoms across a range of birth cohorts and time periods (Keyes et al., 2014). The data included was from the US National Health Interview Study (NHIS) and the Canadian Community Health Survey (CCHS) and covered the period from 1997 to 2011. The results showed that in the CCHS, psychological distress was highest in late adolescence and early adulthood, peaking in the 20–24-year age group, and in the NHIS was highest in the 50–54-year age group. In both surveys the level of psychological distress was highest for the data collections occurring in 2000–2001. In the US, the oldest cohort (both 1912–1914) evidenced the highest level of psychological distress, with another peak for those born in the 1970s. In Canada, there was evidence for an increase in psychological distress from the 1930s to the 1990s.

3. Using the data provided in Figures 11.1 and 11.2, determine:

   a. the risk of PTSD among those deployed to Iraq or Afghanistan (Figure 11.1)

   b. the risk of PTSD among those not deployed to Iraq or Afghanistan (Figure 11.1)

   c. the risk ratio for PTSD (based on a and b). What does this risk ratio tell us?

   d. the risk of PTSD among those deployed in a combat role to Iraq or Afghanistan (Figure 11.2)

   e. the risk of PTSD among those deployed in a non-combat role to Iraq or Afghanistan (Figure 11.2)

   f. the risk ratio for PTSD (based on d and e). What does this risk ratio tell us?

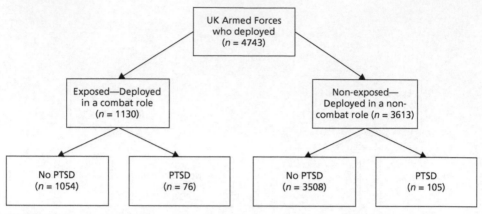

Figure 11.2

Answers

1.

   a. Prospective cohort study (Heikkilä et al., 2011).
      Exposure—breastfeeding and duration of breastfeeding.
      Outcome—behavioural problems in childhood.

   b. Retrospective cohort study (Kesson et al., 2012).
      Exposure—receipt of multidisciplinary care for breast cancer.
      Outcome—breast cancer mortality.

   c. Case–control study (Di Forti et al., 2015).

      Exposure—use of high-potency cannabis.
      Outcome—first-episode psychosis.

2.

   a. Age effects differed between the US and Canada, with young adults having higher levels of distress in Canada and the 50–54-year age group in the US.

   b. The period effects were the same for both countries, with psychological distress highest in 2000–2001.

   c. The cohort effects were examined after accounting for variance attributed to age and period effects. The cohort effects differed between countries, but showed similar increases from the 1930s until the 1970s when the upward trend continued in the Canadian data, but decreased in the US data.

3.

   a. Risk in the exposed = 189/4925 = 0.04.

   b. Risk in the unexposed = 187/4953 = 0.04.

   c. Risk ratio = 0.04/0.04 = 1, the risk of PTSD is no different in the exposed and unexposed groups. Therefore, deployment is not associated with PTSD.

d. Risk in the exposed = 76/1130 = 0.07.

e. Risk in the unexposed = 105/3613 = 0.03.

f. Risk ratio = 0.07/0.03 = 2.33, the risk of PTSD is more than twice as likely in the exposed (combat deployed) group compared to the unexposed (non-combat deployed) group. Therefore, deployment in a combat role is associated with PTSD.

References

Booker, C., Harding, S., and Benzeval, M. (2011). A systematic review of the effect of retention methods in population-based cohort studies. *BMC Public Health*, 11, 249.

Carpenter, L.M., Linsell, L., Brooks, C., Keegan, T.J., Langdon, T., Doyle, P., et al. (2009). Cancer morbidity in British military participants in chemical warfare agent experiments at Porton Down: cohort study. *BMJ*, 338, b655.

Colman, I., Ploubidis, G.B., Wadsworth, M.E.J., Jones, P.B., and Croudace, T.J. (2007). A longitudinal typology of symptoms of depression and anxiety over the life course. *Biological Psychiatry*, 62, 1265–1271.

De Graaf, R., Bijl, R.V., Smit, F., Ravelli, A., and Vollebergh, W.A.M. (2000). Psychiatric and sociodemographic predictors of attrition in a longitudinal study: the Netherlands Mental Health Survey and Incidence Study (NEMESIS). *American Journal of Epidemiology*, 152, 1039–1047.

Di Forti, M., Marconi, A., Carra, E., Fraietta, S., Trotta, A., Bonomo, M., et al. (2015). Proportion of patients in south London with first-episode psychosis attributable to use of high potency cannabis: a case-control study. *Lancet Psychiatry*, 2, 233–238.

Fear, N.T., Jones, M., Murphy, D., Hull, L., Iversen, A., Coker, B., et al. (2010). What are the consequences of deployment to Iraq and Afghanistan on the mental health of the UK armed forces? A cohort study. *Lancet*, 375, 1783–1797.

Gunnell, D., Lopatatzidis, A., Dorling, D., Wehner, H., Southall, H., and Frankel, S. (1999). Suicide and unemployment in young people. Analysis of trends in England and Wales, 1921–1995. *British Journal of Psychiatry*, 175, 263–270.

Hawkes, D. and Plewis, I. (2006). Modelling non-response in the National Child Development Study. *Journal of the Royal Statistical Society: Series A (Statistics in Society)*, 169, 479–491.

Heikkilä, K., Sacker, A., Kelly, Y., Renfrew, M.J., and Quigley, M.A. (2011). Breast feeding and child behaviour in the Millennium Cohort Study. *Archives of Disease in Childhood*, 96, 635–642.

Hotopf, M., Hull, L., Fear, N., Browne, T., Horn, O., Iversen, A., et al. (2006). The health of UK military personnel who deployed to the 2003 Iraq war: a cohort study. *Lancet*, 367, 1731–1741.

Kesson, E.M., Allardice, G.M., George, W.D., Burns, H.J.G., and Morrison, D.S. (2012). Effects of multidisciplinary team working on breast cancer survival: retrospective, comparative, interventional cohort study of 13 722 women. *BMJ*, 344, e2718.

Keyes, K.M., Nicholson, R., Kinley, J., Raposo, S., Stein, M.B., Goldner, E.M., and Sareen, J. (2014). Age, period, and cohort effects in psychological distress in the United States and Canada. *American Journal of Epidemiology*, 179, 1216–1227.

Li, C.-Y. and Sung, E.-C. (1999). A review of the healthy worker effect in occupational epidemiology. *Occupational Medicine*, 49, 225–229.

Lumey, L.H., Stein, A.D., Kahn, H.S., van der Pal-de Bruin, K.M., Blauw, G.J., Zybert, P.A., and Susser, E.S. (2007). Cohort profile: the Dutch Hunger Winter Families study. *International Journal of Epidemiology*, 36, 1196–1204.

Maconochie, N., Doyle, P., Roman, E., Davies, G., Smith, P.G., and Beral, V. (1999). Nuclear Industry Family Study: methods and description of a United Kingdom study linking occupational information held by employers to reproduction and child health. *Occupational and Environmental Medicine*, **56**, 793–801.

Newman, D.L., Moffitt, T.E., Caspi, A., Magdol, L., Silva, P.A., and Stanton, W.R. (1996). Psychiatric disorder in a birth cohort of young adults: prevalence, comorbidity, clinical significance, and new case incidence from ages 11 to 21. *Journal of Consulting and Clinical Psychology*, **64**, 552–562.

Ostamo, A., Lahelma, E., and Lonnqvist, J. (2001). Transitions of employment status among suicide attempters during a severe economic recession. *Social Science & Medicine*, **52**, 1741–1750.

Plewis, I. (2007). Non-response in a birth cohort study: the case of the Millennium Cohort Study. *International Journal of Social Research Methodology*, **10**, 325–334.

Venables, K.M., Brooks, C., Linsell, L., Keegan, T.J., Langdon, T., Fletcher, T., et al. (2009). Mortality in British military participants in human experimental research into chemical warfare agents at Porton Down: cohort study. *BMJ*, **338**, b613.

Chapter 12

Randomized controlled trials

Sube Banerjee, Rod S. Taylor, and Jennifer Hellier*

Introduction

There are three main questions in healthcare: 'What is going on?', 'Why?', and 'What do we do about it?' 'What is going on?' forms the basis for clinical assessment including history taking, examination, and diagnosis as well as descriptive epidemiology. The question 'Why?' underlies all aetiological research from laboratory science to epidemiology. The cross-sectional, case–control, and cohort methodologies discussed in other chapters in this book provide the methodology for addressing 'Why?' questions. However, just as medicine is more than diagnosis, medical research is more than aetiology: it also necessarily extends to the evaluation of interventions.

Aetiological research which cannot be translated into health benefits through new or improved interventions is at best sterile and at worse self-indulgent, begging another important question: 'So what?' Flawed evaluations of interventions can be even more problematic since these may harm as well as help. Randomized controlled trials (RCTs) provide the highest quality of evidence for the impact of interventions.

In this chapter we will consider some of the more important factors in the design, conduct, analysis, and interpretation of RCTs.

What is a randomized controlled trial?

Porta (2014) defines an RCT as:

> A clinical-epidemiological experiment in which subjects are randomly allocated into groups, usually called *test* and *control* groups, to receive or not to receive a preventive or a therapeutic procedure or intervention. The results are assessed by comparison of rates of disease, death, recovery, or other appropriate outcome in the study groups. RCTs are generally regarded as the most scientifically rigorous method of hypothesis testing available in epidemiology and medicine. Nonetheless, they may suffer lack of generalizability due, for example, to the non-representativeness of patients who are ethically and practically eligible, chosen, or consent to participate.[†]

---

* Sube Banerjee originally drafted this chapter. For this new edition, Jennifer Hellier wrote/redrafted the sections entitled 'Analysis strategies' and 'Trial designs and complex interventions' and Rod S. Taylor wrote/redrafted 'Explanatory versus pragmatic trials: efficacy and effectiveness and role of the clinical trials unit'.

† Reproduced with permission from Porta, M. *A Dictionary of Epidemiology*. 6th ed. Oxford University Press (2014). Reproduced with permission of the Licensor through PLSclear.

Box 12.1 The elements of a randomized controlled trial

+ Define the research question.
+ Identify and recruit the sample.
+ Apply the intervention at random.
+ Measure the outcome and compare between intervention groups.
+ Summarize and disseminate findings.

The stages in the RCT process are summarized in Box 12.1. While this process may be clear, it is not necessarily simple. RCTs require a substantial investment of resources in terms of time, expertise, personnel, and finance. This is not to say that the constituent components of assessment, intervention, reassessment, analysis, and interpretation need themselves be complex. Indeed, much of the rigour in trial design revolves around ensuring that these components are simple, meaningful, and explicit before the start of the RCT.

What are randomized controlled trials for?

Treatments are fundamental to the delivery of healthcare and we need information to decide what treatment to give, and to invest in. At its simplest, an RCT answers the question 'Does Treatment A work?'; one level of complexity higher is the design which answers the question 'Does new Treatment B work better than established Treatment A?' Studies that simply observe the effects of treatment without randomization or control groups are subject to bias and confounding and size and direction of their effects need to be interpreted carefully. The use of historical controls (e.g. comparing two case series, one before a new drug and one after) is also problematic (Altman and Bland, 1999), and may lead to an overestimation of the effect of the new intervention (Sacks et al., 1982).

The methodology and practice of RCTs cannot be divorced from their impact upon clinical practice and health policy, and the wider financial and industrial context. There are increasing moves worldwide to base clinical practice on good-quality evidence. This is a reaction to the realization that practice has often varied widely and doctors of all specialties have very often been unable to support their actions with anything other than protestations of established practice, anecdote, or peer group consensus. Quality of evidence for clinical effectiveness forms a hierarchy with consistent findings from several well-conducted RCTs at the top (Centre for Evidence-Based Medicine, 2009).

So on one level the purpose of RCTs is to allow clinicians to select the best treatment for a patient and to allow patients to receive the treatment with the best benefit-to-risk ratio for their condition. However, there are other agencies interested in the data produced by RCTs. Those who purchase healthcare, be they health insurance agencies or governmental health authorities, use evidence of effectiveness to focus or ration care within a limited financial envelope. These agencies therefore factor an assessment of the financial and political costs of sanctioning treatment into their interpretation of RCTs.

The pharmaceutical industry has a particularly strong interest in the findings of RCTs. Billions of dollars are spent in research and development of novel compounds by drug companies each year. It is they who design, conduct, analyse, and promote the vast majority of RCTs, albeit within a framework of governmental control agencies. While the betterment of human health may result, the data from RCTs are the primary channel through which an experimental compound can be turned into a marketable commodity, so that investment can be turned to income, profit, and shareholder value. A desire for a positive result is not restricted to industry, researchers who develop and evaluate complex interventions and psychological treatments fall into similar traps, albeit for less directly financial motives. The complex and competing inter-relationships of clinicians, patients, researchers, health purchasers, and drug companies is of profound importance in any consideration of an RCT. The clear rules and governance structures that have grown up in the past decades along with the strictures of evidence-based medicine are there in part to enable users of trial data to be have greater faith in the results generated. Heathy scepticism remains an important asset in assessing claims and occurrences such as the discontinuation of the FAME trial of a lipid-lowering statin in older adults for commercial reasons raise scientific and ethical issues (Evans and Pocock, 2001; Lievre et al., 2001).

Fundamental design issues

As with all other epidemiological studies, primary objectives in the design of RCTs are to exclude bias and to minimize confounding. Important aspects in the design are summarized in Box 12.2. Lind's elegant mid-eighteenth-century comparative trial of different treatments for scurvy contains many of these methodological components (Lind, 1753; Bull, 1959; Lilienfield, 1982). In this study, he took 12 patients with scurvy on board the *HMS Salisbury* who were 'as similar as I could have them'; he gave them a common diet, divided them into six intervention groups and supplemented the groups' diets in different ways. The two people in each group received either a quart of cider a day; '25 gutts of elixir vitriol'; two spoonfuls of vinegar; a course of sea water; 'the bigness of a nutmeg'; or two oranges and a lemon. After 6 days the group on the oranges and lemon had recovered to such an extent that one returned to duty and the other became the nurse for the remaining patients. However, the translation of research findings into clinical practice was just as much of a problem in the eighteenth century as it is in the twentieth, and it took a further 50 years before the Royal Navy provided its sailors with lemon juice (Pocock, 1983).

One way to understand the particular challenges posed by the carrying out of an RCT is to set up a perfect scenario and then to see just how far this differs from clinical circumstances in general and evaluations of interventions in psychiatry in particular.

Box 12.2 Fundamental design issues

- ◆ Thorough review of existing evidence.
- ◆ Clear hypothesis formulation and statement of objectives.
- ◆ Informed consent.
- ◆ Random allocation of intervention.
- ◆ Use of placebo or active control.
- ◆ Accurate and careful measurement of potential confounding factors.
- ◆ Accurate and careful measurement of outcome.
- ◆ Maximization of follow-up.
- ◆ Blinding.
- ◆ Intention-to-treat analysis.
- ◆ Unbiased dissemination of findings.

'A perfect trial'

The perfect conditions for a trial would involve a disorder (D) which could be diagnosed with absolute precision at minimal cost and whose course was such that it did not matter when it was diagnosed or treatment was started. We would then need a putative treatment (X) which had a compelling scientific basis for its use but whose efficacy was in doubt so that a trial was ethically acceptable. By preference there would be no other active treatment for D so that an inert placebo could be used as a comparator, and X should have no properties by which it could be distinguished from the placebo (e.g. taste, side effects, and perception of effect) either by patient or doctor. D should also be sufficiently common and serious for it to be a good candidate for a clinical trial and full funding should be available.

For ascertaining outcome, we should have a perfect knowledge of the natural history of D and it should consistently lead to an unequivocal outcome, such as a disease-specific death, within a given time (say, 1 year on average). We should then be able to recruit a group of affected people who were absolutely representative of all people with D. These would be randomly allocated on a one-to-one basis to receive a course of X or placebo. We would then follow up all participants in both groups and measure after 1 year the death rate in the intervention and the control groups, comparing the two to ascertain the efficacy of X. The findings would be absolutely unequivocal. Just to make things perfect, X should be a compound which is not under drug company licence and which is cheap and simple to manufacture and distribute so that the whole world can benefit from this work.

Preferably several independent research groups would have carried out separate similar trials at the same time, and they would all be published together. The role of X in the treatment of D would be systematically reviewed showing a consistent and powerful treatment effect in the individual studies and after meta-analysis. The fairy story would end with there being no political or clinical resistance to the introduction of the treatment and the healthcare delivery systems being universally available to make X available to all without prejudice. And we would all live happily ever after in a world without D.

Clearly this is to argue by absurdity but it is important to make the point that the real world is a messy place full of uncertainly and complexity. Diagnosis or case ascertainment may be imprecise and difficult, and it may be modified by help-seeking behaviour which has an influence on outcome. There may be comorbidity with other conditions and the patient may be taking other medication. Recruitment and obtaining informed consent may be difficult. There may be competing treatments and established practice may mean that placebos are not ethically justifiable. Treatments have side effects which may be unpleasant or serious, affecting both compliance and blinding to treatment group. Outcome may be difficult to measure accurately and loss to follow-up may compromise the validity of the study. When translating outcomes from RCTs into clinical practice, issues of cost and practicality invariably need to be taken into account.

Elements of a randomized controlled trial

In this section we will deal sequentially with some of the major practical elements of the design and conduct of RCTs. These cannot be dealt with in detail here due to constraints of space and the reader is referred to comprehensive texts such as Pocock's *Clinical trials: a practical approach* (1983) for further details and Porta's *A dictionary of epidemiology* (2014) for succinct explanations of terms.

Review the literature

Before embarking on a trial there is a need to investigate systematically the existing evidence to ascertain the current state of the therapeutics of the disorder being studied and of the intervention being proposed. If there is already compelling evidence in the public domain then it may not be necessary, and therefore ethical, to carry out a trial. Techniques for the conduct of systematic reviews are increasingly well developed and the methods and outputs of Cochrane (see Chapter 14) should be consulted and used.

Clear formulation of a single primary hypothesis to be tested

RCTs typically need to test a single primary hypothesis. There may be secondary hypotheses but these should be limited to avoid multiple significance testing and 'data dredging'. At this point, the level for statistical significance for the primary (e.g. $p < 0.05$) and secondary hypotheses should be set (e.g. $p < 0.01$).

Specify the objectives of the trial

The hypothesis should be stated clearly and simply, for example, 'The objective of the study is to test if Treatment B is more effective than Treatment A in Disease X'. However, this means that you need to have decided what constitutes 'more effective'. If we know that A gets 30% of people with X better, how much more effective does B need to be? These are complex questions when A is an acceptable, economic, and widely available treatment with known side effects. We may say that we are only interested in B if it gets another 20% of people with X better, but to an extent these figures will always be arbitrary. They are, however, vital to the study design since the effect size being sought will determine the size of the study, with larger studies required to detect smaller differences.

It is at this point that the pre-study power calculations need to be completed. At the least these will require:

- an estimation of the treatment effect of your comparison group (i.e. the percentage of people with X who respond to known Treatment A, or in the case of a placebo-controlled trial the spontaneous recovery rate from X)

- an estimate of the minimum effect size of your new Treatment B for it to be considered useful

- the level of statistical significance required for there to be accepted that there is indeed a true difference between the two groups. This is generally set at a p-value of 0.05—that is, a random 'false-positive' result (type 1 error) is acceptable on 1 in 20 occasions

- the 'power' of the study to detect effect. This is generally set at 80–90%—that is, 'false-negative' results (type 2 error) are acceptable on between 1 in 5 and 1 in 10 occasions.

Power calculations are not generally complex but specialized statistical help is vital. Lower acceptable rates of type 2 error and smaller potential differences in effect require larger numbers of participants. Recruitment targets also need to be inflated to allow for those who will withdraw from the study and those who are lost to follow-up.

The statement of the study objectives should form the start of a detailed study protocol which sets out why the study is being carried out and exactly how the study will be conducted and analysed. This will form the basis for the ethical approval which is necessary for all trials.

Define the reference population

Define the population to which you wish to generalize. In the case of the donepezil trial (Rogers and Friedhoff, 1996) discussed in "'Explanatory' versus 'pragmatic' trials: efficacy and effectiveness", this might have been 'extraordinarily fit and well people with Alzheimer's disease'.

Select study population

It is not generally feasible to create a list of all people in a reference population and randomly select cases for inclusion in the study, unless the disorder is very rare and there are very careful records. It is more common that the trial will be undertaken in a single or a small number of sites for ease of administration and to control quality. These centres should ideally be representative of centres as a whole and their patient's representative of the reference population. Reliance upon research-friendly 'centres of excellence' may compromise this. Even in the most inclusive of effectiveness studies there will be entry criteria to be applied to potential participants: these may be simple (e.g. age) or complex (e.g. stage of disorder). One should be careful not to select a study population which automatically and irrevocably limits the applicability of any findings obtained.

Participant identification and recruitment

In this phase, participants are recruited by the plan set out in detail in the protocol. Since the RCT may be being carried out simultaneously at multiple sites, it is important that the same processes are adhered to in all study centres so that any selection bias can be minimized. Comprehensive and up-to-date lists of possible cases will need to drawn up and used as a sampling frame from which to randomly sample cases for assessment. Those participants who meet the predetermined inclusion and exclusion criteria are eligible for entry into the study. A fairly solid rule is that the more exclusions there are, the more compromised is the generalizability of the study. Most scientific journals require the Consolidated Standards of Reporting Trials (CONSORT) guidelines to be followed before they will publish a trial (Begg et al., 1996). These include a flow diagram summarizing the effect of all inclusion and exclusion criteria and loss to follow-up through the study (Figure 12.1). The presentation of such data is an invaluable aid to assessing generalizability and therefore the clinical robustness of a study. Those studies presented without such data should be appraised with care.

Informed consent

There is insufficient space here for a detailed consideration of ethical issues in RCTs, and major issues are well summarized by Edwards and Lilford (1998). If there is no doubt of the efficacy of an intervention then there is no ethical reason for withholding, and such withholding is implicit in a trial. If there is insufficient evidence of the potential for efficacy then there may be poor ethical grounds for conducting a trial and such evidence should be collected using other methodologies. If a trial has insufficient statistical power to demonstrate the required difference between intervention and control groups then again it is unethical since it cannot provide useful data. Equally, poorly designed trials where any observed difference may be a function of bias or confounding are also unethical on the same grounds.

If the RCT design is satisfactory, there remains the problem of recruiting participants into the study and the dilemma of how to obtained truly informed consent. In this brief discussion the issue of capacity to consent, which is of importance in mental health research, not only for people with dementia and learning disabilities, but also for people with psychotic and other disorders, will be left to one side. Obtaining informed consent may involve a tension between the requirement to provide full information and the objectives for the trial itself. Comprehensive details of every conceivable risk may reduce participation, potentially compromising recruitment, generalizability, and the possibility of important therapeutic advances. Participants will need to receive written and verbal information on the trial and have the chance to discuss any questions they might have; they

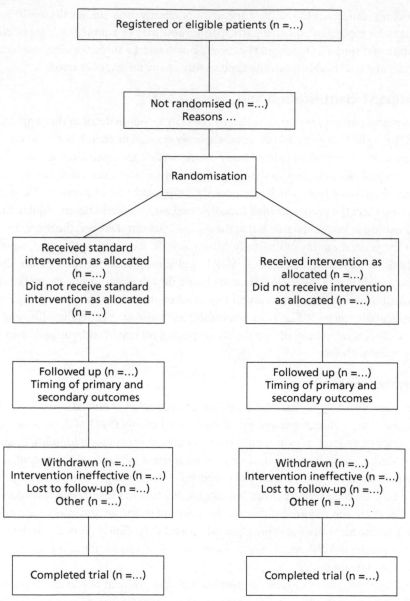

Figure 12.1 Flow diagram summarizing progress of participants through both arms of a randomized controlled trial.

http://www.consort-statement.org/.

might need time to consider and consult with family, all of which is time-consuming and difficult for research teams. Consent will almost always need to be written and witnessed with stipulations of being able to withdraw at any time without giving any reason and without such withdrawal compromising their medical care in any way. These documents need to be submitted to and approved by appropriate research ethics committee.

Silverman and Chalmers (2001) have summarized elegantly some of these ethical issues and the value of random allocation of treatment: 'when there is uncertainty about the relative merits of the double edged swords we wield in medicine today, we are wise to employ this ancient technique of decision making. It is a fair way of distributing the hoped for benefits and the unknown risks of inadequately evaluated treatments.' There is a tension where recruiting physicians stand to gain from recruiting individuals into trials. This gain may be direct, such as a financial payment from the pharmaceutical industry per participant recruited, or indirect, mediated by the scientific kudos of completing a trial or being seen as successful by peers and seniors. In this context it is of great concern that reports from physicians recruiting patients into trials indicate that a half to three-quarters thought that few of the patients they had recruited understood that trial even though they had given written consent (Spaight et al., 1984; Blum et al., 1987; Taylor and Kelner, 1987). In the circumstances that apply in a trial, how good are doctors in protecting their patients' rights?

Baseline measurements

The literature review will have pointed to important possible prognostic variables. These need to be measured with accuracy so that their potential effect on the outcome can be measured, considered as stratification factors, and controlled for in the analysis. At this stage, social, demographic, and other variables of interest (e.g. financial state and service use) which might change as part of the study need to be recorded. In mental health studies, we seldom have hard outcomes such as unequivocal disease-related death. The measurement of the presence and/or severity of the disorder at recruitment is a vital consideration. This must be achieved accurately and dispassionately, without conscious or unconscious bias, and without any knowledge of which treatment group the individual will be randomized to.

Baseline measurements of the outcome variable, if available, can be used in the response variable analyses. Frisson and Pocock (1992) describe three methods: post, change, and analysis of covariance (ANCOVA). ANCOVA accounts for between-subject variation in baseline measurement by using the mean of the baseline values for each subject as a covariate in a linear model for the comparison of post-randomization outcomes. With a single baseline measure of the outcome variable and a degree of correlation between the measures, they show that ANCOVA is more powerful than both analysis of the change scores and analysis of post-randomization means. Furthermore. any potential moderators or mediators of treatment must be recorded at baseline to ensure accurate analyses. Researchers should record variables that may be useful predictors of missing data or inform drop out.

Randomization

Randomization is the single most powerful element of the RCT design. Its purpose is to ensure that all variables which might have an effect on outcome (known and unknown) other than the intervention(s) being studied are distributed as equally as possible between the intervention and the control group so that the effect of the intervention can be accurately estimated.

The application of randomization has developed over the course of the twentieth century. Its roots, however, are deeper; as early as 1662 a chemist named van Helmont advocated the drawing of lots to compare the effectiveness of competing contemporary treatments (Armitage, 1982). His excellent concise protocol suggested: 'Let us take out of the hospitals ... 200, or 500 poor People that have Fevers, Pleurises, etc. Let us divide them into half, let us cast lots, that one half may fall to my share, and the other to yours ... We shall see how many funerals both of us shall have.' Another early proposal for the random allocation of treatments in human health referred to studies of cholera and typhoid in the first decade of the twentieth century (Greenwood and Yule, 1915; Pocock, 1983). While first actually applied in agricultural research in 1926 (Box, 1980), stratified randomization of matched groups was used in a 1931 study by Amberson and colleagues (1931) to investigate the efficacy of a gold compound in pulmonary tuberculosis. However, the first trial to be reported which used full randomization, using in this case sealed envelopes, was the Medical Research Council's (1948) careful and methodologically advanced trial of streptomycin in tuberculosis in the late 1940s. It is interesting to note that this trial was only ethically possible because the 'small amount of streptomycin available made it ethically permissible for the control participants to be untreated by the drug' (D'Arcy Hart, 1999).

Randomization uses individual-level unpredictability to achieve group-level predictability. So if randomization is on a one-to-one basis, we have no idea whether the individual in front of us will be randomized to the intervention or the control group. The result is that there will be a predictably equal distribution between the two groups of known *and unknown* potential confounders.

One of the major objectives in randomizing participants to treatment groups is to achieve between-group comparability on certain relevant participant characteristics known as prognostic factors. Measured prior to randomization, these factors are expected to correlate with subsequent participant response or outcome. Stratified randomization, most relevant in small trials, helps to achieve comparability between study groups for a chosen set of prognostic factors. A stratum for randomization is formed by selecting one subgroup from each factor (continuous variables must be divided into groups). Thus, the total number of strata is the product of the number of subgroups in each factor. The number of strata increases rapidly as factors are added and the levels within factors are refined; only the most important variables should be chosen and the number kept to a minimum. Stratified randomization aims to make treatment groups comparable with respect to specific prognostic factors but it may also lead to increased power if the stratification is taken into account in the analysis reducing variability in group comparison. In many cases it may be more useful to employ a stratified analysis, adjusted for prognostic factors when treatment differences are assessed (Roberts and Torgerson, 1999).

It is vital that the process of randomization is removed entirely from recruiting researchers since any knowing or unknowing compromise of the chance element to group allocation will undermine the whole basis of the study (Schulz, 1995; Altman and Schulz, 2001). This will usually require the involvement of a third party who can assure that strict randomization is implemented (e.g. telephoning with the name/study number and only then being assigned a randomization code). The method of assignment and concealment of allocation are important components. For example, if we were interviewing a woman and felt that she might have a poor response to the treatment we were testing, and we had worked out that (perhaps because she had an even-numbered birthday (or hospital number we had glimpsed on an appointment card) so she would be allocated to the intervention group), we might knowingly or unknowingly, in the process of gaining informed consent, discourage her from participation. Equally, if we knew she would be in the control group then we might knowingly or unknowingly encourage her to participate.

Altman and Schulz (2001) suggest that there are two main requirements for adequate concealment of allocation. First, the person generating the allocation sequence must not be the same person determining whether a participant is eligible and enters the trial. Second, the method for treatment allocation should not include anyone involved in the trial. Where the second is not possible they conclude that the only other plausible method is the use of serially numbered, opaque sealed envelopes although this may still be open to external influence (Schulz, 1995; Torgerson and Roberts, 1999). In practice, given the expense and complexity of trial design and the vital role that randomization and concealment of allocation plays in a trial, it should be a priority to set up an external incorruptible system.

In a useful systematic review, Kunz and Oxman (1998) demonstrated that studies which failed to use adequately concealed random allocation generated distorted effect size estimates with the majority overestimating effect. The effects of not using such concealed allocation were often of comparable size to those of the interventions. Another study by Schulz and colleagues (1995) suggested that RCTs without adequately concealed randomization produce effect size estimates that are 40% higher than trials with good-quality randomization. They concluded that while the main effect was to produce a poorer response in the control group, there were also occasions where effects of interventions were obscured or reversed in direction. These data provide strong support for the use of robust and concealed methods for randomization and the need to be very sceptical about data from trials not using, or not declaring that they used, such methodology.

In this chapter, the focus has been on simple individual intervention and randomization. However, the unit of randomization need not be the individual. In a trial of a general practitioner (GP) psychoeducational package, the unit might be the GP or a group of GPs in an individual practice, even though its efficacy is assessed by measurement of their participants. Equally, where the intervention is population wide, as in trials of water fluoridation to prevent dental caries, the unit of randomization will be the entire catchment area of a reservoir system. Statistical power in such cluster randomization depends more on the number of clusters (i.e. the number of units of randomization) than the numbers within the clusters, as well as the intra-cluster correlation of outcome (Kerry and Bland, 1998).

There are also adaptive randomization procedures such as minimization, where imbalances in the distribution of prognostic factors are minimized according to some criteria. This approach achieves balance between treatment groups on selective prognostic factors: the chance of allocating a new participant to a particular treatment is adjusted according to any existing imbalances in the baseline characteristics of the groups. In practice this method is implemented in situations involving several prognostic factors and participant allocation is then based on the aim of balancing the marginal treatment totals for each level of each factor (Pocock, 1983).

Intervention, control groups, and blinding

At its most simple, participants are randomized into an intervention or a control group. The intervention group receives the novel treatment and the control group a placebo if there is no established treatment—or the best established treatment if there is one. If the study design is sound and the randomization robust, then the control group should differ from the intervention group only in the treatment allocated to it.

The problems start when the participant, the clinical staff, or the researchers can work out which group they are in. There are fewest problems with drug trials. Placebos or active control treatments can be formulated to look like the novel treatment. Inert placebos may, however, be discernible from active interventions if they differ in side effects (e.g. anticholinergic side effects) which may alert a patient or clinician to the intervention status. The use of placebos which contain side effect-mimicking compounds may partially address this difficulty. Problems are far greater when the intervention cannot be concealed—for example, in a trial of psychotherapy. It is comforting to bear in mind Bradford Hill's (1963) defence of not subjecting control patients in the Medical Research Council Tuberculosis Trial to the 4 months of four times daily intramuscular injections which the streptomycin intervention group received, that there was 'no need in the search for precision to throw common sense out of the window'.

Blinding is different from concealment of random allocation, and concerns the degree to which participants and/or researchers are unaware of intervention groups after these have been allocated following randomization. This is an important tool in minimizing potential bias but may not always be possible depending on the nature of the intervention. *Single-blind* studies usually describe a situation where the participant does not know their group but the researcher does. In a *double-blind* study, both the participant and the investigators are unaware of group membership. In a *triple-blind* study, the participants, the researchers, and the statisticians analysing the data are unaware of group membership. In an *open trial*, everybody knows what is going on and making solid inferences can therefore be difficult. Blinding is not only important in RCTs: for example, the performance of diagnostic tests may be overestimated when the test result is known (Lijmer et al., 1999).

A particular issue for RCTs in mental health is the complexity of the intervention. Procedures which we wish to evaluate are often multifaceted and multidisciplinary rather than confined to different tablets (Banerjee and Dickenson, 1997). This compromises blinding and may make intervention seem less precise. Certainly it can be difficult to

Box 12.3 Trial development for complex interventions

- *Theoretical phase*—identifying evidence for the intervention.
- *Phase I*—defining components of the intervention using descriptive studies, and using modelling and qualitative methodologies to understand the components of the intervention and their interaction.
- *Phase II*—defining trial and intervention design including assessment of feasibility, acceptability, what should happen in the control group and even estimating potential effect sizes by carrying out a small-scale exploratory trial where outcome measurement can also be tested.
- *Phase III*—the main trial with a detailed protocol development maximizing generalizability. Concurrent qualitative work can help to understand why things are happening or not happening.
- *Phase IV*—promoting effective implementation putting evidence into practice.

pinpoint what element of intervention may be of help. These are issues across the whole of healthcare and the UK Medical Research Council published a framework for the design and evaluation of complex interventions to improve health (Campbell et al., 2000) and revised these in 2008 (Craig et al., 2008). In these, the authors deal with interventions that are 'made up of various interconnecting parts' citing examples including the evaluation of specialist stroke units and group psychotherapies. They identify a lack of development and definition of the intervention as a frequent difficulty, and propose a five-stage iterative process of trial development (Box 12.3).

Follow-up and reassessment

Given the obstacles to be overcome in getting this far, it is unlikely that assiduous attempts will not be made to follow up all participants in both groups. However, the longer the study, the more likely there are to be drop outs due to defaulters, and people moving or dying. It is important to attempt as complete a follow-up as possible and to get as much information on those lost to follow-up as possible since incompleteness introduces bias. Assessment of outcome may occur continuously during the trial (e.g. mortality in a cancer chemotherapy trial), intermittently at multiple predetermined time points, or simply at the end of the defined period of the trial.

A cardinal rule is that assessment of outcome should be completed by a researcher who is blind to randomization group membership. This requires that personnel for the recruitment and the follow-up stages do not assess the same people if they have any knowledge of randomization group. Also any information which might unblind the assessor should be either collected in a different way or left to the end so as not to influence the assessment of outcome in any conscious or unconsciousness way.

Outcome measures should preferably be understandable if they are to be influential in changing clinical practice. Most drug trials in psychiatry rely on rating scales which generate continuous scores (e.g. of depression or cognitive impairment) where these have been widely used and are held to be sensitive to differential change with treatment. However, it may be difficult to assess, for example, what a two-point change on the Hamilton Depression Rating Scale or the ADAS-Cog actually means in a clinical situation. Clinically relevant outcomes such as recovery from depression need to be used more widely. There is also an increasing role for measures which take a more holistic view of the participant and the impact of the experimental intervention, such as health-related quality of life (Guyatt et al., 1998).

Major trials will generally have a data monitoring committee set up to inspect the data that emerge from the trial before completion. Their remit is to decide whether the trial needs to be stopped early. This may be because of accumulating evidence for a strong benefit from the experimental intervention, or evidence that it appears to be harmful. Trials may also be stopped if they appear to be futile: that is, where interim analyses show that there is no treatment benefit and that the remaining trial would not allow for a benefit to become manifest. An important consideration in setting up such committees is the need for confidentiality, regular review, and pre-agreed criteria for discontinuation (Pocock, 1992; Flemming et al., 1993).

Analysis strategies

The strategy for statistical analysis should be specified prior to the commencement of the study.

The primary and secondary trial objectives are tested by comparing the outcomes of the intervention and control groups. This will normally involve a multivariate analysis. The analysis model should allow for baseline measurements of the outcome being assessed if measured, to control for pretreatment differences (Vickers and Altman, 2001). The analysis can be adjusted for any prognostic baseline clinically relevant covariates or stratification factors. Adjustment for prognostic baseline variables will increase the precision of the treatment estimates if included as covariates in the analysis. Randomization should ensure that all known and unknown baseline variables are balanced over the trial arms; there will be no baseline confounders due to the virtue of randomization. It is important to consider that treatment estimates from multivariate analysis should be presented as 'adjusted' effects, stating the covariates included in the model. For adjusted dichotomous outcomes, if possible, marginal estimates should be given (Greenland et al., 1999).

As with cohort studies, a major concern in RCTs is the completeness of follow-up. It is often hard to persuade participants to stay in the trial, and if they drop out of treatment, it is usual for studies to collect no further information on them. This causes problems, especially if there is differential drop out between the treatment and control groups. If, for example, an antidepressant was highly effective in those who could tolerate it, but caused such unpleasant side effects that over half of participants dropped out of treatment, an analysis which compared outcome on just those who completed treatment and

Box 12.4 Missing data mechanisms

- *Missing completely at random* (MCAR): data are missing independently of both observed and unobserved data.

- *Missing at random* (MAR): given the observed data, data are missing independently of unobserved data.

- *Missing not at random* (MNAR): missing observations related to values of unobserved data

the placebo group (in whom only 10% dropped out of treatment), would tend greatly to exaggerate the effectiveness of the treatment. This would, in effect, be a form of selection bias. To be able to explore the different analysis strategies for RCTs there are three principles of missing data that must first be understood (Carpenter, 2008) (Box 12.4) (also see Chapter 18 for more detail).

In the following sections we expand on the analysis sets commonly used for RCT analysis. We always recommend the guidelines of the CONSORT statement (Moher et al., 2001) and ICH E9 guideline for 'Statistical principles for clinical trials' (European Medicines Agency, 1998) should be closely followed.

Intention to treat

The intention-to-treat (ITT) principle requires all participants in a clinical trial to be included in the analysis in the groups to which they were randomly assigned, regardless of any departures from randomized treatment (Moher et al., 2001). This strategy protects against bias, as participants who depart from randomized treatment are usually a nonrandom subset whose exclusion can lead to selection bias. Full reporting of any deviations from random allocation and missing response is essential in the assessment of the necessity and appropriateness of an ITT. It gives an unbiased estimate of treatment effect and allows the greatest generalizability of the trial results. Missing data must be assessed and a suitable analysis model or method must be implemented. Trialists are expected to justify their handling of missing data and provide valid inferences under missing data assumptions (Carpenter, 2008).

Modified intention to treat

The ITT principle implies that patients are analysed according to their original allocation, regardless of the treatment they actually received. Accordingly, withdrawals, losses to follow-up, and crossovers are ignored in a strict ITT analysis. RCTs that use a modified intention-to-treat (mITT) approach are increasingly being published. White and colleagues (2011) provide a framework for ITT analyses that depends on making plausible assumptions about the missing data and including all participants in a sensitivity analysis. They argue that all observed data should be included in the analysis, but undue focus on including all randomized participants can be unhelpful because participants with no

Box 12.5 Framework for modified intention-to-treat analyses

1. Attempt to follow up all randomized participants, even if they withdraw from allocated treatment.

2. Perform a main analysis of all observed data that are valid under a plausible assumption about the missing data.

3. Perform sensitivity analyses to explore the effect of departures from the assumption made in the main analysis.

4. Account for all randomized participants, at least in the sensitivity analyses.

Reproduced with permission from White, I. R. et al. Strategy for intention to treat analysis in randomised trials with missing outcome data. *BMJ* 2011;342:d40. Copyright © 2011, British Medical Journal Publishing Group. doi: https://doi.org/10.1136/bmj.d40

post-randomization data can contribute to the results only through untestable assumptions. The key issue is therefore not how to include all participants but what assumptions about the missing data are most plausibly correct, and how to perform appropriate analyses based on these assumptions (Box 12.5).

Complier averaged causal effects

A class of methods to deal with non-compliance includes instrumental variable (IV) and complier average causal effect (CACE) approaches (Dunn et al., 2005). These approaches estimate treatment effects, defined as the impact of the intervention compared to the control condition on those who comply with their treatment assignments, by preserving randomization and accounting for potential confounding. Randomization ensures that, on average, the proportion of compliers in the control group is the same as that in the treatment group (Sommer and Zegler, 1991).

Complete case

Complete case (CC) excludes from the analysis all participants for whom the outcome measure is missing. This approach reduces sample size and leads to reduced statistical power (Altman and Bland, 2007) while increasing the potential for bias. Missing not at random data will result in invalid inferences.

Per protocol

Per protocol like complete case focuses on a subset of the trial population, excluding randomized individuals from the analyses. The effects estimated by methods involving analysis 'per protocol' (compares the compliers in the treatment group with all of the controls) or 'as treated' (compares those who receive treatment with those who do not, regardless of random allocation) will not be estimates of valid treatment effects (Sheiner and Rubin, 1995).

All trial analyses should be completed under an ITT or mITT strategy. In addition, trialists may wish to look at CACE to support the results of the ITT analysis.

Interpretation of data

Following analysis, the data need to be presented in a way that can be understood. This is helped by the use of clinically relevant outcome measures, but the paraphernalia of statistical inference can be difficult to penetrate. The presentation of the *number needed to treat* (NNT) may aid comprehensibility. This is the number of patients from your study population who need to be given the new intervention for the study period in order to achieve the desired outcome (e.g. recovery), or to prevent an undesired one (e.g. death). It is calculated as the reciprocal of the risk difference between treatment group and control (Sackett et al., 1991). If, for example, the outcome is recovery from depression, and the risk of recovery at 6 weeks in the treatment group is 0.7, whereas the risk of recovery in the control is 0.5, the risk difference is 0.2, and the NNT is five. To illustrate the meaning of this, one could imagine ten patients receiving the control condition and five of them getting better. If the same number was given the new treatment, seven would get better. Therefore, in two out of ten patients the treatment would have been responsible for recovery (assuming that the results of the trial were valid); in other words, one would need to treat five patients with the treatment, to bring about one recovery attributable to the treatment. The NNT has the unusual characteristic of having a null value of infinity (i.e. one would need to treat an infinite number of patients to bring about a recovery, if the treatment was no better than control), and therefore where a non-significant finding is being reported the 95% confidence intervals will span infinity (e.g. NNT = 40; 95% confidence interval 25, ∞, −50). A negative value on the NNT suggests that the treatment is doing harm.

RCTs typically provide unadjusted comparisons of patient outcomes according to treatment. However, trials often adjust for important predictors of outcome, prognostic factors, to allow for chance imbalances between treatment groups at baseline (Altman, 2001) although such adjustment often makes little difference to the results or conclusions. More recently, it has been proposed that adjustment using appropriate covariates can also be used to improve the power of an RCT irrespective of any baseline imbalance, this is also considered in the context of the potential to reduce the required sample size (Hernándes et al., 2004; Roozenbeek et al., 2009).

Publication, communication, and dissemination

Once a trial has been completed, its findings need to be communicated. The profound importance of all trial data being published and not just the positive is well articulated by Goldacre and his AllTrials (sometimes called All Trials or AllTrials.net) project which supports the principles of open research with 'All trials registered, all results reported' and then following a pre-specified analysis plan (Drysdale et al., 2016). This usually requires the preparation of a scientific paper or series of papers and their submission to peer-reviewed journals. This is a quality control measure, designed to assess the robustness and scientific strength of the study and its conclusions. Unfortunately, publication bias can lead to a tendency for editors and authors to prepare and publish new and significant data rather than replications or negative findings. This can distort an estimation of the true effect of findings and the techniques of systematic review and meta-analysis have developed to attempt to locate unpublished data and to incorporate it into aggregate estimates of effect size. Publication should be seen as the start of a communication strategy for novel findings as it is by drug companies. McCormack and Greenhalgh (2000) have argued powerfully, using data from the UK Prospective Diabetes Study, that there can be a problem with interpretation bias at this stage of a trial with widely disseminated conclusions being unsupported by the actual data presented in the papers. They identified powerful motivations for researchers, authors, editors, and presumably other stakeholders such as the drug industry and the voluntary sector to impart positive spin to trial data. The interpretive biases included the following:

◆ *'We've shown something here' bias*—researcher enthusiasm for a positive result.

◆ *'The result we've all been waiting for' bias*—prior expectations moulding interpretation.

◆ *'Just keep taking the tablets' bias*—overestimating the benefits of drugs.

◆ *'What the hell can we tell the public' bias*—political need for high-impact breakthroughs.

◆ *'If enough people say it, it becomes true' bias*—a bandwagon of positivity preceding publication.

That said, there is a need to ensure that important findings are made available, in a way that is accessible to them, for those who formulate policy and purchase services and also those who use them. Andrews (1999) has argued that mental health services may be particularly resistant to changing practice on the basis of empirical evidence, citing the persistence of psychoanalytic psychotherapy and the lack of implementation of family interventions for people with schizophrenia as examples.

'Explanatory' versus 'pragmatic' trials: efficacy and effectiveness

RCTs minimize the risk of bias (threats to internal validity), particularly selection bias, and are thus the best research design for decisions about the effect of different interventions, be they treatments, therapies, or delivery methods and policies. However, one of the major fault lines in the design of trials is the dynamic between purity in terms of reducing bias and generalizability (or external validity), that is, the degree to which findings of a trial can be extrapolated from the study population to other populations of interest—most often to a much broader range of patients and services in general clinical settings.

RCTs are often described as either explanatory or pragmatic. Rather than a clear divide, the terms reflect different attitudes to many aspects of trial design (MacRae, 1989) and both approaches have strengths and weaknesses. Explanatory trials take the view that it is important to investigate the effect of the intervention in ideal circumstances—so-called efficacy; while pragmatic trials seek to investigate whether the intervention works in real-world settings—so-called effectiveness. There are many ways of highlighting the differences between explanatory and pragmatic trials (Table 12.1).

Exploratory trials are often designed to produce the maximum effect size and so are often smaller that an equivalent effectiveness study, but may take time to recruit participants due to multiple exclusion criteria. Part of their attraction to technology companies and researchers alike lies in this maximization of effect. Efficacy trials are more likely to come up with a positive finding, which is good for marketing a drug and good for the researcher's publication record. In contrast, pragmatic studies generally have to be larger in order to measure smaller effect sizes. They also tend to be more complex to analyse and interpret because more 'typical' groups of participants may be less likely to want to participate in a trial, and more likely to be lost to follow-up. They may also be more likely to have incidental adverse events, such as death, since they are not selected on the basis of being unusually healthy as in many exploratory trials.

Table 12.1 Key differences between trials with explanatory and pragmatic trials

	Explanatory trials	**Pragmatic trials**
Overarching paradigm and question	Efficacy: can the intervention work?	Effectiveness: does the intervention work when used in normal practice?
Setting	'Ideal' setting	Normal or routine practice
Participants	Highly selected; poorly adherent participants and those with conditions which might dilute the effect are often excluded	Little or no selection beyond the clinical indication of interest
Intervention	Strictly enforced ('protocolized') and adherence is monitored closely	Applied flexibly as it would be in normal practice
Comparator	Placebo or no treatment	Usual care or treatment as usual
Outcomes	Often short-term surrogate endpoints, or process measures	Directly relevant to participants, funders, communities, and healthcare practitioners. Often include costs in addition to clinical outcomes
Relevance to practice	Indirect: little effort is made to match the design of the trial to the decision-making needs of those in the usual setting in which the intervention will be implemented	Direct: the trial is designed to meet the needs of those making decisions about treatment options in the setting in which the intervention will be implemented

Adapted from Treweek S and Zwarenstein M (2009). Making trials matter: pragmatic and explanatory trials and the problem of applicability. Trial, *BMJ*, 3, 10–37. DOI: https://doi.org/10.1186/1745-6215-10-37. This article is published under license to BioMed Central Ltd. This is an open access article distributed under the terms of the Creative Commons Attribution License (http://creativecommons.org/licenses/by/2.0).
Source data from Zwarenstein M, Treweek S, Gagnier J, Altman DG, Maclure M, Tunis S, Haynes B, Oxman AD, Moher D: Improving the reporting of pragmatic trials: an extension of the CONSORT Statement. *BMJ*. 2008, 337.

Incidental adverse events are worth dwelling on since they are another reason why drug companies may prefer efficacy trials. Severe adverse events are very problematic in a phase III trial (see 'The phases of pharmaceutical trials' for a description of the drug trial phases) and may occur entirely by chance. However, they are unlikely to be sufficiently common to assort equally across the intervention and control groups. They can get a drug a bad name (giving rival companies ammunition to attack the new drug) and even halt trials, whether or not they have occurred by chance. It is therefore often held that it is more sensible to exclude those with a greater likelihood of such events (e.g. the ill, the disabled, those with comorbid physical disorder, and those who are on other medication) from trials entirely.

In reality, there is a continuum with the gap between efficacy and effectiveness depending on the disorder being studied and the simplicity of the intervention. In our example of the perfect trial, efficacy is the same as effectiveness. However, in many studies the gap between research findings and clinical applicability may be huge. An example of this is provided by a study of donepezil, a treatment for Alzheimer's disease (Rogers and Friedhoff, 1996) whose exclusion criteria are age over 85 years; unable to walk freely or with a cane or walker; vision and/or hearing impairment interfering with testing; psychiatric or neurological disorder; previous or current active gastrointestinal, renal, hepatic, endocrine, or cardiovascular disease; any form of diabetes; obstructive pulmonary disease, or haematological or oncological disorders of onset within the last 2 years; vitamin B_{12} or folate deficiency; and alcohol or drug abuse. However, no mention is made in this paper of exclusions on the grounds of concurrent medication, but this is also likely given that in follow-up trials (Rogers et al., 1998a, 1998b) patients on anticholinergics, anticonvulsants, antidepressants, and antipsychotics were also excluded as well as potentially those taking other drugs with CNS activity. Clinical old age psychiatrists may find these exclusions result in a study population about as far away from those they are called to assess as possible, so bringing into question the applicability of the findings to clinical practice. This is not to say that such drugs are not of use, they may well be, but the evidence that we are often presented with means that real clinical practice is informed by an extrapolation of trial data rather than by its direct application.

Another striking example has been described by Yastrubetskaya and colleagues (1997). In a phase III trial of a new antidepressant, 188 patients were screened and 171 (91%) of them met the inclusion criteria of having sufficiently severe depression for the trial. However, when the multiple exclusion criteria were applied to this real-world sample of people with depression, only eight (4.7%) of those eligible for inclusion could be recruited into the trial. Furthermore, at least 70% of the original sample required antidepressant treatment and were provided with it.

Perhaps the way thorough these conundrums is to acknowledge that each study type has its place and it may be that at times a single study can provide efficacy data which are so clearly generalizable to clinical populations that they are in effect close to effectiveness data. However, clinicians and purchasers need to know whether an intervention works in the real world. It may be that licensing organizations such as the European Medicines

Agency and US Food and Drug Administration can suggest that such data are desirable and base their decisions more directly upon its availability. Alternatively, where there are efficacy data but no data on clinical effectiveness, it may be necessary to commission effectiveness studies, either before or after licensing. This raises questions of who could and should fund such work. Should funding for pragmatic trials be levied from drug companies as a necessary part of the licensing procedure? Or should governmental and private agencies involved in purchasing healthcare fund such work? In either case there is a strong case for such trials being independent of those who stand to gain by the sale of the intervention and also those who stand to pay by purchasing the intervention.

Additional information on randomized controlled trials

In this section we will consider some of the more common supplementary questions raised by RCTs.

Role of clinical trials units

Well-designed, appropriately powered, high-quality RCTs continue to be needed to ensure psychiatry practice is robustly evidence based. Healthcare practitioners and patients are ideally placed to identify the key clinical and service delivery uncertainties to inform the questions that such trials raise. Many well-conducted, high-impact clinical trials may have been undertaken by standalone clinical investigator teams. However, modern clinical trials are often highly complex, with ever increasing levels of methodological sophistication and regulatory requirements, and stringent quality standard processes, and require investigators and therefore require support (McFadden et al., 2015). This complexity is illustrated by the clinical trials route map (http://www.ct-toolkit.ac.uk/routemap). Clinical trials units (CTUs) are multidisciplinary specialist units that have the specific remit to support investigators navigate this complexity and support the design, conduct, and report of clinical trials. CTUs have the expertise to provide statistical, epidemiological, data, and trial management advice to successfully undertake multicentre clinical trials, nationally and internationally. Common services and functions provided by a CTU are summarized in Figure 12.2 (Gale and Juszczak, 2016).

In the UK, the need to ensure national expertise and capacity for the development and delivery of high quality was first identified by the National Cancer Research Network, a network of clinical trials researchers specifically working in cancer trials and supported by the main cancer research funders. Over the last decade, and following the success in cancer trials, the National Institute for Health Research has invested significant resources in initiatives designed to increase participation in high-quality clinical research trials. This has included the formation of disease-specific research networks to improve the recruitment of patients in trials and establishment a country-wide network of 45 UK Clinical Research Collaboration (UKCRC) registered and accredited CTUs to help improve the quality and quantity of clinical trials expertise (McFadden et al., 2015).

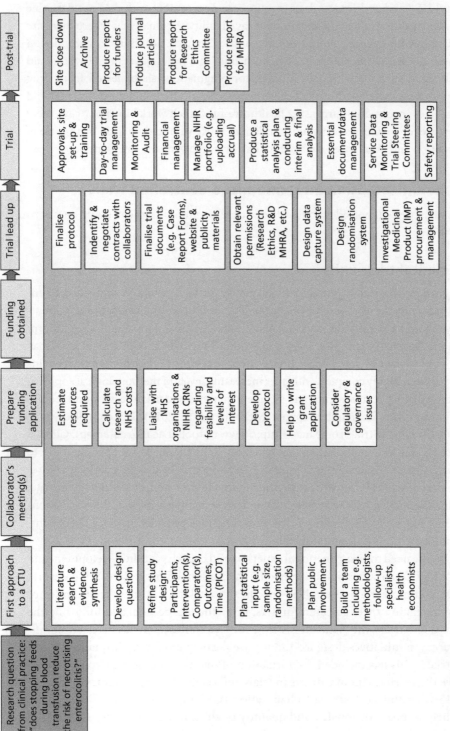

Figure 12.2 Services and functions of a clinical trials unit (CTU). CRN, Clinical Research Network; MHRA, Medicines and Healthcare products Regulatory Agency; NHS, National Health Service; NIHR, National Institute of Health Research; R&D, research and development.

Reproduced from Gale, C., Juszczak, E. A paediatrician's guide to clinical trials units. *Archives of Disease in Childhood: Education & Practice*, 101(5), 265–267. DOI: http://dx.doi. org/10.1136/archdischild-2015-310036. Copyright © BMJ Publishing Group Ltd & Royal College of Paediatrics and Child Health. All rights reserved. This is an Open Access article distributed in accordance with the terms of the Creative Commons Attribution (CC BY 4.0) http://creativecommons.org/licenses/by/4.0/.

So, how do you go about approaching a CTU for support? The first step is to formulate your clinical practice or service delivery uncertainty into a clearly defined research question using the PICO format (Participant, Intervention, Comparator, Outcome). You should also ensure that this research question has not already been answered by checking for recent systematic reviews or performing a literature search. In the UK, your nearest registered CTU can be identified from using the UKCRC CTU website (https://www.ukcrc-ctu.org.uk/search/default.asp). Approaching a CTU for support will usually involve an application form or 'collaboration request'. While it is essential that this process starts at least 3 months before any target funding deadline, the strongest collaborations and proposals often result from an iterative process involving a number of stakeholders including CTUs, patient and public involvement, research networks, study sponsor, and sites that recruit participants, which may often take considerably longer. If your proposed trial is supported, the CTU will then typically work in partnership with you and help build a strong research team to design and deliver the trial, developing the methodological, statistical, organizational, and regulatory components in preparation for the next major hurdle, and apply (where appropriate) for research grant funding.

The phases of pharmaceutical trials

The meanings of and distinctions between the various phases of new drug development can seem opaque. They are best viewed as the necessary processes which need to be completed so that the drug company can satisfy regulatory authorities such as the US Food and Drug Administration or the UK's Medicines Control Agency. These phases explicitly refer only to experiments on human participants, there will have been a substantial programme of *in vitro* and animal experiments which will have been completed before the phase I trials begin, which are beyond the scope of this chapter.

Phase I: clinical pharmacology and toxicology

This represents the first time a drug is given to humans—usually healthy volunteers in the first place followed by patients with the disorder. The purpose is to identify acceptable dosages, their scheduling, and the side effects. These are most often carried out in a single centre, requiring 20–80 patients.

Phase II: initial evaluation of efficacy

These are to determine whether the compound has any beneficial activity. They continue the process of safety monitoring and require close observation; they may be used to decide which of a number of competing compounds go through to phase III trials. They may be single or multicentre, and generally require 100–200 patients.

Phase III: evaluation of treatment effect

This is a competitive phase where the new drug is tested against standard therapy or placebo. There may also be a further element of optimal dose finding. The format for this evaluation is that of an RCT. This phase usually requires large numbers (100s to 1000s) and therefore a multicentre design.

Phase IV: post-marketing surveillance

Once a drug has been put on the market, there is a need to continue monitoring for rare and common adverse effects including mortality and morbidity. These may only become evident when the drug is used in large numbers in real clinical populations.

Complex interventions

Complex interventions are widely used in the health service, in public health practice and areas of social policy that have important health consequences such as education and housing. In 2000, the Medical Research Council published a framework and revised this in 2008 (Medical Research Council, 2000; Craig et al., 2008) to help trialists and researchers to recognize and adopt appropriate methods.

Complex interventions are usually described as interventions that contain several interacting components within the intervention and control groups. There may be many people trained to deliver the intervention and those receiving the intervention could be complex in their needs or behaviours. There may be multiple groups or organization levels targeted by the intervention, the outcomes can be numerous and varied, and a degree of flexibility can be permitted for the delivery of the intervention.

There are two key objectives for trials evaluating complex interventions. Firstly is whether they will be effective and feasible in everyday practice (Haynes, 1999). It is therefore important to understand the whole range of effects and how they vary, for example, among recipients or between sites. A key second question is how the intervention works, understanding the underlying mechanism. This may involve designing research questions targeted at evaluating mediation and moderation (Emsley et al., 2010). A well-designed trial with consideration of mechanism evaluation will lead to more effective interventions.

When developing and evaluating complex studies, trialists must have a good theoretical understanding of how the intervention causes change. Lack of effect may reflect implementation failure rather than genuine ineffectiveness; a thorough process evaluation is needed to identify any implementation problems. Variability in individual-level outcomes may reflect higher-level processes, thus sample sizes need to take into account the extra variability and cluster randomized designs may be required. A range of predefined outcome and process measures will be required to make best use of the data. Remember to always assess levels of potential outcomes, moderators, and mediators at baseline, prior to randomization. Ensuring strict standardization may be inappropriate, the intervention may work better if a degree of adaption to a local setting or participants are allowed but this must be pre-specified in the protocol. Long-term follow-up may be needed to determine whether outcomes predicted by interim or surrogate measures do occur or whether short-term changes persist.

Key elements of development and evaluation process are outlined in the 2000 framework (Figure 12.3).

There are several designs which may be applicable for evaluating complex intervention (Craig et al., 2008), details of trial designs are given in the following section.

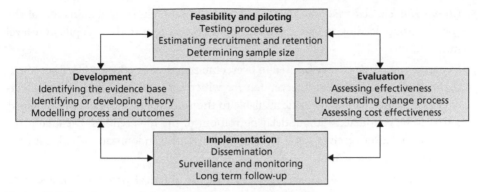

Figure 12.3 Key elements of the development and evaluation process.

Reproduced with permission from Craig, P. et al. Developing and evaluating complex interventions: the new Medical Research Council guidance, *BMJ*. 2008; 337: a1655. doi: https://doi.org/10.1136/bmj.a1655. Copyright © 2008, British Medical Journal Publishing Group.

There are many issues surrounding trials of complex interventions but methods are continuing to be developed. The most important point is the need to consider evaluation requirements in the planning of new initiatives (Dunn et al., 2015):

1. Does it work?

2. How does it work?

3. Who does it work for?

4. What factors make it work better?

Trial designs

1. *Individually randomized trials*: individuals are randomly allocated to receive either an experimental intervention(s) or control treatment.

2. *Crossover trials*: in a crossover trial the intention is that each patient acts as their own control. Randomization is to receipt of the intervention or the control followed by a wash-out period then the treatment not received in the first phase.

3. *Factorial trials*: interventions may be given alone or together so that their individual and joint effects can be evaluated.

4. *Community trials*: sometimes the unit of randomization (i.e. the entity to which the treatment is given) is not an individual but is a community. A good example of this is fluoridation which can only be achieved on a population basis, so that the reservoir and the population it serves becomes the unit of randomization. The number within each community is of secondary importance and may add little to the statistical power of the study. With such interventions there are clear possibilities of problems with compliance (e.g. choosing to drink bottled water only), contamination (travel to fluoridated communities), and blinding (it may be politically unacceptable to prevent the community from knowing what is being done to them).

5. *Cluster randomized trials*: are one solution to the problem of contamination of the control group, leading to biased estimates of effect size, in trials of population-level interventions.

6. *Stepped wedge designs*: may be used to overcome practical or ethical objections to experimentally evaluating an intervention for which there is some evidence of effectiveness or which cannot be made available to the whole population at once. It allows a trial to be conducted without delaying roll-out of the intervention. Eventually, the whole population receives the intervention, but with randomization built into the phasing of implementation.

7. *Preference trials and randomized consent designs*: practical or ethical obstacles to randomization can sometimes be overcome by using non-standard designs. When patients have strong preferences among treatments, basing treatment allocation on patients' preferences or randomizing patients before seeking consent may be appropriate.

8. *N-of-1 designs*: conventional trials aim to estimate the average effect of an intervention in a population. *N*-of-1 trials, in which individuals undergo interventions with the order or scheduling decided at random, can be used to assess between- and within-person change and to investigate theoretically predicted mediators of that change.

9. *Adaptive designs*: an adaptive design is defined as a design that allows modifications to the trial and/or statistical procedures of the trial after its initiation without undermining its validity and integrity (Chow, 2005). The purpose is to make clinical trials more flexible, efficient, and fast.

Other intervention designs

1. *Comparison with historical controls*: in this design, a group of people are treated with a novel intervention and their progress is compared with a group that has been studied in the past with a different or no treatment and whose outcome is known. A major problem with this approach lies in the other changes which may have occurred as well as the intervention (e.g. lifestyle, diet, healthcare delivery, and other risk and prognostic factors). It may be difficult or impossible to adjust for these factors if they have been incompletely recorded or measured in a different way.

2. *Simultaneous comparison of differently treated groups*: this design strategy is subject to bias since there is seldom any element of randomization. The groups for treatment are usually selected either by the treating physicians or by the patients themselves and so are very unlikely to be representative of all individuals with the disorder. It may be impossible to adjust for the effects of variables other than the treatment being studied such as other healthcare provided, illness severity, and concomitant disorders. Inferences concerning the relative efficacy of the interventions may therefore be limited substantially. The same problems are associated with 'waiting list control' evaluations where there is the possibility of any discretion on the part of patients or treating physicians.

3. *Patient preference trials*: in trials of this sort, the patient takes a more or less active role in deciding which of the treatment arms he or she will complete. This clearly compromises the power of randomization and blindness. However, such approaches may be necessary where the belief systems of a study population mean that a standard RCT is not possible. In these trials, patients with strong views as to treatment are given the intervention they want and those without preferences (and those with preferences who still agree) are randomized in the normal way. The data from such studies are often difficult to interpret and they will usually need to be very large to enable adequate statistical power for between-group comparisons.

Conclusion

We hope the reader takes two messages away from this chapter. First, that RCTs are difficult, complicated, and expensive. They are not something that that should be attempted without experienced help and support, and they are not something that can be done 'of a Tuesday' because you have had a good idea for a treatment. Trials almost by definition have the capacity to harm as well as help so they are an ethically serious undertaking. In essence, they are an extremely complicated and expensive way of answering a single question, so you need to have your question right and be sure your trial is really necessary. The second message is that they are also absolutely vital, the nature and quality of inference that can be drawn from well-designed and well-conducted trials is unparalleled and unique. RCTs can tell you what works and what harms. They are among the most important of aids in deciding what we should do for those that seek help from us. As such, we all have a duty to understand them and use their data wisely.

Practical exercises

1. Discuss the following with respect to their implications for a randomized controlled trial:
   a. Extent of exclusion criteria—can you identify a true 'effectiveness' study in your field of research? Is this important?
   b. Randomization—how can this be achieved in service-level research?
   c. Blinding—is this feasible in psychiatry?
   d. Sample size—can a study ever be too large?
   e. Intention-to-treat analysis—what outcomes should be assigned to people who are immediately lost to follow-up?

2. Pick a controversial treatment in a chosen area of practice—ideally an intervention which has positive trials but which is not yet fully accepted by clinicians and/or 'established' as cost-effective. Divide the students into three groups. One group are to represent patients or their advocates, one group are to represent prescribing doctors (or those who will deliver the treatment), and one group are to represent policymakers

(e.g. advisors to a health minister) who have to consider the possible costs of the treatment (and assume that what is spent on this will have to be taken away from other aspects of care). Allow the groups about 30 minutes to prepare a brief presentation and let the fight commence! [Note: the choice of the 'treatment will depend on the nature of the class and current wider debate. Previously successful examples have included atypical antipsychotic agents, anticholinesterase treatments for Alzheimer's disease, and novel pharmacological interventions for smoking cessation. The purpose of the exercise is to emphasize that proof of efficacy is only the beginning ...]

References

Altman, D.G. (2001). Adjustment for covariate imbalance. In: Redmond, C. and Colton, T. (eds.). *Biostatistics in clinical trials*, pp. 122–127. Chichester: John Wiley & Sons.

Altman, D.G. and Bland, J.M. (1999). Treatment allocation in controlled trials: why randomise? *BMJ*, **318**, 1209.

Altman, D.G. and Bland, J.M. (2007). Missing data. *BMJ*, **334**, 424.

Altman, D.G. and Schulz, K.F. (2001). Concealing treatment allocation in randomised trials. *BMJ*, **323**, 446–447.

Amberson, J.B., McMahon, B.T., and Pinner, M. (1931). A clinical trial of sanocrysin in pulmonary tuberculosis. *American Review of Tuberculosis*, **24**, 401–435.

Andrews, G. (1999). Randomised controlled trials in psychiatry: important but poorly accepted. *BMJ*, **319**, 562–564.

Armitage, P. (1982). The role of randomisation in clinical trials. *Statistics in Medicine*, **1**, 345–352.

Banerjee, S. and Dickenson, E. (1997). Evidence based health care in old age psychiatry. *Psychiatry in Medicine*, **27**, 283–292.

Begg, C., Cho, M., Eastwood, S., Horton, R., Moher, D., Olkin, I., et al. (1996). Improving the quality of reporting of randomized controlled trials: the CONSORT statement. *JAMA*, **276**, 637–639.

Blum, A.L., Chalmers, T.C., Deutch, E., Koch-Weser, J., Rosen, A., Tygstrup, N., et al. (1987). The Lugano statement on controlled clinical trials. *Journal of International Medical Research*, **15**, 2–22.

Box, J.A. (1980). RA Fisher and the design of experiments, 1922–1926. *American Statistician*, **34**, 1–7.

Bull, J.P. (1959). The historical development of clinical therapeutic trials. *Journal of Chronic Diseases*, **10**, 218–248.

Campbell, M., Fitzpatrick, R., Haines, A., Kinmouth, L., Sandercock, P., Spiegelhalter, D., and Tyrer, P. (2000). Framework for design and evaluation of complex interventions to improve health. *BMJ*, **321**, 694–696.

Carpenter, J.R. and Kenward, M. (2008). *Missing data in randomised controlled trials—a practical guide*. Publication RM03/JH17/MK. Birmingham: National Institute for Health Research/ http://www.missingdata.org.uk

Centre for Evidence-Based Medicine (2009). Oxford Centre for Evidence-based Medicine – levels of evidence (March 2009). https://www.cebm.net/2009/06/oxford-centre-evidence-based-medicine-levels-evidence-march-2009/

Chow, S.C., Chang, M., and Pong, A. (2005). Statistical consideration of adaptive methods in clinical development. *Journal of Biopharmaceutical Statistics*, **15**, 575–91.

Craig, P., Dieppe, P., Macintyre, S., Michie, S., Nazareth, I., and Petticrew, M. (2008). Developing and evaluating complex interventions: the new Medical Research Council guidance. *BMJ*, **337**, a1655.

D'Arcy Hart, P. (1999). A change in scientific approach: from alternation to randomised allocation in clinical trials in the 1940s. *BMJ*, **319**, 572–573.

Drysdale, H., Slade, E., Goldacre, B., and Heneghan, C. (2016). Outcomes in the trial registry should match those in the protocol. *Lancet*, **388**, 340.

Dunn, G., Emsley, R., Liu, H., Landau, S., Green, J., White, I., and Pickles, A. (2015). Evaluation and validation of social and psychological markers in randomised trials of complex interventions in mental health: a methodological research programme. *Health Technology Assessment*, **19**, 1–115, v–vi.

Dunn, G., Maracy, M., and Tomenson, B. (2005). Estimating treatment effects from randomized clinical trials with noncompliance and loss to follow-up: the role of instrumental variable methods. *Statistical Methods in Medical Research*, **14**, 369–395.

Edwards, S.J.L., Lilford, R.J., and Hewison, J. (1998). The ethics of randomised controlled trials from the perspective of patients, the public, and healthcare professionals. *BMJ*, **317**, 1209–1212.

Emsley, R., Dunn, G., and White, I.R. (2010). Mediation and moderation of treatment effects in randomised controlled trials of complex interventions. *Statistical Methods in Medical Research*, **19**, 237–270.

European Medicines Agency (1998). ICH Topic E9: Statistical principles for clinical trials (CPMP/ICH/363/96). https://www.ema.europa.eu/en/ich-e9-statistical-principles-clinical-trials

Evans, S. and Pocock, S. (2001). Societal responsibilities of clinical trial sponsors. *BMJ*, **322**, 569–570.

Flemming, T.R. and De Mets, D.L. (1993). Monitoring of clinical trials: issues and recommendations. *Controlled Clinical Trials*, **14**, 183–197.

Frison, L. and Pocock, S.J. (1992). Repeated measures in clinical trials: analysis using mean for summary statistics and its implications for design. *Statistics in Medicine*, **11**, 1685–1704.

Gale, C. and Juszczak, E.A. (2016). Paediatrician's guide to clinical trials units. *Archives of Disease in Childhood: Education and Practice Edition*, **101**, 265–267.

Greenland, S., Robins, J.M., and Pearl, J. (1999). Confounding and collapsibility in causal inference. *Statistical Science*, **14**, 29–46.

Greenwood, M. and Yule, G.U. (1915). The statistics of anti-typhoid and anti-cholera inoculations and the interpretations of such statistics in general. *Proceedings of the Royal Society of Medicine, Sections of Medicine, Pathology, and Epidemiology and State Medicine*, **8**, 113–194.

Guyatt, G.H., Juniper, E.F., Walter, S.D., Griffith, L.E., and Goldstein, R.S. (1998). Interpreting treatment effects in randomised trials. *BMJ*, **316**, 690–693.

Haynes, B. (1999). Can it work? Does it work? Is it worth it? The testing of healthcare interventions is evolving. *BMJ*, **319**, 652–653.

Hernández, A.V., Steyerberg, E.W., and Habema, J.D.F. (2004). Covariate adjustment in randomized controlled trials with dichotomous outcomes increases statistical power and reduces sample size requirements. *Journal of Clinical Epidemiology*, **57**, 454–460.

Hill, A.B. (1963). Medical ethics and controlled trials. *British Medical Journal*, **i**, 1943.

Kerry, S.M. and Bland, M. (1998). The intracluster correlation coefficient in cluster randomisation. *BMJ*, **316**, 1455–1460.

Kunz, R. and Oxman, A.D. (1998). The unpredictability paradox: review of empirical comparisons of randomised and non-randomised clinical trials. *BMJ*, **317**, 1185–1190.

Lievre, M., Menard, J., Bruckert, E., Cogneau, J., Delahaye, F., Giral, P., et al. (2001). Premature discontinuation of clinical trial for reasons not related to efficacy, safety, or feasibility. *BMJ*, **322**, 603–606.

Lijmer, J.G., Mol, B.W., Heisterkamp, S., Bonsel, G.J., Prins, M.H., van der Meulen, J.H., et al. (1999). Empirical evidence of design-related bias in studies of diagnostic test. *JAMA*, **282**, 1061–1066.

Lilienfield, A.M. (1982). Ceteris paribus: the evolution of the clinical trial. *Bulletin of the History of Medicine*, **56**, 1–56.

Lind, J. (1753). *A treatise of the scurvy*. Edinburgh: Sands, Murray & Cochran.

MacRae, K.D. (1989). Pragmatic versus explanatory trials. *International Journal of Technology Assessment in Health Care*, **5**, 333–339.

McCormack, J. and Greenhalgh, T. (2000). Seeing what you want to see in randomised controlled trials: versions and perversions of the UKPDS data. *BMJ*, **320**, 1720–1723.

McFadden, E., Bashir, S., Canham, S., Darbyshire, J., Davidson, P., Day, S., et al. (2015). The impact of registration of clinical trials units: the UK experience. *Clinical Trials*, **12**, 166–173.

Medical Research Council (1948). Streptomycin treatment of pulmonary tuberculosis. *British Medical Journal*, **ii**, 769–782.

Medical Research Council (2000). *A framework for the development and evaluation of RCTs for complex interventions to improve health*. London: Medical Research Council.

Moher, D., Schulz, K.F., and Altman, D.G. (2001). The CONSORT statement: revised recommendations for improving the quality of reports of parallel-group randomised trials. *Lancet*, **357**, 1191–1194.

Pocock, S.J. (1983). *Clinical trials: a practical approach*. Chichester: Wiley.

Pocock, S.J. (1992). When to stop a clinical trial. *BMJ*, **305**, 235–240.

Porta, M. (ed.) (2014). *A dictionary of epidemiology*, 6th edn. Oxford: Oxford University Press.

Roberts, C. and Torgerson, D.J. (1999). Baseline imbalance in randomised controlled trials. *BMJ*, **319**, 185.

Rogers, S.L. and Friedhoff, L.T. (1996). The efficacy and safety of donepezil in patients with Alzheimer's disease: results of a US multicentre, randomised, double-blind, placebo-controlled trial. *Dementia*, **7**, 293–303.

Rogers, S.L., Farlow, M.R., Doody, R.S., Mohs, R., and Friedhoff, L.T. (1998a). A 24-week, double-blind, placebo-controlled trial of donepezil in patients with Alzheimer's disease. *Neurology*, **50**, 136–145.

Rogers, S.L., Doody, R.S., Mohs, R.C., Friedhoff, L.T. (1998b). Donepezil improves cognition and global function in Alzheimer's disease. *Archives of Internal Medicine*, **158**, 1021–1031.

Roozenbeek, B., Maas, A.I.R., Lingsma, H.F., Butcher, I., Lu, J., Marmarou, A., et al. (2009). Baseline characteristics and statistical power in randomized controlled trials: selection, prognostic targeting, or covariate adjustment? *Critical Care Medicine*, **37**, 2683–2690.

Sackett, D.L., Haynes, R.B., Gutatt, G.H., Tugwell, P. (1991). *Clinical epidemiology: a basis science for clinical medicine*. Boston, MA: Little Brown.

Sacks, H., Chalmers, T.C., and Smith, H. (1982). Randomized versus historical controls for clinical trials. *American Journal of Medicine*, **72**, 233–240.

Schultz, K.F. (1995). Subverting randomisation in controlled trials. *JAMA*, **274**, 1456–1458.

Schultz, K.F., Chalmers, I., Hayes, R.J., and Altman, D.G. (1995). Empirical evidence of bias. Dimensions of methodological quality associated with estimates of treatment effects in controlled trials. *JAMA*, **273**, 408–412.

Sheiner, L.B. and Rubin, D.B. (1995). Intention-to-treat analysis and the goals of clinical-trials. *Clinical Pharmacology and Therapeutics*, **57**, 6–15.

Silverman, W.A. and Chalmers, I. (2001). Casting and drawing lots: a time honoured way of dealing with uncertainty and ensuring fairness. *BMJ*, **323**, 1467–1468.

Sommer, A. and Zeger, S.L. (1991). On estimating efficacy from clinical trials. *Statistics in Medicine*, **10**, 45–52.

Spaight, S.J., Nash, S., Finison, L.J., and Patterson, W.B. (1984). Medical oncologists' participation in cancer clinical trials. *Progress in Clinical and Biological Research*, **156**, 49–61.

Taylor, K.M. and Kelner, M. (1987). Interpreting physician participation in randomized clinical trials— are patients really informed? *Journal of Health and Social Behavior*, **28**, 389–400.

Torgerson, D.J. and Roberts, C. (1999). Randomisation methods: concealment. *BMJ*, **319**, 375–376.

Treweek, S. and Zwarenstein, M. (2009). Making trials matter: pragmatic and explanatory trials and the problem of applicability. *Trial*, **3**, 10–37.

Vickers, A.J. and Altman, D.G. (2001). Analysing controlled trials with baseline and follow up measurements. *BMJ*, **323**, 1123–1124.

White, I.R., Horton, N.J., Carpenter, J., and Pocock, S.J. (2011). Strategy for intention to treat analysis in randomised trials with missing outcome data. *BMJ*, **342**, d40.

Yastrubetskaya, O., Chiu, E., and O'Connell, S. (1997). Is good clinical research practice for clinical trials good clinical practice? *International Journal of Geriatric Psychiatry*, **12**, 227–231.

Chapter 13

Surveillance, case registers, and big data

Tamsin Ford, Robert Stewart, and Johnny Downs

The application of clinical data to research and why it is important

Health and social care organizations collect a huge amount of data, which are a potentially useful resource for researchers who wish to study clinical issues '*in vivo*'. While administrative datasets are likely to contain more variations in recording and missing information than those completed by small teams working to a clear research protocol, they can afford distinct opportunities that would be difficult to achieve through individually funded research studies—particularly in scale (sample size) and generalizability. This chapter discusses types of research that typically use clinical data in mental healthcare, before considering more broadly the methodological and governance issues that impinge on such use.

Surveillance

What is surveillance?

Surveillance is defined by the 'systematic, ongoing collection, analysis and interpretation of data, closely integrated with the timely and coherent dissemination of the results ... to those who have a right to know so that action can be taken for health improvement or illness prevention' (Porta, 2008). Arguably, surveillance should be 'continuous', which can be used to distinguish it from its more episodic cousin, 'monitoring'. Public health teams often rely on surveillance methods to investigate 'diseases themselves or factors influencing disease' (Porta, 2008), which includes the collection of investigative or control measures in the population. The link to investigative or control measures is also important, while the data collected may pertain 'to diseases themselves or factors influencing disease' (Porta, 2008) language that indicates the prominent role of surveillance to public health. This separates surveillance from screening (testing to detect novel disease at an early stage at an individual level) by its broader focus on factors that may influence prevalence and management at a population level.

History and application of surveillance to mental health

Surveillance was developed as a response to infectious diseases; its application to chronic disease came later. Mental health only became a focus of surveillance in the late 1990s, perhaps as a result of the international recognition of the huge burden of disease related to mental illness and its strong links to physical ill health and premature mortality (Freeman et al., 2010). Much public mental health work involves the collection of mental health data in morbidity surveys or routine health enquiries. Strictly speaking, these represent monitoring rather than surveillance (Singleton et al., 2003), but common examples of continuous surveillance of relevance to public mental health are the collation of data on deaths by suicide and the monitoring of adverse drug reactions, both of which have proved rich sources of data for research (Department of Health, 2014b; Thomas et al., 2014).

The study of rare disorders and events: a special type of surveillance

Rare disorders and events are difficult to study because even large population surveys detect small numbers of affected individuals. For example, the second British Child Mental Health Survey studied 7977 children and reported a prevalence of 0.9% for pervasive developmental disorders (Green et al., 2005) or 67 children; too few for detailed analyses. To study these rare disorders, which are often severe, debilitating, and require extensive support, academics have been exploring methods that minimize the selection biases inherent in clinical samples. However, these biases are lessened for disorders that are so severe that clinical contact is almost inevitable. For example, the British Paediatric Surveillance Unit (http://www.rcpch.ac.uk/bpsu) has applied surveillance methodology to study the clinical management of rare disorders as they present to consultant paediatricians since the 1980s. The results from some of the studies that used the system have changed practice and policy around several conditions; for example, the concentration of care for children with primary biliary atresia within centres of excellence dramatically reduced mortality (Davenport et al., 2004). A more recent psychiatric example is the provision of estimates of the number of young adults who want and need to continue medication for ADHD after the age boundary between child and adult mental health services, which have been shared with commissions and the National Institute of Clinical Excellence (Eke et al., 2019). Similar units are now active in other countries and for other specialties.

In 2005, the Child and Adolescent Psychiatry Surveillance System (CAPSS) was developed to maximize the identification of cases for a study of early-onset eating disorder in the UK and the Republic of Ireland (Nicholls et al., 2011). The pilot system was feasible and acceptable to child and adolescent psychiatrists; 99% of responding psychiatrists supporting the need for surveillance and 95% stating that they would continue to contribute (Lynn et al., 2012). Since that time, further studies have been run (including non-transient conversion disorder, early-onset bipolar disorder, non-affective psychosis, gender identify disorder, childhood disintegrative disorder, early onset depression and Sydenham's Chorea (Sharma et al., 2009; Ani et al., 2013; Tiffin and Kitchen, 2015).

Figure 13.1 illustrates the methodology. A 'card' (now an email) is sent each month to each consultant child and adolescent psychiatrist in the United Kingdom and the Republic of Ireland that lists the conditions currently under study with a reminder of the case definition. Obviously the return of cards, even if no relevant cases have been seen, is essential to separate no contact from non-response. CAPSS notifies the researchers

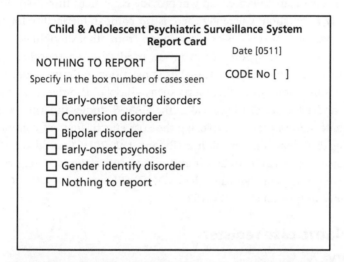

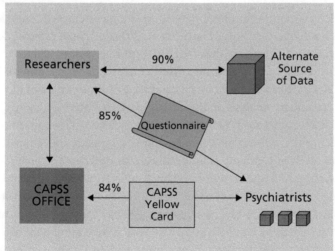

Figure 13.1 Reporting card and illustration of how the Child and Adolescent Psychiatry Surveillance System (CAPSS) works.

- CAPSS sends cards monthly to all consultant child and adolescent psychiatrists listing the conditions under study.
- Psychiatrists return the card reporting which if any conditions they have seen in the last month.
- CAPSS alerts the research team to reported cases; the research team collect data from the reporting psychiatrist.

when a case is reported, and the researchers collect data via questionnaire from the reporting clinician. Studies are kept 'on the card' for a predetermined number of months and provide data on incidence rates, presenting features, and management. Some studies will have a follow-up questionnaire. Incidence calculations are therefore derived from prospective service presentations, with the assumption that such disorders or rare events are likely to come to senior psychiatric attention. This is an important characteristic for events or disorders in surveillance, and will provide equivalent thresholds for detection across the study population. Currently there is no comparable facility for surveillance among other psychiatric specialties or practitioners from other disciplines. While psychiatry deals with fewer rare syndromes than, say, paediatrics or neurology, this type of surveillance is ideal for the study of unusual drug reactions and more common presentations that occur rarely among certain groups, such as bipolar disorder or psychosis among young people under the age of 14 years as in the CAPSS studies described earlier. Other examples include studies that are exploring the cost effectiveness of community-based specialist eating disorder teams for children (Byford et al., 2019; CostEd: http://www.nets. nihr.ac.uk/projects/hsdr/1213670) and transition to adult services among young people with attention deficit hyperactivity disorder (ADHD) (Eke et al., 2019; CATCh-uS: http:// www.nets.nihr.ac.uk/projects/hsdr/142152).

The psychiatric case register

Brief history

The psychiatric case register has been defined as 'a patient-centred longitudinal record of contacts with a defined set of psychiatric services that originates from a defined population' (Horn, 1986). The concept thus overlaps with that of surveillance in clinical settings. Collecting routine clinical data on a disorder to ascertain and monitor its incidence might be called surveillance; assembling a database of people with this disorder for further research (secondary analysis and/or recruitment for interview) would constitute a case register. Case registers are as old as psychiatric research itself—the seminal studies of Kraeplin, Bleuler, and others essentially involved the systematic collection of information on people who received routine mental healthcare in order to characterize and distinguish the presentations and courses of potential underlying disorders. Indeed, it could be claimed that epidemiology itself began with John Snow's 1854 systematic collection of cholera cases. In mental health research, case registers were a major feature for many decades, reaching a peak in the 1960s and 1970s with a large number of regional and national collections. However, this was followed by a rapid decline to near-extinction in the 1980s. External factors such as changes in legal and lay opinion on data protection were likely to have played some role in the decline, underlining the importance of achieving effective governance models in the future (Strobl et al., 2000). However, to some extent case registers simply sank beneath their own bureaucracy because of a reliance on routine data collection in clinical settings for research purposes. This is an important lesson for sustainability. Without a clear clinical academic drive (e.g. because of a shift towards other interests), enthusiasm wanes, funding falls away, and health services rapidly return to collecting information for clinical rather than research priorities. Finally, a third reason for the decline in case registers during the 1980s is that information technology was not adequate at that time, particularly as health records were paper based and manual data entry was required for any derived information resource.

The advent of electronic health records has been described as providing the opportunity for a 'next generation' of case registers (Perera et al., 2009), primarily because the computerization of clinical information means that clinical databases used for research no longer have to involve additional manual creation. In addition, there have been substantial hardware and software advances which allow the storage and manipulation of hitherto unrealized volumes of data, coupled with 'big data' initiatives in wholly unrelated fields which can be adapted and harnessed. These do not solve all the challenges faced by the case register—governance and source data quality are still major considerations—however, they do at least remove some of the obstacles. Most importantly they provide the potential for sustainability because data accrue naturally over time with no necessity for additional impositions on clinical services.

Applications

Before considering the challenges and methodological considerations further, it is helpful to summarize the potential contributions of these types of data to health research. These can be broadly grouped as follows:

1. *Descriptive studies: case characteristics.* At their most basic level, surveillance and case registers are simply the extension of the case series—that is, a means of collecting descriptive data for hypothesis generation. The distinction is in sample size, coverage, and representativeness, rendering more robust conclusions.

2. *Descriptive studies: community prevalence and incidence.* If a case register can claim to refer to a definable source population (i.e. primarily if it is a collection of all cases within a defined geographic catchment), then it can be used to calculate disorder prevalence, although it is important to bear in mind that these statistics apply to clinically diagnosed cases. True community prevalence estimation requires a cross-sectional survey of a community sample applying research instruments and/or diagnostic assessments to ascertain disorders, and the difference between the two approaches depends on the 'penetrance' of the disorder (i.e. what proportion of community cases are likely to receive a clinical diagnosis and thus appear in the case register). For case registers with continued data collection, incidence rates can similarly be calculated, and clearly this overlaps with surveillance.

3. *Analytic studies: disease risk factors.* Case registers can be used to provide cases for case–control studies, and community cohort studies might conceivably use a local or national register for ascertaining disease incidence as an outcome—for example, an important early study of urban environment and schizophrenia risk linked conscription records with a national mental healthcare registry to compare incidence rates by

exposure status (Lewis et al., 1992). The value of a case register for this purpose depends on the disorder in question; it is most likely to be advantageous for studies of rare and severe disorders—that is, where screening would be impractical and where most cases in the population will receive a clinical diagnosis.

4. *Analytic studies: disease outcomes.* Arguably the most important application of the case register is to support cohort studies describing the course and prognosis of mental disorders, and investigating factors predicting these outcomes. Case registers are also a near-essential resource for investigating predictors of response to interventions (including adverse events) because randomized controlled trials rarely have sufficiently large or generalizable samples, even when combined and meta-analysed, to address these questions. Primarily the role of the case register is to provide appropriately representative clinical samples for these cohort studies. Outcome ascertainment might then be carried out by re-contacting participants for formal follow-up, as in a study of psychiatric outcomes of childhood depression (Fombonne et al., 2001). Routine data accruing in records-derived registers potentially allow very large historic cohort studies to be assembled at relatively little cost, their applicability depending on the research question and the nature of the routine data available. Surveillance studies that include a follow-up questionnaire can similarly provide information on outcomes.

5. *Randomized controlled trials.* Case registers theoretically allow targeted sample recruitment for trials, providing a pre-characterized population of people with given disorders and thus minimizing the burdensome screening of clinical samples for inclusion and exclusion criteria. A prerequisite is usually that patients present on the register have provided prior agreement to be contacted in this respect. Records-derived registers also potentially allow routine outcome ascertainment, further increasing the cost-efficiency of the trial, although this depends on data availability and quality (Richards et al., 2014). Finally, records-derived case registers are increasingly recognized as sources of information for pilot investigations of trial feasibility—for example, modelling the potential impact on recruitment of applying different inclusion and exclusion criteria.

Methodological considerations with routine clinical data

The primary methodological challenge for both surveillance and case registers lies in the availability and/or quality of information which can be derived from routine sources.

Data availability

A key decision in setting up a data resource for surveillance or a case register is whether component information will be obtained from what is routinely available or whether it will be specifically collected. Apart from suicide rates, there are few routinely collected statistics for mental health; surveillance and other mechanisms have therefore had to be put in place to monitor conditions of interest. Surveillance units for rare syndromes, such as CAPSS, apply a surveillance definition on the reporting card, which provides operationalized criteria to allow psychiatrists to assess if any child that they have seen should be reported. This is broader than the analytical definition of a case applied by the research team to reported cases and verified by responses to the initial questionnaire. The development of these definitions requires a great deal of thought to avoid clinicians completing questionnaires for cases that do not meet criteria if the surveillance definition is too broad as well as missing cases if either definition is too narrow. For all kinds of surveillance, it is good practice to try and triangulate findings from different sources of data to verify findings, because as mentioned previously, the coding and completeness of data collected routinely will be more varied than that completed purely for research. It is key that studies are clinically salient and avoid over-burdening clinicians, as widespread opt-outs and/or failure to return questionnaires may introduce bias and undermine the generalizability of the data.

Case registers have ranged from those involving in-depth specific data collection to those relying on information collected in routine clinical practice, models which have been considered in depth in a pair of editorials on the 'small' and 'big' case register (see 'Further Reading'). Considering data availability, there has been a long-held (and probably long-true) assumption that the size of an information resource is inversely proportional to the depth/detail of information available. Research cohorts are small but well characterized; administrative data are large but with few variables. However, electronic health records databases present an opportunity for collections that have both very large samples and very large volumes of information on individual cases: a classic big data challenge.

From a research perspective, the 'depth' of information from health records has until recently been theoretical rather than actual. Health records have always contained a great deal of information on individual cases, but only a tiny proportion of this has been available as structured data amenable to statistical analysis. In this respect, earlier registers were limited by the requirement for manual data entry: whether transferring information from paper-based structured fields or extracting interpreted and assimilated information from text. Electronic health records allow structured fields to be extracted and transformed into databases without additional data entry, but also potentially allow at least some degree of automated text processing. At the most basic level, simple keyword searches can be used to identify rare syndromes from large databases, although they may well require supplementary manual coding of text for final definition (Su et al., 2014). More potentially transformative has been the application of natural language processing to provide automatically structured data on a range of constructs. Given the very large volumes of detailed text contained in a standard mental health record (e.g. case summaries, outpatient reviews, medico-legal reports, etc.), this could conceivably revolutionize the potential of the case register for in-depth characterization of clinical course and outcome, particularly as natural language processing techniques are developing rapidly in other data domains. The field is in its infancy in mental health research, but examples of applications include the characterization of bipolar disorder (Castro et al., 2015), and the ascertainment of negative symptoms of schizophrenia (Patel et al., 2015). Recent enhancements in a case register sourced from electronic mental health records using natural language processing, as well as data linkages, have recently been described in detail (Perera et al., 2016).

Data quality

The preeminent consideration with any routine data is that they are not collected for research purposes. Even when a research instrument has been incorporated into clinical care and forms a component of information derived for surveillance or a case register, it is unlikely to be as standardized in its application as the same measure administered by a small group of trained researchers. Data quality considerations can be grouped as follows:

1. *Accuracy*. As described in Chapter 15, non-differential measurement error biases findings towards the null, and true associations may be missed as a consequence. Routine data tend to be collected by large numbers of staff with limited scope for specific training on any incorporated measurements, and accuracy is inevitably compromised. Clearly the more complex or ambiguous the instrument, the more vulnerable it will be to measurement error.

2. *Standardization*. Careful definitions are important but researchers may have little control over these. For example, suicide verdicts are not returned for children under 10 years of age and statistics on 10–14-year-olds do not include deaths with an undetermined cause (seven in 2011 and ten in 2012 in England) that may relate to neglect or abuse as well as self-inflicted injury in this age group. In contrast, self-inflicted injury is assumed for indeterminate deaths in those over 15 years (Department of Health, 2014a). For all age groups, different practices across regions and countries in the recording of death by suicide complicate research in this field.

3. *Provenance*. Deficient accuracy and standardization (within or between data sources) are important considerations but can potentially be overcome in large registers—that is, where sample sizes are sufficient to identify associations of interest despite shortcomings in measurement accuracy. More challenging are intrinsic biases arising from the way in which information is recorded, and the importance of understanding source data provision cannot be emphasized enough. For example, in databases derived from remunerated health services, diagnoses may be recorded in order to justify an insurance payment or to justify a particular treatment being given (Jensen and Weisz, 2002); this clearly compromises any attempt to investigate differences in treatment profiles between diagnoses. Where routinely administered scales are used to justify funding to services then there is clearly an incentive for staff to maximize severity measures at initial assessment (justifying the acceptance of a referral) and to minimize them at the point of discharge (justifying the treatment given). Ultimately, the best measures for secondary analyses are those which are relatively unambiguous (such as demographic factors) and those where there are clinical incentives to maximize accuracy and no administrative biases. For example, the routine recording of cognitive function scores in the context of dementia care is primarily carried out by clinicians because they know that they or their colleagues may reassess the same patient in future and will appreciate

an accurate previous measure. The same can be said for a lot of information recorded in text fields, further underlining the potential value of its extraction through natural language processing.

4. *Missing data*. As well as the problem with unfilled fields within records systems, which may limit the scope for analyses and will be more frequent than with data collected specifically for research, there are also more intrinsic issues concerning the nature of the services providing data. For example, a case register drawing information from a mental healthcare provider will only be able to describe characteristics and occurrences occurring during periods when someone is receiving care from that provider. There are thus 'windows' of time when information is available on that person, interspersed with data-free periods following discharges, which, of course, are not random events but contingent on clinical improvement or disengagement. These need to be factored into the design of analyses—for example, cases with longer periods of available data may become an increasingly unrepresentative subgroup. Clearly this is only a consideration where information depends on a case receiving active care from a provider and does not, for example, apply to mortality data collected at a population rather than service level.

Data availability and quality are to some extent overlapping constructs (e.g. the problem of missing data can be described under either heading) and are both fundamental to the way in which case registers and surveillance initiatives have been designed over the years. A common point of discussion concerns the extent to which clinical services might be incentivized or required to generate more complete or accurate data. However, although a high-quality clinical service with seamless incorporation of research instruments is an attractive concept, it has yet to be demonstrated that these models are applicable beyond specialist centres with strong leadership or that they have long-term sustainability following changes in leadership. Furthermore, there is a frequent assumption that improvements in source data have to be achieved through increasing the structure of the health record. This does potentially increase the volume of immediately-accessible data points for analysis, provided that clinical staff can be persuaded to complete structured instruments. However, data are *not* intrinsically more accurate just because they are pre-structured and alternative approaches with less obvious impositions on clinicians (e.g. through language processing) may be more fruitful in the longer term. Key developments which may revolutionize this field are the development of portals for patients to provide their own information, as well as the wealth of wearables and other devices which may provide important ancillary information (albeit requiring considerable processing and integration). Applicability and acceptability of these initiatives have not yet been demonstrated on a wide scale in mental healthcare but clearly it is an area to watch closely.

Governance

The development of routine data resources for research is as much about achieving a sufficiently robust governance structure as about computational capacity or analytic skills.

The importance of data governance cannot be overemphasized; however, it is beyond the scope of this chapter to provide a full review, particularly as attitudes and practices vary widely between countries. In general, the use of large-scale routine healthcare data for research can only be carried out where there is a legal framework allowing appropriately controlled and justified access to such data without consent. Clearly there are substantial sensitivities around healthcare data and a variety of structures have been set up to ensure that research represents an appropriately justified use of such data (e.g. a requirement to demonstrate that it would not be feasible to recruit a consenting research sample), and that appropriate measures are adopted to preserve anonymity and maintain data security. As well as the removal or masking of personally identifying information from datasets, these include limited release of variables to reduce the risk of identification by data combinations. Achieving wider transparency and acceptability is equally important, and the South London and Maudsley Clinical Record Interactive Search (CRIS) data resource, containing full but de-identified information from electronic mental health records, additionally developed a patient-led security model with an oversight committee reviewing and approving all projects using the data (Fernandes et al., 2013). Additional considerations apply to the use of identifier fields required to create linkages between databases, particularly concerning the justification of such use and the demonstration of techniques and security models which protect anonymity during the process.

In the case of surveillance units, as different jurisdictions will have different types of ethical permissions that change with time, researchers should seek advice from the unit that they are working through and with their own institution. At the time of writing, CAPSS has a rigorous two-stage application process that guarantees fast-track approval with the Health Research Authorities Confidentiality Advisory Group that covers England and is accepted by the other countries in the UK and Ireland. On the understanding that researchers will not know the identity of children and families, and that the latter are never contacted directly, this authority can provide ethical permission for researchers to ask clinicians to complete questionnaires from the clinical records without consent. This necessarily places some limits on what studies conducted using this method can explore.

Big data

What are big data?

The growing digitization of global health information presents a rich opportunity to study risk factors and patterns of disease across very large populations, and provide precise estimates on outcomes for healthcare interventions. There is no rigorous definition for 'big data', but at its simplest, big data refers to any electronic data that cannot be feasibly stored or processed by standard desktop computers or fit into a standard relational database (Dutcher, 2014). The main features are high volume, variety, and velocity: the 'three Vs' (Raghupathi and Raghupathi, 2014). Volume refers to the size of the data, where it is not uncommon for terabytes or petabytes to be available for analyses. Variety refers to the different types of data format (structured fields, free text, images, video, etc.) and multiple contributing sources, for example, health-related data could be derived from both social media and clinical notes.

Velocity indicates the dynamic nature of data, where the volume and types of the data held are changing or evolving—for example, in a database derived from electronic medical records that updates in real time. 'Veracity' has been proposed as a fourth 'V', particularly in relation to social media data (e.g. see http://www.pheme.eu), underlining the challenges in ascertaining the truthfulness of information recorded in these large-volume sources.

The term big data also concerns the tools used to interpret these complex structures. Over the years these have been referred to as data mining, analytics, and, more recently, data science (Royal Society, 2012). These terms describe the development and application of analytical techniques that can integrate and extract meaning from massive datasets. A common feature of these technologies is the capability to interrogate data using automated procedures, or algorithms, replacing the need for resource-intensive manual extraction or interpretation—a healthcare example includes the detection of symptoms from unstructured text as described previously (Patel et al., 2015). Beyond deciphering clinical data, big data technologies can also be used to conduct 'agnostic' analyses, where statistical algorithms process huge volumes of data in order to detect previously unrecognized relationships or hidden signals between exposures and disease outcomes. In this process, analyses are looking to generate new hypothesis or predictive models, rather than test existing theories of causal relations between exposure and outcome variables. These 'hypothesis-free' analyses are now an integral part of the post-marketing safety evaluation performed by pharmaceutical regulators, who scan huge volumes of surveillance data to detect correlations between drugs and adverse events (Harpaz et al., 2012).

Psychiatric epidemiology and big data linkage

Epidemiologists may reasonably argue that big data approaches are not novel. As described in earlier chapters, for decades Scandinavian countries have led the way in the development of whole population data repositories all linked via common identification number, acquired at birth or migration to these countries. These repositories can index on an individual level an array of clinical and social information including birth details, school performance, secondary healthcare use, and social and criminal justice involvement (Munk-Jørgensen et al., 2014). However, for many countries, although equivalent individual-level data exist, these are contained in separate repositories with no common identification number to facilitate linkage between them (Downs et al., 2019). To overcome this, a number of probabilistic linkage methodologies have been developed (Tromp et al., 2011) which use specified identifiers common to each record in both datasets (e.g. surname, post code, and date of birth) and generate a probability estimate of the match being a true one by comparing each set of identifiers in one record against all other records provided. Matches are then ranked in probability and a cut-off determined, often through manual review, to select the lowest probability score taken to represent a positive match for a record pair. Understandably, this process is computationally intensive, and efficient probabilistic linkages across different health and social domains have only become feasible over the last decade (Holman et al., 2008). Figure 13.2 provides an UK example of the potential database linkages that would permit routine analysis of the impact of

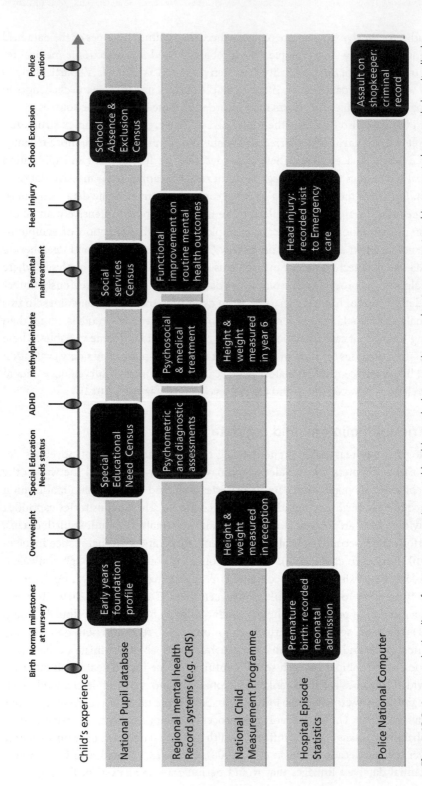

Figure 13.2 An example timeline of a young person's mental health needs, interventions, and outcomes captured in separate large-scale longitudinal data sources amenable to probabilistic data linkages.

interventions on key childhood mental health risk factors and outcomes (Holman et al., 2008; Administrative Data Taskforce, 2012; Ford et al., 2012).

Examples of methodologies

A number of big data approaches are being tested to see whether they can provide time-efficient methodologies in mental health research, for example, in the measurement of psychiatric symptom prevalence, trends, and treatment outcomes. To give a few examples: the Durkheim Project is attempting to measure the prevalence of suicidal feelings in army veterans from text mining within clinical notes and social media (Poulin et al., 2014). Online resources, such as PatientsLikeMe (Frost et al., 2011) and myhealthlocker (Ennis et al., 2014) are assessing the safety and effectiveness of treatments related to a number of psychiatric disorders using patient-reported outcome data. Mobile phones are being used for continuous monitoring, via their internal accelerometers, to detect abnormal movement patterns in patients with ADHD (Young et al., 2014) and Parkinson's disease (Arora et al., 2015). The hope for these projects, and many similar, is that big data methodologies may eventually be integrated into clinical records to enhance the evaluation of clinical interventions and service provision.

Developing a big data project using routine healthcare data

Large-scale healthcare data resources amenable to big data approaches are increasing, and present tremendous opportunities for tackling a wide range of clinical research questions. However, they often involve information which is both personally sensitive and complex to analyse. In addition to the methodological considerations described earlier in this chapter, there are a number of steps to consider when developing a big data project, using routine healthcare data:

1. *Defining and justifying study objectives*. In the past, patients and healthcare organizations have been reluctant to support projects where the immediate output of big data initiatives were not clear to them (Kirby, 2014). The onus is on the researcher to demonstrate the public benefit of a big data project, and the *justification* for needing high volumes of potentially sensitive healthcare data. For example, NHS Digital (the Health and Social Care Information Centre), a public body responsible for the management of England's secondary healthcare data sets, will only provide data to researchers whose projects they consider will provide value to the health and social care of National Health Service (NHS) patients (Health and Social Care Information Centre, 2015).

2. *Understanding the data*. It is important to ensure *understanding* of how source data are collected and defined, and ascertain where inconsistencies may emerge. For example, when using longitudinal records, classifications of disorders and hospital procedural codes can change over time. Also, the delivery and recording of healthcare is heterogeneous even within one healthcare organization (Chan et al., 2010). If the healthcare context is not well understood, even the highest levels of computational and statistical proficiency will not prevent spurious findings arising. An effective research team is therefore likely to incorporate a range of disciplines, from those who understand the nature of mental health conditions and the way they are described/categorized in

routine healthcare settings, to specialists in database assembly and analysis. Alongside such a team, it is important to have sufficient data-processing resources and to operate within a robust data governance structure. Without explicit and clear governance frameworks, data custodians are likely to be unwilling or unable to release data for analysis (Department for Education, 2015; Health and Social Care Information Centre, 2015).

3. *Validation*. Considerable care needs to be applied to understand the *validity* of the data, particularly where clinical data are being entered by staff removed from the clinical process. For example, the NHS Hospital Episode Statistics (HES) database which adds 125 million admitted patient, outpatient, and accident and emergency records each year to its database, is reliant on hospital data submissions provided by expert coders rather than clinicians. As a result, some aspects of HES data have been critiqued for their inaccuracies (Spencer and Davies, 2012). To manage this, researchers will need to determine the extent of misclassification and whether it is systematic, by undertaking a validation exercise with subset of patients. This may involve cross checking the same clinical variables using linked patient-level data across databases (Morley et al., 2014). As clinical electronic record systems are dynamic, it is also important to bear in mind that prior assumptions about data may become incorrect with updates. Similarly, it is essential to remain aware of local changes to electronic records used in routine clinical care or administrative data collection, and to continue systematic revalidation of any automated data extraction or analytical algorithms (Chan et al., 2010).

Conclusion

Routinely collected healthcare records, case registers, and surveillance provide huge opportunities for mental health researchers, but as with all other types of research, it is essential to understand the strengths and weaknesses of a particular source of data, and to carefully define the research questions, outcomes, and exposures under study. Surveillance, case registers, and big data also involve additional attention to the governance covering access and use, as well as issues of data accuracy, validity, and completeness.

Practical exercises

1. What follows is an example of a broad surveillance definition for a study of transition among young adults with ADHD; the aim of the study is to identify the number of young adults requiring ongoing medication monitoring in relation to ADHD in adult mental health services.
   - A young person with a clinical diagnosis of ADHD who is reviewed within 6 months of reaching the services' age boundary.
   - The young person is considered to require continued drug treatment for their symptoms of ADHD after crossing the service age boundary.
   - Young people with ADHD and comorbid diagnoses, including learning/developmental disabilities, should be reported ONLY if it is their ADHD for which ongoing drug treatment in adult services is required.

a. What exclusion criteria should you include with this definition?

b. List the questions that you would need to ask in your questionnaire to verify that reported cases met the above-listed definition?

c. How would you improve the case definition?

2. You have been asked to set up a register of dementia cases in your locality. The budget is limited, but you are expected to maximize the volume and quality of research utilizing this resource.

a. Thinking about your local resources and any restrictions or limitations, how would you set up such a register? How would the cases be ascertained and included? What measurements would be available and/or administered and how would this be funded and supported?

b. What would be the most important limitations of such a data resource? What would be its strengths? What research would it allow which would not otherwise have been possible?

c. Your funders will want a report within a year after setting up the database. What type of research questions might you seek to address as an 'early win' (bearing in mind the information most immediately available)?

d. A neighbouring locality would like to set up a similar register. How 'portable' is your proposed resource (i.e. how easily could it be set up elsewhere)?

e. If the study lead left their job next year, how sustainable would the register be without their involvement? Roughly what level of funding and clinical support would it require to continue?

3. You are designing a study in children with ADHD that examines the effect of co-morbid physical health problems on school attendance. You do not have the resources to undertake a sufficiently powered cohort study, so you wish to utilize big data resources. You have permission to link a primary care records dataset containing 5 million individuals, and a nationally held administrative dataset of all children's school attendance records. Both databases contain longitudinal individual-level data from 2008 to the present day but do not have a common identification number.

a. Before you link this data, what could you do to reduce the chance of false-positive matches?

b. List the key exposure, outcomes, and potential confounding variables you are interested in. How are you going to extract these from the data? Given the data sources, are there any concerns you have about the quality of these data? What steps could be taken to validate some of these variables of interest?

c. Describe the research team you would assemble to help with this study, and what tasks they would support you with.

d. What ethical or governance issues may arise in the course of this work?

Further reading

Amaddeo F. (2014). The small scale clinical psychiatric case registers. *Acta Psychiatrica Scandinavica*, 130, 80–82.

Lynn, R., Viner, R.M., and Nicholls, D.E. (2012). Ascertainment of early onset eating disorders; a pilot for developing a National Psychiatric Surveillance System. *Child and Adolescent Mental Health*, 17, 109–112.

Nuffield Council on Bioethics (2015). The collection, linking and use of data in biomedical research and healthcare: ethical issues. http://nuffieldbioethics.org/project/biological-health-data/

Munk-Jørgensen, P., Okkels, N., Goldberg, D., Ruggeri, M., and Thornicroft, G. (2014). Fifty years' development and future perspectives of psychiatric register research. *Acta Psychiatrica Scandinavica*, 130, 87–98.

Royal Society (2012). Science as an open enterprise. https://royalsociety.org/policy/projects/science-public-enterprise/Report

Stewart, R. (2014). The big case register. *Acta Psychiatrica Scandinavica*, 130, 83–86.

References

Administrative Data Taskforce (2012). UK Administrative Data Research Network: improving access for research and policy. Economic and Social Research Council. http://www.esrc.ac.uk/_images/ADT-Improving-Access-for-Research-and-Policy_tcm8-24462.pdf

Ani, C., Reading, R., Lynn, R., Forlee, S., and Garralda, E. (2013). Incidence and 12-month outcome of non-transient childhood conversion disorder in the U.K. and Ireland. *British Journal of Psychiatry*, 202, 413–418.

Arora, S., Venkataraman, V., Zhan, A., Donohue, S., Biglan, K.M., Dorsey, E.R., and Little, M.A. (2015). Detecting and monitoring the symptoms of Parkinson's disease using smartphones: a pilot study. *Parkinsonism & Related Disorders*, 21, 650–653.

Byford, S., Petkvoa, H., Stuart, R., Nicholls, D., Simic, M., Ford, T., et al. (2019). Alternative community-based models of care for young people with anorexia nervosa: the CostED national surveillance study. *Health Serv Deliv Res*, 7(37). https://www.journalslibrary.nihr.ac.uk/hsdr/hsdr07370/#/abstract

Castro, V.M., Minnier, J., Murphy, S.N., Kohane, I., Churchill, S.E., Gainer, V., et al. (2015). Validation of electronic health record phenotyping of bipolar disorder cases and controls. *American Journal of Psychiatry*, 172, 363–372.

Chan, K.S., Fowles, J.B., and Weiner, J.P. (2010). Review: electronic health records and the reliability and validity of quality measures: a review of the literature. *Medical Care Research and Review*, 67, 503–527.

Davenport, M., De Ville de Goyet, J., Stringer, M., Mieli-Vergani, G., Kelly, D., McClean, P., and Spitz, L. (2004). Seamless management of biliary atresia in England and Wales (1999–2002). *Lancet*, 363, 1354–1357.

Department for Education (2015). National Pupil Database user guide. UK Government. https://www.gov.uk/government/uploads/system/uploads/attachment_data/file/261189/NPD_User_Guide.pdf

Department of Health (2014a). *Statistical update on suicides (revised)*. London: Department of Health.

Department of Health (2014b). *Chief Medical Officer (CMO) annual report: public mental health*. London: Department of Health.

Downs, J., Ford, T., Stewart, R., Epstein, S., Shetty, H., Little, R., et al. (2019). An approach to linking education, social care and electronic health records for children and young people in South London: a linkage study of child and adolescent mental health service data. *BMJ Open*, 9, e024355.

Dutcher, J. (2014). What is big data?—blog. https://datascience.berkeley.edu/what-is-big-data/

Eke, H., Ford, T., Newlove-Delgado, T., Price, A., Young, S., Ani, C., Sayal., K., Lynn, R., Paul, M. and Janssens, A. (2019). Transition between child and adult services for young people with attention-deficit hyperactivity disorder (ADHD): findings from a British national surveillance study. *British Journal of Psychiatry*, 1–7. doi:10.1192/bjp.2019.131

Ennis, L., Robotham, D., Denis, M., Pandit, N., Newton, D., Rose, D., and Wykes, T. (2014). Collaborative development of an electronic personal health record for people with severe and enduring mental health problems. *BMC Psychiatry*, 14, 305.

Fernandes, A.C., Cloete, D., Broadbent, M.T., Hayes, R.D., Chang, C.-K., Jackson, R.G., et al. (2013). Development and evaluation of a de-identification procedure for a case register sourced from mental health electronic records. *BMC Medical Informatics and Decision Making*, 13, 71.

Fombonne, E., Wostear, G., Cooper, V., Harrington, R., and Rutter, M. (2001). The Maudsley long-term follow-up of child and adolescent depression. *British Journal of Psychiatry*, 179, 210–217.

Ford, T., Edwards, V., Sharkey, S., Ukoumunne, O.C., Byford, S., Norwich, B., and Logan, S. (2012). Supporting teachers and children in schools: the effectiveness and cost-effectiveness of the incredible years teacher classroom management programme in primary school children: a cluster randomised controlled trial, with parallel economic and process evaluations. *BMC Public Health*, 12, 719.

Freeman, E., Colpe, L., Strine, T., Dhingra, S., McGuire, L., Elam-Evans, L., and Perry, G. (2010). Public health surveillance for mental health. *Preventing Chronic Disease*, 7, A17.

Frost, J., Okun, S., Vaughan, T., Heywood, J., and Wicks, P. (2011). Patient-reported outcomes as a source of evidence in off-label prescribing: analysis of data from PatientsLikeMe. *Journal of Medical Internet Research*, 13, e6.

Green, H., McGinnity, A., Ford, T., and Goodman, R. (2005). *Mental health of children and young people in Great Britain 2004*. Basingstoke: Palgrave Macmillan.

Harpaz, R., DuMouchel, W., Shah, N.H., Madigan, D., Ryan, P., and Friedman, C. (2012). Novel data mining methodologies for adverse drug event discovery and analysis. *Clinical Pharmacology and Therapeutics*, 91, 1010–1021.

Health and Social Care Information Centre (2015). Data access request service. https://digital.nhs.uk/services/data-access-request-service-dars

Holman, C.D.J., Bass, A.J., Rosman, D.L., Smith, M.B., Semmens, J.B., Glasson, E.J., Stanley, F.J. (2008). A decade of data linkage in Western Australia: strategic design, applications and benefits of the WA data linkage system. *Australian Health Review: A Publication of the Australian Hospital Association*, 32, 766–777.

Jensen, A.L. and Weisz, J.R. (2002). Assessing match and mismatch between practitioner-generated and standardized interview-generated diagnoses for clinic-referred children and adolescents. *Journal of Consulting and Clinical Psychology*, 70, 158–168.

Kirby, T. (2014). Controversy surrounds England's new NHS database. *Lancet*, 383, 681.

Lewis, G., David, A., Andreasson, S., and Allebeck, P. (1992). Schizophrenia and city life. *Lancet*, 340, 137–140.

Lynn, R., Viner, R.M., and Nicholls, D.E. (2012). Ascertainment of early onset eating disorders: a pilot for developing a national child psychiatric surveillance system. *Child and Adolescent Mental Health*, 17, 109–112.

Morley, K.I., Wallace, J., Denaxas, S.C., Hunter, R.J., Patel, R.S., Perel, P., and Hemingway, H. (2014). Defining disease phenotypes using national linked electronic health records: a case study of atrial fibrillation. *PLoS One*, 9, e110900.

Munk-Jørgensen, P., Okkels, N., Golberg, D., Ruggeri, M., and Thornicroft, G. (2014). Fifty years' development and future perspectives of psychiatric register research. *Acta Psychiatrica Scandinavica*, 130, 87–98.

Nicholls, D.E., Lynn, R., and Viner, R.M. (2011). Childhood eating disorders: British national surveillance study. *British Journal of Psychiatry*, **198**, 295–301.

Perera, G., Soremekun, M., Breen, G., and Stewart, R. (2009). The psychiatric case register: noble past, challenging present, but exciting future. *British Journal of Psychiatry*, **195**, 191–193.

Patel, R., Jayatilleke, N., Broadbent, M., Chang, C.K., Foskett, N., Gorrell, G., et al. (2015). Negative symptoms in schizophrenia: a study in a large clinical sample of patients using a novel automated method. *BMJ Open*, **5**, e007619.

Perera, G., Broadbent, M., Callard, F., Chang., C.-K., Downs, J., Dutta, R., et al. (2016). Cohort profile of the South London and Maudsley NHS Foundation Trust Biomedical Research Centre (SLaM BRC) Case Register: current status and recent enhancement of an Electronic Mental Health Record derived data resource. *BMJ Open*, **6**, e008721.

Porta, M. (ed.) (2008). *A dictionary of epidemiology*, 5th edn. Oxford: Oxford University Press.

Poulin, C., Shiner, B., Thompson, P., Vepstas, L., Young-Xu, Y., Goertzel, B., et al. (2014). Predicting the risk of suicide by analyzing the text of clinical notes. *PLoS One*, **9**, e85733.

Raghupathi, W. and Raghupathi, V. (2014). Big data analytics in healthcare: promise and potential. *Health Information Science and Systems*, **2**, 3.

Richards, D.A., Ross, S., Robens, S., and Borglin, G. (2014). The DiReCT study-improving recruitment into clinical trials: a mixed methods study investigating the ethical acceptability, feasibility and recruitment yield of the cohort multiple randomised controlled trials design. *Trials*, **15**, 398.

Royal Society (2012). Science as an open enterprise: final report. https://royalsociety.org/policy/projects/science-public-enterprise/Report

Sharma, A., Neely, J., Le Couteur, A., Grunze, H., Nicholls, D., James, A., et al. (2009). Study of pediatric bipolar disorder in UK and ROI: development of a case definition and pilot data from North East England. *Bipolar Disorders* **11** (Suppl. 1), 79.

Singleton, N., Meltzer, H., and Jenkins, R. (2003). Building a picture of psychiatric morbidity in a nation: a decade of epidemiological survey in Great Britain. *International Review of Psychiatry*, **15**, 19–28.

Spencer, S.A. and Davies, M.P. (2012). Hospital episode statistics: improving the quality and value of hospital data: a national internet e-survey of hospital consultants. *BMJ Open*, **2**, e001651.

Strobl, J., Cave, E., and Walley, T. (2000). Data protection legislation: interpretation and barriers to research. *BMJ*, **321**, 890–892.

Su, Y.P., Chang, C.K., Hayes, R.D., Harrison, S., Lee, W., Broadbent, M., et al. (2014). Retrospective chart review on exposure to psychotropic medications associated with neuroleptic malignant syndrome. *Acta Psychiatrica Scandinavica*, **130**, 52–60.

ten Horn, G.H.M.M. (1986). *Psychiatric case registers in public health: a worldwide inventory, 1960–1985*. New York: Elsevier.

Thomas, K.H., Martin, R.M., Potokar, J., Pirmohamed, M., and Gunnell, D. (2014). Reporting of drug induced depression and fatal and non-fatal suicidal behaviour in the UK from 1998 to 2011. *BMC Pharmacology & Toxicology*, **15**, 54.

Tiffin, P.A. and Kitchen, C.E.W. (2015). Incidence and 12-month outcome of childhood non-affective psychoses: British national surveillance study. *British Journal of Psychiatry* **206**, 517–518.

Tromp, M., Ravelli, A.C., Bonsel, G.J., Hasman, A., and Reitsma, J.B. (2011). Results from simulated data sets: probabilistic record linkage outperforms deterministic record linkage. *Journal of Clinical Epidemiology*, **64**, 565–572.

Young, Z., Craven, M.P., Groom, M., and Crowe, J. (2014). Snappy app: a mobile continuous performance test with physical activity measurement for assessing attention deficit hyperactivity disorder. In: Kurosu, M. (ed.). *Human-computer interaction: applications and services*, pp. 363–373. Heidelberg: Springer International Publishing.

Chapter 14

Research synthesis: Systematic reviews and meta-analyses

Marianna Purgato, Giovanni Ostuzzi, and Corrado Barbui

Introduction

Clinical decision-making is a key component in daily clinical practice. The choice of the best treatment to be delivered to patients should always be based on the integration of three closely dependent and related factors: patient values, clinical experience, and the current best evidence available in the literature about efficacy and tolerability of each treatment. The approach that integrates individual clinical expertise with scientific evidence is known as *evidence-based medicine* (Sackett et al., 1996), which consists of a conscientious, explicit, and judicious use of current best evidence in making decisions about the care of individual patients (Akobeng, 2005). Evidence-based practice is based on four basic contingencies: recognition of the patient's problem and construction of a structured clinical question; comprehensive search of the medical literature to retrieve the best evidence to answer the question; critical appraisal of evidence; and integration of the evidence base with the clinical context (Akobeng, 2005; Manchikanti et al., 2008).

One challenge in applying this approach is that, with an increasing number of quantitative and qualitative studies being published in health sciences, it is not easy for busy clinicians and researchers to keep up with the literature. In particular, it may be very difficult to identify studies of good quality, and also interpret data that are often controversial or explicitly conflicting. This has led to the development of methodologies to systematically collect, analyse, and critically appraise all relevant studies on a specific topic, in order to produce a description of the evidence and, if possible, to calculate overall estimates of the outcomes of interest. The term 'systematic review' (SR) refers to the procedure of collecting all studies meeting predefined inclusion and exclusion criteria (Garg et al., 2008; Purgato et al., 2012). Such study designs can present a complete framework of what is known about a specific topic responding to clinically relevant questions (Bero and Rennie, 1995; Cipriani and Barbui, 2006b). Specific tools are used for summarizing outcomes from available studies in order to obtain accurate information which may inform clinical practice (Uman, 2011).

However, various methodological approaches can be used to frame different topics of interest. Some phenomena, such as the frequency of a disease, its impact on survival, or the efficacy of one treatment over another, can be described in terms of quantitative data. At the same time, phenomena such as patients' and caregivers' experiences and attitudes and other possible barriers and facilitators to treatments, cannot be easily and consistently measured, but can be approached with a qualitative analysis.

The statistical procedure for combining results of quantitative studies is known as 'meta-analysis'. For example, when answering questions about the efficacy of interventions the randomized design is considered to be at the pinnacle of the evidence hierarchy (Figure 14.1), not forgetting that such a ranking may change when considering, for example, tolerability outcomes (Ho et al., 2008) and the quality of the study.

However, research synthesis is not necessarily only about randomized controlled trials (RCTs) and, despite intrinsic limitations of observational designs, many efforts have been made for developing proper procedures for selecting, evaluating, and pooling observational data (Higgins and Greene, 2011). Such data may play a relevant role when assessing the epidemiology of a condition, the consequences of exposure to risk factors, or even the efficacy of interventions in community populations or in patients for whom exposure to experimental designs would be difficult to study (e.g. pregnant women). As quantitative data cannot exhaustively frame the complexity of some clinical topics, specific techniques for reliably synthesizing qualitative data have been gradually developed. The most relevant examples are approaches

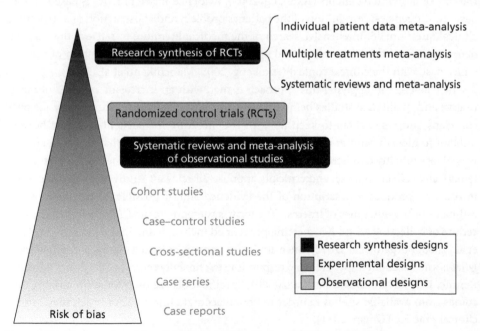

Figure 14.1 Diagram describing the hierarchy of evidence for efficacy outcomes.

called 'meta-ethnography' and 'grounded theory', which not only aim to summarize the current knowledge provided by qualitative studies, but also at interpreting data and developing explanatory frameworks through an inductive process (Britten et al., 2002; Campbell et al., 2011). Data from these studies may in turn be an excellent basis for planning new observational and experimental studies. Thus, both quantitative and qualitative research may be helpful for characterizing different aspects of a given condition of interest. It has long been acknowledged that the development of reliable methodologies for blending quantitative and qualitative data and for conducting mixed designs of research would be of great value in both research and clinical practice (Morgan, 1998; Creswell et al., 2004).

A detailed description of the appraisal and synthesis of qualitative data is not covered in this chapter, which is focused on quantitative data. The aim of this chapter is to describe how results from quantitative studies can be effectively included in SRs and combined in meta-analyses to provide useful information for everyday practice.

Systematic reviews

As with primary research, each phase of a good SR needs to be well planned, well conducted, and well reported. The first step is the definition of research hypotheses and the preparation of a protocol, which should report the eligibility criteria for including studies. The protocol should also specify the search strategies that investigators planned to run for the identification of studies and any efforts that will be made to identify unpublished data, as well as strategies for data analysis (Cipriani and Barbui, 2006b).

To deal with the complexity underlying this process, international networks of researchers from different countries of the world were established with the aim of undertaking and maintaining SRs. Some of the most authoritative networks aimed at research synthesis are the Centre for Reviews and Dissemination (CRD) of the University of York (https://www.york.ac.uk/crd/), the National Institute for Health and Care Excellence (NICE) (https://www.nice.org.uk/), the Campbell Collaboration (http://www.campbellcollaboration.org/), and Cochrane (http://www.cochrane.org/). These are national and international non-profit organizations, which aim to collect and maintain up-to-date information not only on healthcare interventions, but also health policy, research methodology, education, and social welfare. These organizations also make available the results from research synthesis, by building comprehensive databases. For example, full texts of Cochrane SRs are recorded in the Cochrane Database of Systematic Reviews, available online as part of the Cochrane Library, an electronic library which collects both Cochrane protocols and reviews (http://www.cochranelibrary.com). Moreover, these represent a resource for providing researchers with guidance for the development of robust SRs. One paradigmatic example of that is the 'Cochrane Handbook for Systematic Reviews of Interventions', which is an official document (freely downloadable online and periodically updated) that describes in detail the process that should be followed for preparing and maintaining SRs on the effects of healthcare interventions (Higgins et al., 2011a, 2011b). Several detailed instruments have been developed in order to help researchers rigorously conducting and reporting a SR of quantitative data (Table 14.1).

Stages for conducting a systematic review

The steps required for the production of a SR are illustrated in Figure 14.2.

Study protocol

The methodological aspects outlined previously should be described in detail in the study protocol. The protocol of a SR is a formal document that describes the objectives, methods, statistical considerations, and all aspects related to the organization of a review. This instrument acts as guidance against arbitrary decisions during the conduct of the review, enables readers to assess for the presence of selective reporting against completed reviews, and reduces duplication of efforts. The protocol contains the theoretical background and the rationale that have generated the review question(s), and defines a priori methodological and analytical approaches such as inclusion/exclusion criteria, data collection and analyses, published versus unpublished studies, and language restrictions (Moher et al., 2015). These elements may be operationally defined in a format called PICO, which stands for Population (i.e. type of patients, age range, and diagnosis), Intervention (i.e. type of treatments and route of administration: timing, dose, and duration of follow-up), Comparator, and Outcomes (primary and secondary outcome measures) (Uman, 2011). Also, the roles of investigators in each step have to be specified in advance.

The protocol is usually disseminated on dedicated websites or may become a publication (Moher et al., 2015). Online repositories of review protocols for SRs, such as the Cochrane Library (http://www.cochranelibrary.com/) and the International Prospective Register of Systematic Reviews (PROSPERO) (http://www.crd.york.ac.uk/PROSPERO/), have been developed in order to enable a transparent comparison between what is reported in the review methods and what was actually planned in the protocol.

Search strategy

After deciding on the question and scope of a SR, the subsequent step is to try to identify all studies that are eligible for inclusion (Figure 14.2 and Table 14.1). Eligibility criteria inform how the search will be conducted. Depending on the review question, it is possible to search only for the types of designs, participants, or intervention and, in less common cases, the types of outcomes to be addressed. Usually, the final search strategies are published in the review. The inclusion of search strategies using the appropriate and database-specific search terms and syntax increases transparency and facilitates future updates (Hausner et al., 2012) (https://chmg.cochrane.org). The importance of a comprehensive search for both published and unpublished trials has been stressed many times in relation to SR of effects of healthcare interventions. We are aware that retrieving unpublished materials represents a compelling issue and that there are no standardized ways to collect them (Trespidi et al., 2011). However, the problem of 'publication bias', which

Table 14.1 Some examples of documents and tools designed to help researchers properly conduct and report systematic reviews and meta-analyses

Tool	Description	Website
RevMan	Free software for conducting SRs and MAs of both experimental and observational studies. It includes the risk of bias tool for assessing the quality of included studies	http://tech.cochrane.org/revman/download
Cochrane Handbook for Systematic Reviews of Interventions	A theoretical and pragmatic guide for conducting each phase of SRs and MAs of both experimental and observational studies. It includes guidelines for assessing the risk of bias	http://handbook.cochrane.org/
Campbell Collaboration Systematic Reviews: Policies and Guidelines	A practical guide which informs on the requirements for Campbell SRs and provides guidelines for producing them	http://www.campbellcollaboration.org/lib/project/328/
Centre for Reviews and Dissemination: guidance for undertaking reviews in healthcare	A practical guide for conducting SRs and MAs. It includes specialized topic areas, including research synthesis on clinical tests (diagnostic, screening, and prognostic), public health, adverse effects, costs, and incorporating qualitative evidence in effectiveness reviews	http://www.york.ac.uk/crd/guidance/
Methodological Expectations of Cochrane Intervention Reviews (MECIR)	A document where methodological expectations for conducting and reporting Cochrane protocols, reviews, and updates of reviews are described	http://editorial-unit.cochrane.org/mecir
Methodological Expectations of Campbell Collaboration Intervention Reviews (MEC2IR)	A document where methodological expectations for conducting and reporting Campbell protocols, reviews, and updates of reviews are described	http://www.campbellcollaboration.org/Methods_Resources/MEC2IR.php

(continued)

Table 14.1 Continued

Tool	Description	Website
PRISMA Statement	A checklist which guides the reporting of SRs and MAs of RCTs and other study designs aimed at evaluating the effect of interventions	http://www.prisma-statement.org/statement.htm
MOOSE Checklist	A checklist which guides the reporting of SRs and MAs of observational studies	https://www.editorialmanager.com/jognn/account/MOOSE.pdf
GRADE Pro—Guideline Development Tool (GDT)	Web-based software for summarizing all key information from SRs and MAs and for transparently assessing their quality	http://www.guidelinedevelopment.org

MAs, meta-analyses; RCTs, randomized controlled trials; SRs, systematic reviews.

refers to the fact that whether or not a trial is published depends on its results, has to be carefully considered by systematic reviewers, in order to avoid the risk that the review presents only a proportion of the evidence base, systematically ignoring the results of studies that are not published, which usually are negative studies (Clarke, 2005). An

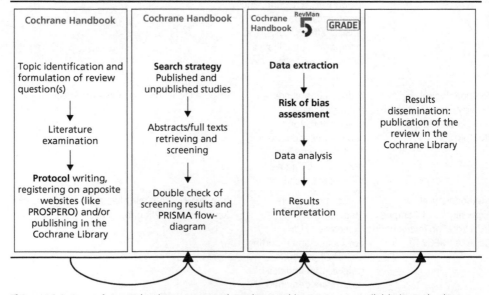

Figure 14.2 Steps for conducting a systematic review and instruments available in each phase.

analysis restricted to only the published literature is likely to overestimate the efficacy of a given intervention (Turner et al., 2008).

Study selection and data extraction

Once a comprehensive list of abstracts has been retrieved and reviewed, studies meeting inclusion criteria are obtained in full. It is recommended that authors keep a log of all reviewed studies with reasons for inclusion or exclusion. The next stage is data extraction (Figure 14.2—third step). It is essential to create a simple data extraction form to collect and organize information extracted from each reviewed study (i.e. authors, publication year, number of participants, age, and outcomes). Both study selection and data extraction should be made by two reviewers independently, to establish inter-rater reliability and avoiding data extraction/entry errors.

Risk of bias assessment

Many tools have been proposed for assessing risk of bias of studies. For example, Cochrane recommends simple approaches for assessing methodological quality of RCTs using specific tools, such as the risk of bias tool (Higgins et al., 2011; Savovic et al., 2014). This tool is a domain-based evaluation, in which critical assessments are made separately for the following domains: randomization, sequence generation, allocation concealment, blinding, incomplete data, and outcome reporting (Higgins et al., 2011). Items are assessed by providing a description of what is reported in the study (it is preferred to use quotations from reports) and providing a judgement on the adequacy of the study with regard to each item. The judgement is formulated by answering a pre-specified question, such that an answer of 'Yes' indicates low risk of bias, an answer of 'No' indicates high risk of bias, and an answer of 'Unclear' indicates unclear or unknown risk of bias (Higgins et al., 2011a, 2011b). Often an 'Unclear' risk of bias reflects a common lack of exhaustive reporting of published trials, despite the availability of instruments designed to help transparent reporting, such as the Consolidated Standards of Reporting Trials (CONSORT) statement (Turner et al., 2012). Many other tools have been developed for assessing the risk of bias of observational studies. For example, the Newcastle–Ottawa Scale (NOS) is frequently used in SRs of cohort studies (Higgins and Green, 2011).

Meta-analysis

Where appropriate, SR includes a meta-analysis, which involves the use of statistical procedures to synthesize data by calculating an overall quantitative estimate of the average treatment effect (Naylor, 1997). Meta-analysis calculates an aggregate 'weighted average' of results of individual studies, generated by the sum of individual RCTs. The 'weight' in the overall estimate is determined by the sample size of each study (RCTs with larger populations have more weight) and by the frequency of events (RCTs with higher rates of events have more weight). The advantage of this technique is that it calculates estimates from large samples of patients that have more statistical power than each single trial (Haidich, 2010).

The results of meta-analysis are usually represented graphically through a forest plot (Cipriani and Barbui, 2006a), which provides both a graphical representation of the results of each study, and a general estimate derived from the sum of the results of each trial included in meta-analysis (Figure 14.3) (Cipriani and Barbui, 2006a).

Limitations and challenges of systematic reviews and meta-analyses

Even though SR and meta-analysis are considered the best instrument for obtaining a definitive answer to specific research questions, there are certain inherent limitations associated with it. First, the process of conducting a SR is time-consuming. Second, the value of a SR depends on what was done, what was found, the quality of included studies, and the clarity and completeness of reporting. Another problem is publication bias, which occurs when negative studies are less likely to be published than positive ones. This poses a serious threat to the ability of syntheses of published research to reach unbiased conclusions, although through searching may help locate some unpublished material (Trespidi et al., 2011).

Heterogeneity is another challenge inherent to meta-analysis rather than a problem to solve (Berlin and Golub, 2014). When there is variation in the findings from trials included in the analysis, there may be a certain degree of heterogeneity, and researchers or clinicians should explore what this implies in terms of diversity and generalizability of results. Homogeneity, especially in human research, is not necessarily more desirable than heterogeneity, considering that highly homogeneous results may suggest over-selection of participants and therefore low applicability in the real world (Purgato and Adams, 2012). Certainly, perceptions of diversity or its lack may influence meta-analysis on what data to combine, what data to avoid combining, what methods to use to combine, and how to interpret results they eventually get (Ioannidis, 2008). There are three main types of heterogeneity: clinical heterogeneity refers to variability in participants, types of intervention, and outcomes (Fletcher, 2007). Methodological heterogeneity refers to variability in study design, conduct, and risk of bias. Finally, statistical heterogeneity exists when the observed intervention effects are more different to each other than one would expect due to random error (chance) alone (Higgins and Thompson, 2002). Statistical heterogeneity can often be spotted by simple visual inspection of forest plots: when confidence intervals overlap, heterogeneity is lower than when they do not overlap (Figure 14.3—E1). Viewing data on graphs helps to have an immediate understanding, but formal inferences should not depend only on visual impressions (Ioannidis, 2008). Statistical approaches may help to quantify some elements of heterogeneity, including the Q statistic (a measure of total within-study variance), $I2$ statistic (the ratio of variability of results among studies to total observed variation) (Figure 14.3—E2) and the τ (a measure of between-studies variance) (Berlin and Golub, 2014).

The results of a meta-analysis should always be interpreted and discussed in light of the above-discussed limitations. A useful tool for assessing and summarizing the quality of a body of evidence and therefore the reliability of a given estimate of effect or association is the GRADE approach, which is nowadays broadly used and recommended (Guyatt et al.,

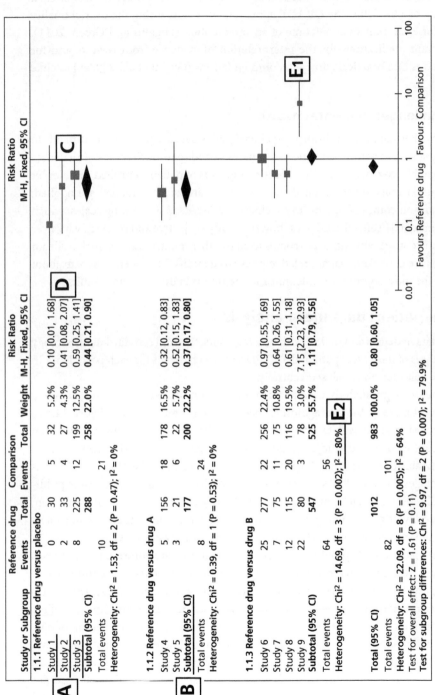

Figure 14.3 Graphical representation of meta-analysis—a forest plot. The left column (A) lists the names of included studies. Results of each subgroup of studies can be collected as a subtotal (B). The diamond at the bottom represents the pooled point estimate and the horizontal line its confidence interval (CI). In the column corresponding to the number of events, results of each study are pooled, reporting the number of events out of the total number of subjects randomized to each treatment. Individual studies are represented graphically (C) as squares but also numerically (D). The horizontal line running through the square is the CI, which is shown in parentheses in numerical representation. The vertical line indicates the absence of differences between treatments.

2008b). The Cochrane risk of bias tool focuses on the possible sources of bias of each included study of a SR, while the GRADE approach aims at assessing the overall quality of evidence for each individual outcome of an intervention (Higgins and Green, 2011). This has relevant implications for the interpretation of evidence from reviews and for their translations into practical clinical recommendations (Guyatt et al., 2008a; Jaeschke et al., 2008).

Specific challenges in mental health

Compared to other medical conditions, psychiatric disorders are particularly difficult to describe, diagnose, and assess over time in a consistent and reproducible way. As a consequence, clinical heterogeneity is likely to occur, as groups of patients enrolled in different studies may differ considerably even if the same standardized parameters are applied. Moreover, many outcomes of interest in psychiatry are assessed with rating scales, which are usually considered 'soft' outcomes, as they are highly subjective and prone to vary over time. This is in contrast with 'hard' outcomes used in other medicine areas, such as death or major events (e.g. stroke), that are relatively easy to quantify. This opens a debate about the choice of the most appropriate outcome and the interpretation of study results.

Individual-patient data meta-analysis

To examine data in details and to deal with heterogeneity, the gold standard methodology is a meta-analysis of individual patient data (IPD), in which details for each participant in every trial are collected and analysed centrally.

While standard meta-analysis uses aggregate data from different trials to provide a more precise estimate of the average difference between interventions (Figure 14.4a), IPD meta-analysis combines data from the central collection of raw information from each participant to included studies (Figure 14.4b) (Clarke, 2005). This approach requires considerable time and effort (especially in requesting and collecting data) but has several advantages. First, it allows the examination of data in detail and removes publication bias. The IPD approach can also help to identify eligible studies (van Walraven, 2010), because investigators may provide information about trials otherwise not identified with standard searching that they have done or that they know (Clarke, 2005). In addition, IPD meta-analysis provides the opportunity to explore additional hypotheses and to measure treatment effects in important subgroups of patients or the influence of characteristics such as age, severity, and gender (Cipriani and Barbui, 2007). IPD meta-analysis allows the harmonization of outcomes across studies (e.g. some studies collect data on a particular outcome but do not report it in publications, or the definition of outcomes may be different across studies), data analyses, and time points. Finally, it allows the effects of competitive treatments over time to be described (van Walraven, 2010). Information that refers to the outcome of each included subject is usually collected not only at endpoint but also at various time intervals after random allocation (Cipriani and Barbui, 2007).

(a) Standard meta-analysis with data aggregated

(b) Individual patient data meta-analysis

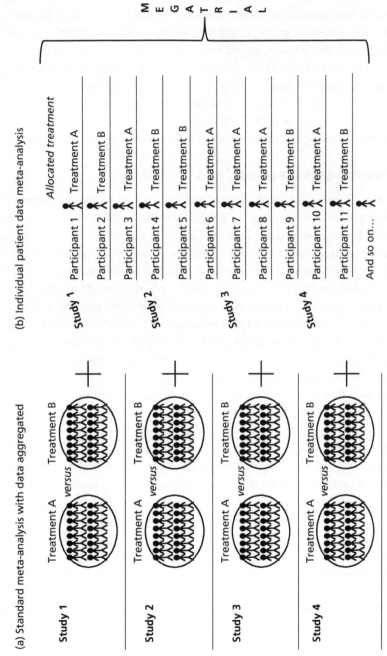

Figure 14.4 Standard meta-analysis on the left (a), in which every row corresponds to a study, and individual patient data meta-analysis on the right (b), in which every row corresponds to an individual randomized participant.

However, this methodology is complex and not always feasible (Stewart and Tierney, 2002). One of the most challenging parts of IPD meta-analysis is the collection of IPD: trialists may be reluctant to share data from their studies, and even when they are willing to share it, there are practical difficulties to be managed. For example, the harmonization of data from each trial into a common, standard dataset is a complex procedure, considering the variations between studies in data formats, data structure, and variable definition (van Walraven, 2010). To overcome these problems reviewers usually are flexible, and try to collaborate regularly with trial investigators, involving them in the IPD project, sharing authorship, and assuring that all data will be kept anonymized (Clarke, 2005; Salanti et al., 2008). Having the collaboration of these investigators has the additional advantage of creating a scientific group of experts with content knowledge.

Multiple treatments meta-analysis

Methods for data collection and analysis described so far focus on the evaluation of one or two treatments at a time, providing a partial view of the possible wealth of treatment options available for a given clinical condition (Salanti et al., 2008). Advanced statistical techniques have been developed to provide inferences on the comparative effectiveness of interventions even when they have never been evaluated directly in clinical trials (Mills et al., 2011). This method allows the estimation of the relative efficacy of multiple treatments simultaneously, using treatments 'in common' to create an indirect comparison (the so-called multiple-treatments meta-analysis or network meta-analysis) (MTM) (Caldwell et al., 2005). Moreover, even when a direct estimate is available, MTM contributes to improve the precision of this estimate by reducing the width of confidence intervals (Salanti et al., 2008).

Given its complexity, before conducting an MTM, some assumptions have to be satisfied. The first is that eligible trials have to be similar in terms of clinical and methodological characteristics, interventions tested, and expected direction of effects (Mills et al., 2011; Cipriani et al., 2013b). In addition to similarity, transitivity is the extension of clinical and methodological homogeneity to comparisons across groups of studies that in turn compare treatments. In complex network structures, the transitivity assumption should hold for all cases where indirect or mixed estimates are derived (Cipriani et al., 2013b), taking into account all possible modifiers that may vary across comparisons (i.e. type of comparator, way of administration, and type of population). Another important assumption is 'consistency' or 'coherence', which is the statistical representation of transitivity and can be evaluated when direct and indirect evidence for an interventions comparison is available (Veroniki et al., 2013; Tricco et al., 2014). Inconsistency is measured by differences between direct and indirect estimates beyond what chance can explain (Cipriani et al., 2013b).

We might wish to compare different interventions against each other, but only studies comparing each of these interventions versus placebo are available (Figure 14.5—1). MTM allows us to obtain an indirect estimate considering the treatment in common ('common comparator') (Figure 14.5—2) and improves the precision of the direct estimate where this is available (Figure 14.5—3). This type of comparison is extremely useful to interpret evidence from RCTs comparing network of different types of intervention, different types of classes of drugs, and different doses of the same drug. When many RCTs were under- taken for different treatment options for the same conditions, it is important to understand the pattern of these comparisons. This pattern represents the geometric configuration that the networks of studies may assume (Salanti et al., 2008). The evaluation of network geometry helps to achieve a global view of all the comparisons that were made in meta- analysis since it provides a graphical representation of them, and informs about how many treatments were compared and if some of them were studied preferentially than others. In fact, networks can assume different configurations according to the type of compari- sons and number of treatments (diversity), and frequency with which different treatments are compared to each other (co-occurrence) (Salanti et al., 2008). For example, when dif- ferent treatments are compared with a single comparator, the network assumes a 'star' shape (Figure 14.5—1). Results of MTM are extremely useful in clinical practice. However,

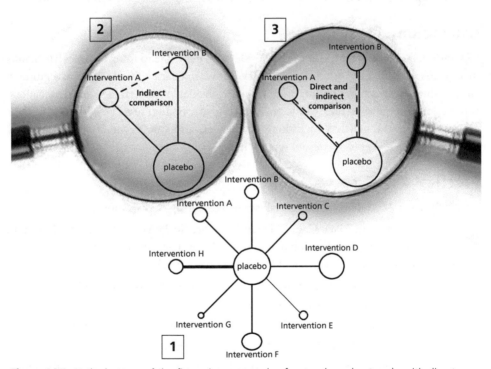

Figure 14.5 At the bottom of the figure is an example of a star-shaped network, with direct comparisons (1). The thickness of each line represents the number of trials, while the size of each node represents the number of randomized patients. The top of the figure demonstrates how multiple treatment meta-analysis works, using the treatment 'in common' (placebo) to create a comparison between intervention A and intervention B (2) and increasing precision in direct comparison (3).

expert statistical support together with subject expertise are required for carrying out this complex type of meta-analysis. Nowadays, the MTM approach is broadly used in different areas of medicine. In the field of mental health, the MTM approach has been particularly helpful in shedding light on some controversial issues, including, for instance, the choice of antipsychotics for schizophrenic patients (Leucht et al., 2013), the therapy of acute mania episodes (Cipriani et al., 2011), the comparative efficacy of new-generation antidepressants (Cipriani et al., 2009), and the efficacy of different psychotherapeutic approaches for depressive disorders (Barth et al., 2013). In the study by Leucht and colleagues (2013), for example, the efficacy of 15 antipsychotic drugs and placebo for the acute treatment of schizophrenia was compared. The analysis included 212 RCTs and therefore a very large population of patients (about 43,000 individuals). Particular analyses allowed treatments to be ranked according to their probability of being effective or harmful when compared to each other. Such rankings provide a detailed framework of each antipsychotic's efficacy and tolerability profile, which is extremely useful for informing daily clinical choices. Furthermore, this also has theoretical implications, as it strongly challenges the assumption of a relevant class effect within both first- and second-generation antipsychotics.

Conclusion

SRs and meta-analysis represent the highest level of evidence to inform clinical decisions in all fields of medicine, including psychiatry. They can be used by clinicians as a guide to choose the best treatment option from the many available. Nevertheless, evidence alone is not enough to guide action. Clinicians should incorporate research evidence with their experience and the patient's condition, preferences, and values. Medical evidence may supplement clinical judgement, not replace it.

Practical exercises

Critically assess the following meta-analyses by answering the questions:

1. Cortese, S., Moreira-Maia, C.R., St Fleur, D., Morcillo-Peñalver, C., Rohde, L.A., and Faraone, S.V. (2016). Association between ADHD and obesity: a systematic review and meta-analysis. *American Journal of Psychiatry*, 173, 34–43.

   a. Comment on the search strategy used. In particular, were unpublished studies searched? Which resources were used for this purpose?

   b. What were the inclusion criteria and were these appropriate to the objectives?

   c. Discuss the way the quality of included trials was assessed.

   d. How was the process of the selection of outcome measures for use in the meta-analysis justified?

   e. Discuss the way in which heterogeneity was managed. Do you think this was adequate?

   f. What statistical methods were used to combine results?

   g. Which types of subgroup analyses were performed?

2. Murphy, S.M., Irving, C.B., Adams, C.E., and Waqar, M. (2015). Crisis intervention for people with severe mental illnesses. *Cochrane Database of Systematic Reviews*, 12, CD001087.

   a. Comment on the inclusion and exclusion criteria. How representative of the research were the included trials?

   b. How was heterogeneity detected? Are there other statistical measures of heterogeneity?

   c. What are the main methodological limitations of included studies?

   d. Discuss the clinical implications of this review.

Further reading

Koopman, L., van der Heijden, G.J., Glasziou, P.P., Grobbee, D.E., and Rovers, M.M. (2007). A systematic review of analytical methods used to study subgroups in (individual patient data) meta-analyses. *Journal of Clinical Epidemiology*, **60**, 1002–1009.

Salanti, G., Del Giovane, C., Chaimani, A., Caldwell, D.M., and Higgins, J.P. (2014). Evaluating the quality of evidence from a network meta-analysis. *PLoS One*, **9**, e99682.

Whiting, P., Savović, J., Higgins, J.P., Caldwell, D.M., Reeves, B.C., Shea, B., et al. (2016). ROBIS: a new tool to assess risk of bias in systematic reviews was developed. *Journal of Clinical Epidemiology*, **69**, 225–234.

References

Akobeng, A.K. (2005). Principles of evidence based medicine. *Archives of Disease in Childhood*, **90**, 837–840.

Barth, J., Munder, T., Gerger, H., Nüesch, E., Trelle, S., Znoj, H., et al. (2013). Comparative efficacy of seven psychotherapeutic interventions for patients with depression: a network meta-analysis. *PLoS Medicine*, **10**, e1001454.

Berlin, J.A. and Golub, R.M. (2014). Meta-analysis as evidence: building a better pyramid. *JAMA*, **312**, 603–605.

Bero, L. and Rennie, D. (1995). The Cochrane Collaboration. Preparing, maintaining, and disseminating systematic reviews of the effects of health care. *JAMA*, **274**, 1935–1938.

Britten, N., Campbell, R., Pope, C., Donovan, J., Morgan, M., and Pill, R. (2002). Using meta ethnography to synthesise qualitative research: a worked example. *Journal of Health Services Research & Policy*, **7**, 209–215.

Caldwell, D.M., Ades, A.E., and Higgins, J.P. (2005). Simultaneous comparison of multiple treatments: combining direct and indirect evidence. *BMJ*, **331**, 897–900.

Campbell, R., Pound, P., Morgan, M., Daker-White, G., Britten, N., Pill, R., et al. (2011). Evaluating meta-ethnography: systematic analysis and synthesis of qualitative research. *Health Technology Assessment (Winchester, England)*, **15**, 1–164.

Cipriani, A. and Barbui, C. (2006a). What is a forest plot? *Epidemiologia e Psichiatria Sociale*, **15**, 258–259.

Cipriani, A. and Barbui, C. (2006b). What is a systematic review? *Epidemiologia e Psichiatria Sociale*, **15**, 174–175.

Cipriani, A. and Barbui, C. (2007). What is an individual patient data meta-analysis? *Epidemiologia e Psichiatria Sociale*, **16**, 203–204.

Cipriani, A., Barbui, C., Salanti, G., Rendell, J., Brown, R., Stockton, S., et al. (2011). Comparative efficacy and acceptability of antimanic drugs in acute mania: a multiple-treatments meta-analysis. *Lancet*, 378, 1306–1315.

Cipriani, A., Furukawa, T.A., Salanti, G., Geddes, J.R., Higgins, J.P., Churchill, R., et al. (2009). Comparative efficacy and acceptability of 12 new-generation antidepressants: a multiple-treatments meta-analysis. *Lancet*, 373, 746–758.

Cipriani, A., Higgins, J.P., Geddes, J.R., and Salanti, G. (2013b). Conceptual and technical challenges in network meta-analysis. *Annals of Internal Medicine*, 159, 130–137.

Clarke, M.J. (2005). Individual patient data meta-analyses. *Best Practice and Research: Clinical Obstetrics and Gynaecology*, 19, 47–55.

Cortese, S., Moreira-Maia, C.R., St Fleur, D., Morcillo-Peñalver, C., Rohde, L.A., and Faraone, S.V. (2016). Association between ADHD and obesity: a systematic review and meta-analysis. *American Journal of Psychiatry*, 173, 34–43.

Creswell, J.W., Fetters, M.D., and Ivankova, N.V. (2004). Designing a mixed methods study in primary care. *Annals of Family Medicine*, 2, 7–12.

Fletcher, J. (2007). What is heterogeneity and is it important? *BMJ*, 334, 94–96.

Garg, A.X., Hackam, D., and Tonelli, M. (2008). Systematic review and meta-analysis: when one study is just not enough. *Clinical Journal of the American Society of Nephrology*, 3, 253–260.

Guyatt, G.H., Oxman, A.D., Kunz, R., Falck-Ytter, Y., Vist, G.E., Liberati, A., et al. (2008a). Going from evidence to recommendations. *BMJ*, 336, 1049–1051.

Guyatt, G.H., Oxman, A.D., Vist, G.E., Kunz, R., Falck-Ytter, Y., Alonso-Coello, P., et al. (2008b). GRADE: an emerging consensus on rating quality of evidence and strength of recommendations. *BMJ*, 336, 924–926.

Haidich, A.B. (2010). Meta-analysis in medical research. *Hippokratia*, 14 (Suppl. 1), 29–37.

Hausner, E., Waffenschmidt, S., Kaiser, T., and Simon, M. (2012). Routine development of objectively derived search strategies. *Systematic Reviews*, 1, 19.

Higgins, J.P., Altman, D.G., Gøtzsche, P.C., Jüni, P., Moher, D., Oxman, A.D., et al. (2011a). The Cochrane Collaboration's tool for assessing risk of bias in randomised trials. *BMJ*, 343, d5928.

Higgins, J.P.T., Douglas, A., and Sterne J. (2011b). Chapter 8: Assessing risk of bias in included studies. In: Higgins, J.P.T. and Green, S. (eds). *Cochrane Handbook for Systematic Reviews of Interventions*. Version 5.1.0 [updated March 2011]. The Cochrane Collaboration. https://training.cochrane.org/handbook

Higgins, J.P.T. and Green, S. (eds). (2011). *Cochrane Handbook for Systematic Reviews of Interventions*. Version 5.1.0 [updated March 2011]. The Cochrane Collaboration. https://training.cochrane.org/handbook

Higgins, J.P. and Thompson, S.G. (2002). Quantifying heterogeneity in a meta-analysis. *Statistics in Medicine*, 21, 1539–1558.

Ho, P.M., Peterson, P.N., and Masoudi, F.A. (2008). Evaluating the evidence: is there a rigid hierarchy? *Circulation*, 118, 1675–1684.

Ioannidis, J.P. (2008). Interpretation of tests of heterogeneity and bias in meta-analysis. *Journal of Evaluation in Clinical Practice*, 14, 951–957.

Jaeschke, R., Guyatt, G.H., Dellinger, P., Schünemann, H., Levy, M.M., Kunz, R., et al. (2008). Use of GRADE grid to reach decisions on clinical practice guidelines when consensus is elusive. *BMJ*, 337, a744.

Leucht, S., Cipriani, A., Spineli, L., Mavridis, D., Orey, D., Richter, F., et al. (2013). Comparative efficacy and tolerability of 15 antipsychotic drugs in schizophrenia: a multiple-treatments meta-analysis. *Lancet*, 382, 951–962.

Manchikanti, L., Hirsch, J.A., and Smith, H.S. (2008). Evidence-based medicine, systematic reviews, and guidelines in interventional pain management. Part 2: randomized controlled trials. *Pain Physician*, **11**, 717–773.

Mills, E.J., Bansback, N., Ghement, I., Thorlund, K., Kelly, S., Puhan, M.A., and Wright, J. (2011). Multiple treatment comparison meta-analyses: a step forward into complexity. *Clinical Epidemiology*, **3**, 193–202.

Moher, D., Shamseer, L., Clarke, M., Ghersi, D., Liberati, A., Petticrew, M., et al. (2015). Preferred reporting items for systematic review and meta-analysis protocols (PRISMA-P) 2015 statement. *Systematic Reviews*, **4**, 1.

Morgan, D.L. (1998). Practical strategies for combining qualitative and quantitative methods. applications to health research. *Qualitative Health Research*, **8**, 362–376.

Murphy, S.M., Irving, C.B., Adams, C.E., and Waqar, M. (2015). Crisis intervention for people with severe mental illnesses. *Cochrane Database of Systematic Reviews*, **12**, CD001087.

Naylor, C.D. (1997). Meta-analysis and the meta-epidemiology of clinical research. *BMJ*, **315**, 617–619.

Purgato, M. and Adams, C.E. (2012). Heterogeneity: the issue of apples, oranges and fruit pie. *Epidemiology and Psychiatric Sciences*, **21**, 27–29.

Purgato, M., Cipriani, A., and Barbui, C. (2012). [Randomized trials, systematic reviews, meta-analyses: basic criteria in the world of scientific evidence]. *Rivista di Psichiatria*, **47**, 21–29.

Sackett, D.L., Rosenberg, W.M., Gray, J.A., Haynes, R.B., and Richardson, W.S. (1996). Evidence based medicine: what it is and what it isn't. *BMJ*, **312**, 71–72.

Salanti, G., Higgins, J.P., Ades, A.E., and Ioannidis, J.P. (2008). Evaluation of networks of randomized trials. *Statistical Methods in Medical Research*, **17**, 279–301.

Savovic, J., Weeks, L., Sterne, J.A., Turner, L., Altman, D.G., Moher, D., and Higgins, J.P. (2014). Evaluation of the Cochrane Collaboration's tool for assessing the risk of bias in randomized trials: focus groups, online survey, proposed recommendations and their implementation. *Systematic Reviews*, **3**, 37.

Stewart, L.A. and Tierney, J.F. (2002). To IPD or not to IPD? Advantages and disadvantages of systematic reviews using individual patient data. *Evaluation and the Health Professions*, **25**, 76–97.

Trespidi, C., Barbui, C., and Cipriani, A. (2011). Why it is important to include unpublished data in systematic reviews. *Epidemiology and Psychiatric Sciences*, **20**, 133–135.

Tricco, A.C., Ashoor, H.M., Antony, J., Beyene, J., Veroniki, A.A., and Isaranuwatchai, W., et al. (2014). Safety, effectiveness, and cost effectiveness of long acting versus intermediate acting insulin for patients with type 1 diabetes: systematic review and network meta-analysis. *BMJ*, **349**, g5459.

Turner, E.H., Matthews, A.M., Linardatos, E., Tell, R.A., and Rosenthal, R. (2008). Selective publication of antidepressant trials and its influence on apparent efficacy. *New England Journal of Medicine*, **358**, 252–260.

Turner, L., Shamseer, L., Altman, D.G., Weeks, L., Peters, J., Kober, T., et al. (2012). Consolidated standards of reporting trials (CONSORT) and the completeness of reporting of randomised controlled trials (RCTs) published in medical journals. *Cochrane Database of Systematic Reviews*, **11**, MR000030.

Uman, L.S. (2011). Systematic reviews and meta-analyses. *Journal of the Canadian Academy of Child and Adolescent Psychiatry*, **20**, 57–59.

van Walraven, C. (2010.). Individual patient meta-analysis--rewards and challenges. *Journal of Clinical Epidemiology*, **63**, 235–237.

Veroniki, A.A., Vasiliadis, H.S., Higgins, J.P., and Salanti, G. (2013). Evaluation of inconsistency in networks of interventions. *International Journal of Epidemiology*, **42**, 332–345.

Chapter 15

Inference 1: Chance, bias, and confounding

Robert Stewart

Introduction

Inference is the 'process of passing from observations to generalizations', and is a key activity in all research—fundamentally guiding study design as well as interpreting findings. An observed *association* between two factors does not mean that one definitely caused the other. In epidemiology, the roles of chance, bias, and confounding need to considered, as well as any ambiguity in the direction of causality, before any conclusions can be drawn about potential implications (Box 15.1). If an association is observed, might it have occurred by chance? Might it have arisen because of error intrinsic to the study design (bias)? Might the association have arisen because of other factors (confounding)? Has an association between factors A and B arisen because A has caused B or because B has caused A (direction of causation)?

The vast majority of research is carried out within a defined sample but seeks to uncover broader truths about a wider 'source' population from which the sample is derived (whether this is the 'community' or whether it is a defined clinical population). Without that wider applicability, findings are only relevant to the sample and the research team, and are of no interest to anyone else. Chance and bias should be the first considerations in study design and critical appraisal because they address the 'translation' of inference from the *sample* to the *population*. For example: 'Here is an association between two factors in a sample. But can I assume that this is true for the source population?' Confounding and direction of causation on the other hand address potentially more complex issues: 'Here is an association which I believe to be present in the source population (having considered the roles of chance and bias), but what does this tell me about how this disease or event is caused?' Confounding will be considered with chance and bias out of convention, but the issue of inferring cause and effect will be then be taken up in more detail in Chapter 16.

Chance

The role of chance in explaining an observed association is assessed in the statistical analysis of results. Statistical inference involves generalizing from sample data to the wider population from which the sample was drawn (whether a community or clinical

Box 15.1 Inference

Chance

What is the likely value in the population (95% confidence intervals)?
What is the probability of chance (p-value)?

Bias

Through sampling/participation/follow-up (selection bias)
Through measurements applied/information obtained (information bias)
From participants/from observers
Differential/non-differential

Confounding

'An alternative explanation'
Addressed in the study design (by restriction/matching/randomization)
Addressed in the analysis (by stratified/multivariate analysis)

Further considerations

Relationship between prevalence, incidence, and survival
Relationship between the ecological level and the individual level
Direction of causation
Mediating factors
Effect modification
Background literature
Implications for research/clinical practice/public health

population). Inferences are made by calculating the range around an observed property of the sample within which the 'true' property of the population is likely to lie (confidence intervals) or, less commonly now, the probability that chance alone might have accounted for a given observation (the p-value).

Sampling error and sampling distributions

Chance operates through sampling error. If we wanted to estimate the mean alcohol intake in people aged 16 years and over in the United Kingdom, we would not go to the trouble of interviewing the whole nation. We would instead draw a representative sample, possibly from a population register. Non-random selection might give rise to unrepresentative samples—this situation is considered in the later 'Bias' section. For the moment, a random and entirely representative sample is assumed. If, say, 100 people were interviewed we would have a mean alcohol intake for that sample. Assuming a symmetrical 'normal' distribution for alcohol intake, 95% of people in the sample will have intakes within approximately two (actually 1.96) standard deviations either side of this mean (because this is a property of the normal distribution). If, however, we were to interview another random sample of 100 people, the mean intake would not be exactly the same. Which one should we believe? If we were to repeat the study over and over, we would end up with a distribution of mean intakes. This hypothetical distribution is referred to as the *sampling distribution*. The observed means from repeated sampling will be normally distributed. This tends to be true even if the trait itself is not normally distributed in the population (the proof is referred to as the *central limit theorem*). The mean of the sampling distribution will be the population mean; sample estimates for the mean which deviate considerably from the true population mean will be observed much less commonly, appearing in the tails of the distribution. Note that if the size of the samples were to be increased (i.e. above 100 in this example), then the variance (i.e. spread) of these means would decrease. This is because larger samples give more precise estimates.

Standard errors and confidence intervals

The standard deviation for the sampling distribution is known as the *standard error* of the mean—so 95% of *sample means* obtained by repeated sampling will lie within approximately two *standard errors* either side of the population mean (because of this property of the normal distribution). This information can therefore be used to estimate limits of uncertainty around an observed *sample* mean, giving the range of likely values for the *population* mean. These limits of uncertainty are referred to as *95% confidence intervals*. They represent the range in which 95% of mean values would lie if sampling was repeated indefinitely under identical conditions.

Confidence intervals for other types of observations in a sample are calculated in a similar way (by estimating the standard error)—such as proportions (e.g. the prevalence of depression), mean differences (e.g. gender differences in alcohol intake), odds ratios (e.g. for associations between gender and alcoholism), or rate ratios (e.g. for male/female incidence rates of alcoholism). The calculation of standard errors is relatively simple for many situations and some formulae are given in Box 15.2. For small sample sizes, other formulae may have to be used and these are described in most generic statistics guides (e.g. Kirkwood and Sterne, 2016). A pocket calculator is sufficient but computers generally 'take the strain' and there are a variety of online calculators available for more complex functions, easily identified through searches. The principle is still that 'out there' in the whole source population (e.g. UK adults) is a true proportion, mean difference, odds ratio, rate ratio, etc. These cannot be directly measured without recruiting the whole population but, for a representative sample, 95% confidence intervals give a range of values within which the true value will lie on 95% of occasions. The choice of '95%' for defining confidence intervals is entirely arbitrary, but there is generally little reason to stray beyond convention.

Box 15.2 Formulae for calculating standard errors and confidence intervals

Situation 1: a single proportion 'p' in a sample of size 'n':

$$\text{SE} = \sqrt{\{p(1-p)/n\}} \quad 95\% \text{ CI} = p \pm 1.96 \times \text{SE}$$

where SE is standard error and CI is confidence interval (suitable when np and $n - np$ are 10 or more).

Situation 2: a mean for a sample of size 'n' and standard deviation 's':

$$\text{SE} = s/\sqrt{n} \quad 95\% \text{ CI} = \text{mean} \pm 1.96 \times \text{SE}$$

(suitable for sample sizes above 20).

Situation 3: the difference between two proportions 'p_1' and 'p_2' in samples with sizes 'n_1' and 'n_2' respectively:

$$\text{SE} = \sqrt{\{p_1(1-p_1)/n_1 + p_2(1-p_2)/n_2\}} \quad 95\%\text{CI} = \text{difference} \pm 1.96 \times \text{SE}$$

(suitable when both samples fulfil criteria for situation 1).

Situation 4: the difference between two means in samples with sizes of n_1 and n_2 and a standard deviations of s_1 and s_2 respectively:

$$\text{SE} = \sqrt{(s_1/n_1 + s_2/n_2)} \quad 95\%\text{CI} = \text{difference} \pm 1.96 \times \text{SE}$$

(suitable when both samples fulfil criteria for situation 2).

Statistical tests and p-values

Statistical procedures are used to test whether a hypothesis about the distribution of one or more variables should be accepted or rejected. In the case of a hypothesized association between a risk factor and a disease, we can estimate the probability of an association of at least a given size being observed if the *null hypothesis* were true (i.e. that there is no real association and the observed association merely arose through chance). Conventionally, the threshold for statistical significance is taken to be 0.05—that is, findings are accepted as present if the probability that they occurred by chance is 5% or less. As with confidence intervals, it is important to remember that there is nothing magical about the $p = 0.05$ threshold. It represents nothing more than a generally agreed acceptable level of risk of making what is known as a *type 1 error*, that is, falsely rejecting a null hypothesis when it is true (a 'false-positive' finding). This is generally based on the assumption that a two-tailed statistical test will be used (see 'A note on p-values'). The probability of rejecting the null hypothesis when it is indeed false (i.e. detecting a true association) is the study's *statistical power* (although conventionally expressed as a percentage). The converse scenario, accepting a null hypothesis when it should have been rejected (i.e. failing to detect a true association) is referred to as a *type 2 error*.

For differences in proportions and mean values between two groups, estimating the p-value for a given observation is, like confidence intervals, relatively simple since it just involves calculating the number of standard errors the observed difference is away from the null value. For these estimations, the null hypothesis is that there is no difference between group A and group B (e.g. men and women) with respect to a mean value or a proportion (e.g. mean alcohol consumption or prevalence of depression). For example, you might observe that men drank 4 units of alcohol per week more than women. You might then calculate that the standard error for that difference was 1 unit/week. The observed difference is therefore four standard errors away from the null. This is called a 'z-score'. We know already that 1.96 standard errors away from the null give 95% confidence intervals—and are therefore equivalent to a p-value of 0.05 (for a two-tailed test—see 'A note on p-values'). So the p-value for a difference of four standard errors is considerably less than 0.05—therefore 'highly significant'. We really knew this anyway because 95% confidence intervals for the mean difference would have been approximately 2–6 units/week (i.e. nowhere near the null value of zero). The equivalent z-score for a p-value of 0.01 is 2.58, for 0.001 is 3.29, and for 0.0001 is 3.89. So for our analysis, the p-value is less than 0.0001. Tables linking z-scores more precisely to p-values are given in most statistics textbooks or online resources. In general, a computer will come up with a needlessly precise estimate. The calculation of p-values for other situations (e.g. odds ratios) are slightly more complex, although with similar underlying principles, and are described in other texts (e.g. Kirkwood and Sterne, 2016).

The relationship between *p*-values and confidence intervals

There are therefore two ways in which the role of chance can be estimated for a given association. One is the probability that the association might have arisen through chance (the p-value); the other is the range of values within which the true strength of association is likely to lie (confidence intervals). The problem with p-values is that they only give a single probability (related to whether the null hypothesis is true or not). The size of the p-value gives little indication of the strength of association (e.g. a weak association of little clinical significance may be detected with a 'highly significant' p-value if the sample is very large). Confidence intervals on the other hand describe both the likely magnitude of an association as well as giving an idea of whether it can be concluded to be present or not (i.e. for a significance cut-off of 0.05, whether 95% intervals overlap the 'null' value of 1.0 for a ratio, or 0.0 for a difference). Confidence intervals are therefore preferred and there are now a decreasing number of circumstances where calculation of a p-value is considered helpful or necessary.

A note on hypotheses

It is important to bear in mind that two different sorts of hypothesis are referred to in research methods literature. In research papers and funding applications, one or more 'positive' hypotheses are generally required—that is, that X and Y will be associated, or that X will occur at a greater frequency in group Y than group Z. A requirement for the paper or funding application is to demonstrate that the design and sample size are sufficient to test these propositions. In order to carry this out in statistical analysis, the starting point is always from the opposite point of view—that is, that there is no association between X and Y (the 'null hypothesis'). The task is then to establish whether this can be disproved and with what degree of certainty. Distinctions are also sometimes made between *a priori* and *post hoc* hypotheses. These refer to the timing of the hypothesis in relation to the experiment or research study. The strongest approach (for reasons that will be discussed further in Chapter 16) is for a hypothesis to be articulated first (*a priori*), followed by an experiment to test this—this leads the researcher naturally on to the development of an appropriate study design, the sample size calculation, and the appropriate analysis. It also keeps the study focused on a single question and renders the findings and statistical tests much more credible and more likely to have wider scientific impact. Weaker hypotheses are those which are derived from the findings of a study (*post hoc*)—while these might turn out to be genuine, they have not strictly speaking been tested experimentally and there is a much higher risk of 'false-positive' findings, particularly if analyses have been exploratory and have involved multiple statistical tests. Therefore, *post hoc* hypotheses should be treated with a lot more caution and as requiring further testing and verification before inferences and implications can be considered.

A note on *p*-values

It is customary practice to apply what are known as *two-tailed* statistical tests for significance. These test whether an observation is *different* from the null rather than specifically whether it is either *greater* or *less*—that is, it concerns both tails of the normal distribution. A common misinterpretation of the two-sided *p*-value is that it represents the probability that the point estimate is as far or further from the null value as was observed. For large samples, this probability is approximately the square of the *p*-value (i.e. considerably lower). This problem with interpreting two-sided *p*-values is another reason to focus on confidence intervals instead.

A note on confidence intervals

In the absence of bias, 95% confidence intervals will, over unlimited repetitions of the study with a given sample size, include the true parameter on at least 95% of occasions. A common misinterpretation of confidence intervals is that there is a 95% *probability* that they contain the true parameter. This situation only applies to confidence intervals derived using Bayesian analysis, and cannot be assumed for those calculated using standard procedures.

Bias

Bias refers to systematic error arising from the design or execution of a study. It is an entirely undesirable feature which, unlike confounding (see 'Confounding'), cannot be 'adjusted for' once data have been gathered. Most of the thought put into study design is aiming to limit bias. Bias can be broadly categorized into that which arises from deriving the sample or comparison groups from the 'base' population (*selection bias* as well as bias arising from incomplete sampling and differential attrition) and that which arises from the measurements taken (*information bias*). Different study designs are more or less prone to particular sources of bias, and readers are also referred to the respective chapters for a more detailed account.

Information bias

Information bias arises from any error in the measurements applied in a study. All measurements are potentially subject to error, whether they are an assay for cholesterol levels, a genetic test, a questionnaire assessment of personality traits, or a structured clinical interview diagnosis of major depression. Error in categorical measures such as diagnoses is conventionally referred to as misclassification. The effect of the bias depends upon whether the error is *differential* or *non-differential*. In *differential misclassification*, the misclassification in the measured variable is different between the groups being compared—that is, when misclassification of exposure is affected by the known outcome, or when outcome status misclassification is different between known exposure groups. For example, in an unblinded clinical trial, knowing what intervention someone has received might influence a clinician's assessment of their clinical improvement; or people who are cases may be more likely to remember a particular exposure than someone who is a control. Where differential misclassification has occurred, *bias might operate in either direction*—that is, the 'true' strength of the association may be over- or underestimated.

On the other hand, most misclassification tends to be *non-differential*—that is, occurs to the same extent in all participants (e.g. because of a faulty blood pressure machine used by all participants, or because of a sub-optimally designed questionnaire). This is sometimes simply called *measurement error* and is predictable in its effects, always biasing results *towards the null*. This means that the 'true' strength of association is underestimated, and it does not give rise to spurious associations (i.e. if an association is found to be present, it cannot be explained by non-differential bias).

Information bias may be derived from either participants or assessors. Participant-derived information bias is a frequent consideration in case–control studies, often called *recall bias*, where information on previous exposure relies on someone remembering it, but where cases may be more or less likely to recall and/or report this information than controls. For example, people with multiple episodes of major depression as an adult (cases) may be more likely to recall and report childhood abuse (the exposure of interest) than people with no history of mental health problems (controls). This will give rise to a spuriously strong association between abuse and depression unless measures are taken to prevent this bias (not always simple or even possible). The experience of disease encourages an 'effort after meaning' whereby the participant has already thought through their life history in an attempt to understand why they have become ill. Investigator-derived information bias in the above-mentioned case–control study might arise if an investigator puts extra effort into obtaining disclosure of abuse from major depression cases than from controls. In a randomized controlled trial, investigators' judgements concerning side effects or clinical improvement may be influenced if they are aware of, or can guess, whether a participant is receiving a treatment or placebo.

The key solutions to information bias in study design are firstly to maximize the accuracy of a measurement (because something which is 100% accurate cannot give rise to error), but also to minimize its ambiguity and susceptibility to influence. For example, attempts are made to conceal allocation from participants in *single-blind trials*, and from both participants and investigators in *double-blind trials* (see Chapter 12). In case–control studies, participants may be blinded to the hypothesis under investigation, and investigators may be blinded to a participant's case status, as well as to the study hypothesis. Clearly neither of these procedures is universally feasible.

Selection/inclusion bias

Selection bias is again a particular problem in case–control studies. Cases selected for the study should be representative of all cases from the base population and controls should be representative of all controls. Clearly there is some degree of selection in any recruitment process, because participants both have to be identified and agree to take part; however, selection *bias* occurs where the selection of cases and/or controls is influenced by the exposure under investigation. For example, take a primary care-based case–control study comparing people with and without depression on recent life events. It might be reasonable to recruit cases from people known to have depression and compare them to other registered patients with no depression. However, we know that many cases of depression remain unidentified, and depression might be more likely to be picked up in primary care when someone has had a recent life event—thus exaggerating the association of interest. On the other hand, it is possible that general practitioners might be reluctant to make a depression diagnosis after certain events (e.g. bereavement), which would have the opposite influence. For a case–control study, cases and controls should be drawn from the same base population (one useful check is to ask yourself the question 'If this control had developed the disease could he/she have been included in the case group?'). Inclusion and exclusion criteria need to be examined carefully to ensure that they are the same for case and control groups. In the earlier example, selection bias would be much less likely if cases were identified from a screened community population; it would also be unlikely if a genetic factor, rather than life events, was the exposure of interest (because it is difficult to think of a way in which the exposure could influence selection).

Bias may also arise because of less avoidable reasons. Cross-sectional surveys rarely if ever have 100% participation rates, and even then may be incompletely sampling the source population of interest (e.g. relying on people answering the door to household enumerators). If non-inclusion is random then this will only have an impact on statistical power; however, if non-inclusion is influenced either way by the outcome that is being measured in a survey (e.g. people with depression more likely to be at home, or less likely to be willing to participate) then clearly this will influence an observed prevalence. In a cohort study or trial, loss to follow-up ('attrition') is the main source of inclusion bias, as there needs to have been at least some follow-up for an original cohort member to contribute to the analysis. As with survey participation, if attrition is random then this only influences statistical power; it becomes problematic if it is affected by both exposure and outcome. Because the outcome is unknown (by definition) in people lost to follow-up, the focus is on evaluating whether there are any exposures influencing attrition (e.g. differences between randomization groups in a trial). The solutions to inclusion bias are primarily logistic—that is, simply trying one's utmost to achieve high participation rates in a survey and to maximize follow-up rates in a trial. Readers are referred to the relevant chapters on these study designs for more detailed consideration.

Other bias

Two other situations are commonly described as sources of bias although are better considered as limitations of individual study designs rather than arising from an error in their application.

Prevalence bias refers to the fact that prevalence (the proportion of people having a disease at a particular time) is a product both of the rate at which new cases arise (the incidence) and the rate at which cases cease to have the condition (e.g. through recovery or death). Factors identified in a cross-sectional study as positively associated with a disorder will include those which are associated with increased incidence, and those associated with increased duration (or 'maintenance') of that disorder state. This is a particular issue with fluctuating disorders such as depression where prevalence is strongly influenced by time to recovery. One approach, used particularly in case–control studies is to restrict 'case' participants to those with a recent-onset disorder, 'incident cases', hence limiting the influence of duration.

A fundamental limitation of ecological studies (described in Chapter 8) is that it cannot be inferred that associations observed at a group level also apply at an individual level. This is referred to, somewhat confusingly and apparently interchangeably in many texts, as '*ecological bias*', 'ecological confounding', and the 'ecological fallacy'. However, individual-level generalizations from ecological data are better described as 'fallacy' than bias since they represent a failure to draw appropriate inferences rather than an error in the methodology of the study itself.

Confounding

The term confounding derives from the Latin *confundere*, meaning to mix up. Confounding describes a situation in which the measured effect of an exposure is distorted because of the association of that exposure with other factors that influence the disease or outcome under study. A confounding variable might cause or prevent the outcome of interest, is not an intermediate variable (on the causal pathway between the exposure and the outcome), and is independently associated with the exposure under investigation. As discussed earlier, consideration of confounding factors represents an intermediate step between relatively simple questions of whether an association is true or not and the nature of the causal pathways under investigation.

A hypothetical illustration of confounding would be an observed association between grey hair and increased mortality. This observation might have arisen from a rigorously designed study with a representative sample, perfect outcome ascertainment, and with statistical tests indicating a strong association with narrow confidence intervals. The association in the sample therefore appears to be entirely valid—that is, true for the source population as well as the sample. However, it quite obviously does not imply that grey hair *causes* mortality. The limitation in the inferences which can be drawn is that increased age is a likely confounding factor which has not been taken into account. Increased age is associated with grey hair and is more likely to be a cause of mortality. It therefore represents an *alternative explanation* for the observed association. Confounding may be addressed either in the design of a study or, more usually, in the statistical analysis of results, and it is important to remember that confounding, like bias, may lead to true associations being missed as well as false associations being identified. It may even lead to an association being reversed in its direction. For example, driving a fast car might be found to be associated with lower mortality. However, people who drive fast cars are also likely to have higher incomes and socioeconomic status. If the association was adjusted for income, driving a fast car might instead be associated with higher mortality.

Addressing confounding through study design

Strategies in the study design to limit confounding operate by removing variation in confounding factors between comparison groups of interest. A potential confounding factor cannot influence an observed association if it is evenly distributed between the groups compared. An extreme method is sample *restriction*—that is, the sample is limited so that the confounding factor does not vary at all. For example, if gender was believed to be an important confounder, a study might be carried out only in men or only in women. This removes confounding by gender, although obviously limits generalizability (results in women could not be assumed to be the same as results in men). A second approach for case–control studies is *matching*. In this method, control participants are specifically chosen to be as similar as possible to cases with respect to a given confounding factor. In the earlier example, for each person with grey hair, another person without grey hair might be recruited with the same age (one-to-one matching) or within a similar age range (restriction matching). However, there are obvious logistical difficulties with matching on more than one or two factors and there is a danger of 'over-matching' (i.e. creating groups which are so similar that they are partially matched on the exposure of interest). Matched designs have limitations and tend to be restricted to small case–control studies. An exception is a growing recent interest in *propensity score matching*, particularly in large historic cohort designs where exposed and unexposed groups are matched on a score derived from multiple covariates associated with exposure status.

Ultimately, the best method for removing confounding effects is through *randomization*. If an intervention is randomly assigned then all other factors should be evenly distributed between intervention and control groups (given reasonable sample sizes). Any difference in outcome between comparison groups can therefore be reasonably attributed to the intervention. An important advantage is that randomization *controls for both measured and unmeasured confounding factors*. However, randomization is limited ethically to interventions which might be beneficial but where no strong evidence exists one way or another. Where only observational cohorts are available, propensity score matching (as previously described) provides probably the closest possible alternative.

Addressing confounding through statistical analysis

The simplest and most appropriate 'first stage' for investigating confounding is the *stratified analysis*. For the grey hair–mortality example, if we had a sufficiently large sample, and were to subdivide it into 5-year age bands, we would probably find that the association between grey hair and mortality was no longer present (or at least substantially reduced) within each of these bands. Relatively simple statistical equations (e.g. for odds ratios, the *Mantel–Haenszel procedure*) allow stratum-specific estimates to be combined to produce an 'adjusted' estimate (in this case, an age-adjusted association between grey hair and mortality). The limitation is that only one, or at the most two, confounding factors can be considered before strata become too small. More advanced *multivariable analyses* (discussed in more detail in Chapter 18) allow associations of interest to be adjusted simultaneously for multiple potential confounding variables. The choice of analysis depends on the nature of the outcome (or 'dependent') variable. Linear regression and analysis of variance (ANOVA) are used for continuously distributed outcomes (e.g. level of alcohol intake), logistic regression for binary outcomes (e.g. presence or absence of depression), and Cox proportional hazards models where the outcome is a rate or 'survival' (e.g. onset of depression or mortality). Multivariable analyses need to be used with caution and careful forethought. Most importantly, effect modification may be missed if stratified analyses are not first carried out (discussed in Chapter 16), and there is a danger that confounding and mediating factors may not be distinguished (discussed in 'Confounding factors, causal pathways, and planning a statistical analysis').

Confounding, inference, and critical appraisal

The example of grey hair and mortality is a simple one with a clear single confounding factor. 'Real-world' situations are inevitably more complicated, particularly in psychiatric research. An important first step for evaluating the role of a potential confounding factor is interpreting adjusted values. There is no 'test' for confounding and the judgement is a subjective one on the part of the author and the reader of a research report. The focus should be on the estimated strength of an association—for example, an odds ratio, a mean difference, or a correlation coefficient. The extent to which this estimate changes following adjustment, gives the best idea of the extent to which the association was explained by a confounding factor. For example, if the rate ratio for mortality associated with the presence of grey hair was 7.0 (i.e. a sevenfold higher mortality rate in people with grey hair than those without), and if after adjustment for age this ratio was reduced to 1.0 (i.e. equal mortality rates), it would imply that all of the association was 'explained' by age as a confounder. If the age-adjusted rate was reduced to 2.0, the situation would be less clear and would raise the possibility of another confounder accounting for the remainder of the association (e.g. mental or physical stress independently causing both premature physiological ageing and mortality).

The concept of *residual confounding* is an important consideration at this stage of appraisal. Any measurement error in a confounding factor will reduce the effect of adjustment on the association of interest. In the grey hair–mortality example, adjustment for age would have less effect on the rate ratio of interest if age was entered into the multivariate analysis in 10-year categories rather than 1-year units. However, some degree of measurement error or misclassification is inevitable for most potential confounding factors. Furthermore, even with the most rigorous study, it is likely that there is a cluster of unmeasured confounding factors which cannot be taken into account. The combination of unmeasured factors and error in measured factors is known as residual confounding and there is no means of removing it, apart from randomization in intervention studies as discussed earlier. Statistical adjustments therefore should always be assumed to *underestimate* confounding. The decision about residual confounding is entirely subjective in critical appraisal and again depends on the difference between the adjusted and unadjusted strengths of association and how extensively potential confounding factors have been measured and controlled for. If an association is little changed (e.g. an odds ratio changes from 5.0 to 4.8) following adjustment for all conceivable major confounding factors (and if these have been measured satisfactorily), it is unlikely that residual confounding will explain a substantial further proportion. If an association is markedly reduced in strength (e.g. an odds ratio changes from 5.0 to 1.5) following adjustment, residual confounding is more of a concern even if the adjusted association remains 'significant'.

A frequently confusing issue in critical appraisal is whether the role of chance should be considered before or after confounding. If a 'significant' association is 'no longer significant' after adjustment, what should be concluded? This is again subjective, since there is no consensus. As mentioned earlier, if an association remains statistically significant but substantially reduced following adjustments, there is the concern of residual confounding. If on the other hand an odds ratio and 95% confidence intervals were to change from 3.3 (1.4–7.8) to 3.2 (0.9–10.8) following adjustment for all major potential confounding factors, it might be reasonable to assume a true association which was not substantially explained by confounding (NB the widening of the confidence intervals might reflect missing data on some confounding factors, and most regression procedures will exclude cases with missing data on any entered variable, so the sample at the end of an analysis may be different from that at the beginning). In general, the problem with this aspect of appraisal is imparting too great an importance to the arbitrary 5% significance cut-off. For the adjusted odds ratio given earlier, 90% confidence intervals might well have excluded the null value. Would inferences have been any different?

Confounding factors, causal pathways, and planning a statistical analysis

In considering confounding factors, and particularly in planning the statistical analysis of a study, it is important to develop first an idea of potential causal pathways. This is discussed in more detail towards the end of Chapter 16. The principal danger is to confuse confounding and *mediating* factors—since the results of statistical 'adjustment' appear the same. For example, lower social class is generally found to be associated with increased depression. Part of that association may be because people with lower status are more likely to suffer traumatic life events. The association between social class and depression might therefore be reduced after adjustment for recent life events. However, life events are not a confounding factor because they probably lie on the causal pathway between the exposure and outcome of interest. Life events are not an *alternative* explanation for the association of interest. Instead, they provide *additional* information on why risk of depression is higher in people with lower status. If the association between social class and depression were to 'disappear' (i.e. return to the null value) after adjustment for life events, this would not imply that lower social class was not a risk factor. It would instead imply that any causal link was *mediated* by life events—that is, that the effect of social class on life events entirely explained the effect of social class on depression. If the association remained present but reduced after adjustment, the residual association would be that which was not mediated by life events (i.e. operating along other causal pathways—e.g. reduced access to healthcare, family tensions, substandard accommodation, or occupational strain). Causal pathways are potentially complex in psychiatric research. For example, particular life events might conceivably cause a downward social drift as well as later depression (and therefore be confounding rather than mediating factors). For both cross-sectional and prospective research, there are often difficulties in inferring the direction of causation because of the nature of the disorders which we study. These issues will be discussed in Chapter 16.

Conclusion

A fundamental process in interpreting one's own or another's research is to consider what the observations 'mean'—that is, what can be *inferred* from them. This involves a series of questions and considerations (Figure 15.1). The first step theoretically is to decide whether observations can be believed in the first place. It is the duty of the guarantor for any submitted research paper to ensure that the data and results derived from analyses are valid—and to withdraw a submission promptly if there are any concerns over this. Readers have no choice but to assume the integrity of the raw data. The first formal stage of appraisal is therefore to decide to what extent the observations in the *sample* are likely to apply to the source *population*. The principal considerations here are chance and

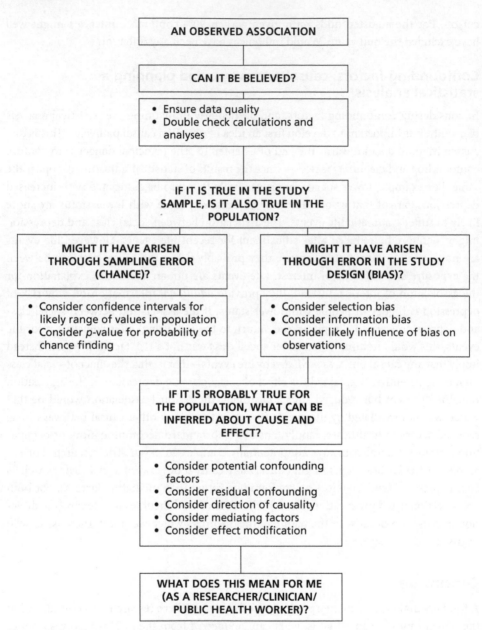

Figure 15.1 Inference—questions and considerations.

bias. If the reader is happy that a population-level association is likely, the next stage is to consider what can be inferred concerning cause and effect. This begins with considering whether the association between proposed exposure and outcome is a direct one and not confounded by other factors. After this point, there are a series of more complex decisions regarding causal pathways, which may not always be inferred from a single study but may require a more broad knowledge of the background literature. These are discussed in Chapter 16 and include the direction of causality (whether an association between A and B is because A causes B or vice versa), mediating factors (does A cause C because A causes B which in turn causes C, or are there other pathways by which A and C are related?), and effect modification (does A cause B to a uniform extent across the population or does the strength of association depend on other factors being present?). Finally, the implications of these inferences need to be considered with respect to developing new hypotheses and investigations, as well as for clinical practice and public health.

Practical exercises

An understanding of chance, bias, and confounding is vital for interpreting most forms of research. This is best assessed through the critical appraisal of a research paper. Students should be able to define confidence intervals; *p*-values; selection and information bias; the relationship between prevalence, incidence, and duration; and confounding factors. They should also be able to define the meaning of these concepts in relation to a given research paper. The paper under discussion should be of reasonable quality so that students can discuss the strengths as well as the weaknesses of the study. They should also be encouraged to discuss ways in which weaknesses might be addressed in a future study (how they would do things differently) and the 'real-world' logistical issues involved in setting up such a 'perfect' study. In an extension to the critical appraisal exercise, a literature search might be carried out to investigate how different study designs (with their strengths and weaknesses) have been used to address the research question of interest.

Further reading

Kirkwood, B.R. and Sterne, J.A.C. (2016). *Essential medical statistics*, 2nd edn. Oxford: Wiley-Blackwell.

Chapter 16

Inference 2: Causation

Robert Stewart

Introduction

The study of cause and effect forms the basis for most human interaction. The repetitive investigation of actions and their consequences can be readily seen in children's behaviour. Adult behaviour may be more complex but essentially involves identical principles. When we speak to someone for the first time, an initial impression is formed. If the conversation proceeds, the impression (hypothesis) is tested and refined through evaluating actions (what we say) and their consequences (the reaction or reply this provokes). If an unknown factor is present (e.g. the other person is preoccupied with something else), the relationship between cause and effect may be misinterpreted resulting in a false impression (e.g. that they are rude or unfriendly). The process can be seen as a repeated series of experiments, albeit unconscious. All of us are therefore involved in active cause–effect research for most of our waking lives. However, the inferences (whether true or false) derived from these day-to-day experiments apply only to ourselves. Science and philosophy on the other hand seek to uncover truths that are generalizable beyond the individual. Because of this, their experiments require greater scrutiny.

Research may be divided into that which is observational (describing what is there) and that which is analytic (explaining why it is there). Deducing cause-and-effect relationships is central to analytic research. The 'result' of any given experiment is indisputable. What is open to interpretation is what caused that result. As discussed in Chapter 15, a series of questions have to be asked. What is the likelihood of it having occurred by chance? Was it caused by problems in the design of the study (bias), by the influence of a different factor to that hypothesized (confounding), or by a cause–effect relationship in the opposite direction to that anticipated ('reverse' causality)? If the anticipated cause–effect relationship is supported, what precise cause and effect were being measured in the study and how might other factors contribute to this? And what are the implications of the findings? The focus for critiquing a research report (apart from allegations of deliberate falsification) strictly speaking should not be the reported 'Results' but the 'Discussion' and 'Conclusions'—the inferences (particularly regarding cause and effect) which can be drawn from the results and therefore the generalizability of findings beyond the experimental situation.

Determinism and the boundaries of cause–effect research

Is it possible that one day we will be able to explain the causes of all diseases in all people? This is surely the ultimate objective of all risk factor research. However, it is fair to say that, for many of the more common non-infectious disorders, analytic research is beginning to 'run dry'—that is, the major risk factors have already been identified and what is left may take considerably more effort to clarify. Possible new directions for epidemiological research will be discussed in the final chapter of this book (Chapter 25) and it is likely that there are important risk factors still 'out there' and unidentified. There will also be large numbers of risk factors (such as specific gene polymorphisms) accounting for much more minor degrees of variation, and undoubtedly complex risk factor interactions which will keep researchers busy for a long time to come. However, what is the final target? How much of the variation for a given disorder might ultimately be explained by identifiable causes and their interactions? The determinist viewpoint is that all variation can ultimately be explained. In epidemiology, this attitude became prominent with the original focus on infectious diseases. Smallpox is caused by a single identifiable 'cause' and vaccination (i.e. in effect, the removal of the cause) has resulted in the complete eradication of this disease, a situation which would have been viewed as nothing short of miraculous two centuries ago. For many other infectious diseases, the principal obstacles to eradication are logistical rather than fundamental.

Many disorders were once viewed as essentially random occurrences with only limited modification by external influences. Optimism arising from infectious disease research was carried over to other disorders and supported by early findings for clear risk factor–outcome associations (e.g. smoking and lung cancer). Science will undoubtedly continue to uncover important causal processes, even if newly identified risk factors are steadily weaker in their influence and interactions more complex. However, it cannot be assumed that outcomes will ever be predicted with 100% accuracy and there are many examples in the natural world (for instance in weather systems) where early optimism about ultimate predictability has been challenged by 'chaos theory'. Random events may therefore substantially limit the extent to which 'causation' can be investigated.

In psychiatry, a deterministic view has been particularly prevalent, possibly because disorders affecting a person's thoughts and behaviour are intuitively felt to be 'explainable'. The tradition of the psychiatric formulation, for example, has required generations of psychiatrists to provide sufficient reasons why *this* person developed *this* disease at *this* time. However, even if a disorder is readily attributable to a discrete cause, the cause itself (e.g. an adverse life event) may have considerably less predictable origins. This is important from a preventative point of view—how do you stop people having adverse life events? Determinism is understandably popular in research because it implies that further discoveries are 'out there'. However, there are dangers in over-optimism and a lack of awareness of science's limitations. Where discoveries within a field prove elusive, demoralization can result in important areas of research (and important opportunities for prevention/treatment) becoming sidelined in favour of 'easier targets'.

Principles underlying cause–effect research

Inductivism

So how then should cause and effect be investigated? Inductivism describes a conceptual framework going back to Francis Bacon's writings in the seventeenth century, a time when science and philosophy were closely and openly interrelated. From a scientific viewpoint, an often quoted example of induction concerns Jenner's observation that smallpox occurred less frequently than expected in milkmaids. From this observation, Jenner surmised that cowpox (to which milkmaids had a high exposure) might confer immunity to smallpox. From an observed relationship between two factors, an interpretation is therefore made concerning cause and effect. Taking another example, if a light comes on after a switch is flicked, an interpretation is made, particularly after repeated trials, that the switch controls the light. However, there are obvious unsatisfactory elements to this approach. The observation that two events occur together in temporal succession does not necessarily imply cause and effect. If dawn is always preceded by a rooster crowing, does this imply that the rooster causes the sun to rise?

Refutationism

Dissatisfaction with inductivism, raised particularly by David Hume in the eighteenth century, led to the alternative theoretical framework of refutationism (aka deductivism or hypotheticodeductivism), refined and championed in the twentieth century by Karl Popper, although not a million miles away from Socratic dialogue in ancient Athens where proposed ideas would be put under pressure by counter-argument. A central tenet is that cause and effect can never be proved but only refuted. For example, the rooster is silenced and the sun still rises; water heated at altitude shows that its boiling point is not always 100°C; and Newtonian principles are superseded by those of relativity. Popper proposed that good science advances through conjecture and refutation. Through this process, a hypothesis should always lead to predictions which can be tested through experiment. The hypothesis may be supported but never proved absolutely. On the other hand, it may be refuted by inconsistent observations and replaced by another hypothesis which explains these more satisfactorily. As Einstein said: 'No amount of experimentation can ever prove me right; a single experiment can prove me wrong'.

Hypothesis generation

Refutationism at its extreme is disparaging of inductivism, pointing out that it consists of little more than assumption and circular argument. However, an important deficiency in refutationist theory is that it assumes that a hypothesis is already there to be tested. Where should hypotheses come from in the first place? An optimistic viewpoint is that they arise *de novo* from a good scientist's intuition or 'brainwaves'. However, any worthwhile intuition is likely to be grounded in experience and observation—that is, inductivism. From a clinical perspective, it is important to bear in mind that most modern medical knowledge has its origins in careful observation and induction—and also that important treatments, for disorders from psychoses to male erectile dysfunction, have arisen out of chance observations in entirely different circumstances. Inductivism is therefore fundamental to hypothesis generation. However, causal inferences are limited and refutationism provides the most appropriate framework for testing and refining hypotheses. A certain amount of induction may also be involved in interpreting results and considering ways to refine hypotheses, particularly in epidemiology as will be discussed. The process of hypothesis formulation and testing is therefore a cyclical process involving both inductivist and refutationist principles as described in Figure 16.1.

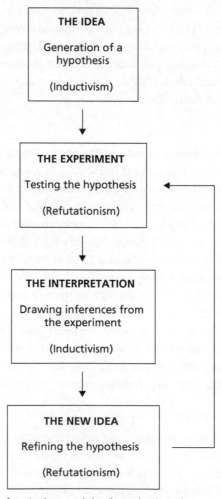

Figure 16.1 Inductivism, refutationism, and the 'hypothesis cycle'.

Limitations for refutationist epidemiology

A hypothesis concerning the causal relationship between two factors, according to refutationist theory, should lead to predictions which can be tested through an appropriate experiment. Epidemiological research faces two difficulties in this respect. The first is that there is no 'clean' experimental environment. Epidemiology is carried out in the natural world with all its random occurrences. If experimental observations support a hypothesis, all well and good but, as discussed earlier, hypotheses can never be proved. More importantly, if observations are inconsistent with the study hypothesis, it is unlikely to be possible to refute this absolutely in the natural world. If a different population had been sampled, would a different association have been observed? There are therefore obvious difficulties in determining cause-and-effect relationships if a hypothesis can neither be proved nor disproved. A second, but related difficulty is that epidemiology is largely an observational science and interventional research is substantially limited by ethical considerations. People cannot be randomly exposed to a hypothesized risk factor and, once there is a suspicion that something may be a risk factor (or a certainty that it is beneficial), it becomes steadily less ethical to observe the 'natural' course of events.

Causal criteria

If hypotheses cannot be proved or disproved absolutely and research findings are principally derived from observation rather than experiment, causal inference in epidemiology comes perilously close to pure inductivism with all of its associated shortcomings. One attempt to remedy this situation has been the use of 'causal criteria', particularly those drawn up by Bradford Hill (the origins of which lie in the work of Hume) although Hill actually referred to these as 'standards' rather than 'criteria'. The intention was to provide a framework for judging causality with respect to an observed association. A prior assumption is that competing explanations for the association such as chance, bias, and confounding have already been considered. Limitations of individual criteria are outlined in Table 16.1 and a more comprehensive critique is given by Rothman and Greenland (1998). An overriding difficulty is that these standards do not move very far beyond inductivism since they rely heavily on the subjective judgement of the reviewer. The criterion of temporality can be reasonably claimed to be the most important—hence the weight given to evidence from prospective research. However, as described in Table 16.1, it should not be taken to indicate that cause and effect are always in one direction. A particularly dangerous criterion is that of biological plausibility. A degree of speculation as to biological mechanisms underlying observations has become acceptable and possibly even expected in epidemiological research reports. However, with a vast and expanding biomedical literature and sophisticated search engines, it is not difficult to find evidence from basic science which backs up any association found (in whatever direction it happens to be) conferring a spurious respectability.

Table 16.1 Criteria for causation

Criterion	Description	Limitations
1. Strength	A strong effect size for an association	This reduces the chance of minor unmeasured confounding, but assumes that major confounding factors have been accounted for. Weak associations may also be causal
2. Consistency	Repeated observations of an association in different populations/circumstances	This assumes that all necessary causal factors are evenly distributed between populations. If a risk factor–outcome association were present only in men, would this imply non-causality?
3. Specificity	A risk factor leads to a single outcome	There is no reason why a risk factor should be associated with a single disorder (e.g. multiple disorders associated with alcohol misuse)
4. Temporality	The cause should precede the effect	A study should ideally demonstrate this. However, the fact that one event follows another does not rule out the opposite direction of causation in other circumstances. For example, depression may cause physical ill health, but physical ill health may also cause depression
5. Biological gradient	A 'dose–response' relationship	This assumes that the 'ceiling' of risk has not been reached. A single life event may be sufficient to cause depression with no influence of further events. Of little use for cross-sectional associations since a 'dose–response' pattern of association could be predicted with either direction of causation
6. Plausibility	That the hypothesis is biologically plausible	Frequently a highly subjective judgement, given the volume of the biological literature. There are many historical examples of important findings rejected on the ground of implausibility at the time (e.g. Darwin's theory of evolution in 'On the Origin of Species')
7. Coherence	That the interpretation does not conflict with the known biology of the disease	This depends heavily on the quality of the ancillary information. It also is not entirely consistent with the principle of refutationism
8. Experimental evidence	Evidence from interventional research	Experimental evidence should be sought where possible, but interventional research may not be ethical and/or feasible for many cause–effect investigations. The intervention may not be sufficiently discrete to infer causation
9. Analogy	Similar associations in other fields	A highly subjective judgement

Reproduced from Hill AB (1965). The environment and disease: association or causation? *Proceedings of the Royal Society of Medicine*, 58, 295–300. Copyright © 1965, © SAGE Publications. DOI: https://doi.org/10.1177/003591576505800503

Bayesianism

Epidemiology is therefore caught between the ideal of pure refutationist science and the real world of chaotic natural processes, observational research with sampling error, and conclusions which are derived to a large part through inductivist principles. Like many areas of science, it is also saddled with a regular flow of seemingly important findings which attract interest but which cannot subsequently be replicated. Inductivism and refutationism alone may be an insufficient framework for clarifying causation. A third approach, Bayesianism, again rooted in eighteenth-century philosophy (and seen by some as inductivism's twenty-first-century heir), has been used to address some of these difficulties. There is insufficient space in this chapter to discuss this theoretical framework in detail but essentially it espouses a more transparent acceptance of probability rather than certainty both in observations from a study and in the assumptions which underlie those observations, relieving scientists of a perceived responsibility to provide absolute proof/disproof. A more detailed discussion of Bayesian theory in epidemiology can be found in the textbook by Haynes and colleagues (2006).

Consensus

Perhaps the most important force underlying causal inference in health research is that of consensus: that is, the gradual accumulation of individual studies resulting in a shift of scientific opinion on a causal question of interest (for example, the move from social to biological theories for schizophrenia aetiology, followed by the more integrated recent models). In the broader field of science, the concept of truths held and evaluated by the academic community is most strongly associated with the writings of Thomas Kuhn. This issue is particularly pertinent in epidemiology because of the above-mentioned difficulties with 'pure' refutationist research. Ideally, observations from a single study are not viewed in isolation but in the context of other findings and broader opinion: hence the rapid recent expansion of research synthesis. An advantage of consensus is that the interpretation of causation becomes less dependent on an individual's subjective judgement. Also, heterogeneity in findings can be taken into account, or even (ideally) investigated in its own right as a clue to other causal processes. Disadvantages, as with all consolidation, are that anomalous findings which challenge a prevailing hypothesis may be ignored as 'outliers', and originality in research design may be stifled. A narrow focus on the quality of the evidence may also ignore the restricted populations from whom the evidence base is derived.

The *a priori* hypothesis

Consensus therefore acts to limit speculative interpretation of research findings. On a more individual level, the approach to the research project is also important. If observations are 'explored' without clear forethought, it is much more likely that inferences will be biased and causation misrepresented. 'Negative' findings, which might have been important refutationist contributions to a particular field of interest, may be glossed over and a large number of between-variable correlations filtered for those which are positive and 'significant'. Having drawn inferences (and this process may be as easy for a finding in one direction as another) it is not difficult, as discussed previously, to find other data to back up a finding that may well have arisen through chance. The more interesting the finding, the more demoralizing the consequences for other research teams who are unable to replicate the result. Causal inferences in this situation are derived entirely through induction, although the sample size and meticulous study design may mask the fact that no hypothesis was being tested when the data came to be analysed. A much more satisfactory approach is to formulate the hypothesis (through insight, intuition, observation, background reading, etc.) before the study is designed, or at the very least before the data are analysed. A certain amount of subjectivity may still be involved in the process of drawing conclusions; however, this is likely to result in a substantially more reliable interpretation (Box 16.1). A useful and popular procedure is to draw up and label 'dummy' tables for results before commencing data analysis. Minor revisions may still be needed but most of the thought and work will have been done and the quality of the resulting report will have been improved.

Box 16.1 Principles underlying cause-and-effect research

Underlying principles

+ Inductivism—from an observed co-occurrence of two factors, a cause-and-effect relationship is inferred.
+ Refutationism—a hypothesis is generated. Predictions are made which are tested in an experimental situation.

Limitations in epidemiology

+ No 'clean' experimental environment. Difficult to test hypotheses with absolute certainty.
+ Principally an observational science. Interventional research limited substantially through ethical considerations.
+ Therefore inductivism strongly involved in interpreting cause-and-effect relationships.

Solutions

+ Causal criteria—but these still require a considerable degree of subjective judgement.
+ Bayesianism—allows cause-and-effect relationships to be considered in terms of probabilities rather than absolutes.
+ Consensus—synthesizing research findings to reduce subjectivity.
+ The *a priori* hypothesis—limiting post hoc subjective inference.

The role of research without hypotheses

The objectives of epidemiology are to describe as well as to explain the distributions of health states. A study describing the prevalence of depression or the performance of a screening instrument does not have a hypothesis. Furthermore, where a disorder is being investigated in a new population which differs substantially from other samples, pre-formed hypotheses about cause-and-effect relationships may be counterproductive since they will narrow the focus of the investigation and ignore potentially important influences. In these cases, it may be preferable to begin with a 'clean slate', and describe relationships in order to generate rather than test hypotheses. However, it is important that this approach remains transparent in any research report and that caution is exercised in drawing causal inferences until hypotheses have been tested. Another requirement for exploratory analysis is in genetic epidemiology where it is mathematically inappropriate to test 1–2 million individual hypotheses. Probabilistic modelling is used instead, coupled with a requirement from many journals for independent replication prior to publication.

A structure for cause–effect relationships

Induction and latent periods

The assumption behind causation is that there are factors which contribute towards the probability of an 'outcome' such as a disease. The outcome therefore requires a sufficient number or combination of these factors to have exerted their influence. (For non-determinists this position remains tenable if random occurrences are allowed to contribute.) The period during which causal factors operate is referred to as the *induction period*. Once the final factor has exerted its influence, the outcome becomes inevitable. The ensuing period from this point until the clinical manifestation of the disease is the *latent period*.

This framework has been useful for describing causal processes in many areas of health research, including cancer and infectious disease. However, the focus on disease 'onset' has obvious limitations for psychiatric epidemiology. For mental disorders manifesting in early adulthood, distinctions with abnormal mental states in adolescence or childhood may be difficult to draw because of changing symptom patterns (such as in schizophrenia) or a longstanding fluctuating 'subclinical' course (such as in affective disorder). When then do these disorders have their onset (i.e. become inevitable)? For Alzheimer's disease, where underlying pathological processes are at least more clearly defined, an induction/latency model was proposed as a framework for discussing causation (Mayeux and Small, 2000). The 'onset' in this case was defined as the first appearance of characteristic pathological changes. This is believed to occur a decade or more before clinical manifestations and hence a long latent period is proposed. However, the distinction between these periods probably cannot even be applied to Alzheimer's disease since many people with Alzheimer pathology do not develop symptoms of dementia. Onset is not therefore inevitable at early pathological stages and other 'causal' factors must continue to operate. Survival is also an important issue. A factor may act to reduce the probability of dementia occurring by postponing its onset to a later date. By this time a person may have died from another disorder and dementia can be said to have been prevented. Whatever caused the earlier mortality is also in theory preventative in this respect. If dementia is not inevitable until the onset of symptoms, it has no latent period.

The time course of causation

An induction/latency distinction may be of little use for outcomes (i.e. most, if not all psychiatric disorders) which are defined in terms of clinical symptoms, since causal influences will always operate up to the time of manifestation. Contributing causes are instead sometimes subdivided into 'predisposing' and 'precipitating' factors on the basis of the believed proximity between their influence and the outcome event, although distinctions may not always be clear—for example, when does an adverse life event become a precipitating rather than predisposing factor for depression? However, some idea of the time course over which causes exert their influence is important in drawing inferences from observed relationships between two or more potentially causal factors. In Figure 16.2, four examples are given with respect to two hypothetical risk factors (A and B) and an outcome (C). The associations shown in the results tables illustrate the importance of thinking through potential causal pathways (and developing hypotheses) before analysing the data. For scenarios 2, 3, and 4, identical results might have been obtained if the association between B and C had been 'adjusted' for A in a regression analysis (i.e. the association between B and C would be reduced in strength after adjustment). Conducting a stratified analysis is sufficient to illustrate *effect modification* (scenario 4) but will not distinguish between confounding and mediation, even in prospective studies. Statistical procedures such as lag time analyses may be of assistance but require large sample sizes and multiple examination points. For most studies, the distinction can only be made through considering what is known about A and B—in particular, the relationship between them and the likely timings of their influence on C. As emphasized in Chapter 15, these questions are far better considered before approaching the data, rather than in a *post hoc* discussion of puzzling findings.

Interactions and effect modification

Taking the scenarios in Figure 16.2, a hypothetical situation can be imagined where A and B are only two possible causes for outcome C. The simplest situation is that each cause exerts its influence independently (scenario 1). This implies that A and B are both in themselves sufficient to cause outcome C. Assuming no random occurrences were involved, everyone with *either* A *or* B would develop C. An example of this situation might be certain conditions with a very strong genetic influence, such as Huntingdon's chorea or early-onset Alzheimer's disease, where the presence of particular mutations are in themselves sufficient to make the disease inevitable and where the occurrence of the disease is stereotyped with respect to the age of onset (i.e. nothing short of early mortality will prevent its occurrence). However, these examples are (fortunately) rare. An alternative scenario is that causes combine in their influence on the outcome. Therefore, C depends

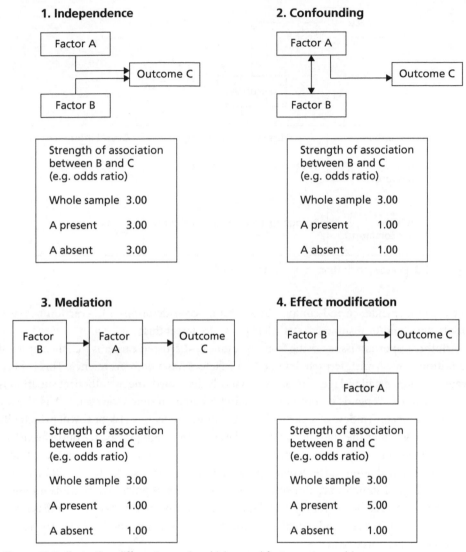

Figure 16.2 Illustrating different ways in which causal factors may combine.

on both A and B being present. This is illustrated by scenario 4 (effect modification). B is therefore only associated with C if A is also present (and the results of the analysis in the table would be the same if the association between A and C was stratified by B). The importance of effect modification is inherently acknowledged in the traditional psychiatric formulation which proposes causation at the level of the individual patient. In particular, the concept of predisposing and precipitating factors acknowledges that single causes are usually insufficient to bring about the outcome and that 'precipitants' may require a 'predisposition' in order to exert their effects (and *vice versa*). However, despite this, statistical analyses for the majority of studies appear to be carried out entirely to distinguish

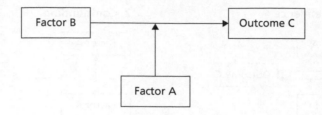

Situation	Observed relationship	Causal inference
A is common B is rare	Frequency of C will depend on B	B causes C
A is rare B is common	Frequency of C will depend on A	A causes C

Figure 16.3 Effect modification and assumed causation.

between independence and confounding, with no consideration of interaction between risk factors (and/or insufficient statistical power to detect this).

Another important issue arising from the example discussed earlier is that the nature of causation may be misinterpreted if one of the factors has a high prevalence. This is illustrated in more detail in Figure 16.3. As previously described, the hypothetical situation is that outcome C depends on both causes A and B being present. However, if A is already present in most members of a particular population, someone's risk of C will principally depend on whether they have B. For a population with a high prevalence of B, the risk of C will depend on A. An often quoted example of this principle is Rose's comment that if everyone smoked, lung cancer would appear to be a genetic disease (Rose, 1985). Where epidemiological samples are drawn from homogeneous populations, there is a danger that important risk factors for a particular disorder may be missed because there is insufficient variation between individuals—a good scientific reason, if nothing else, for a more international research field.

Practical exercises

1. Why are hypotheses important? Discuss.
2. How can we get beyond guesswork in interpreting cause and effect? Discuss with respect to epidemiology in general and then specifically with respect to psychiatric research.
3. Choose a cause–effect relationship of interest in psychiatric research, review two or three key papers, and apply Bradford Hill's criteria. Discuss their implications with respect to improving the evidence base through future research (considering the feasibility of proposed studies).

4. Take an example of two causes and an outcome. Think of as many ways as possible in which these causes might plausibly interact in their influence (with reference to Figures 16.2 and 16.3). This should be done without considering evidence for any particular combination. For many areas of psychiatry confounding, mediation and effect modification can be considered with the causal factors arranged any way around. Possible examples might be diabetes and depression as risk factors for dementia; family strain and socioeconomic deprivation as risk factors for schizophrenia; and poor health and social isolation as risk factors for depression.

5. For the example in question 4, try swapping around the 'outcome' with one of the causes (e.g. diabetes and dementia as risk factors for depression; schizophrenia and family strain as risk factors for socioeconomic deprivation; or depression and poor health as risk factors for social isolation). Repeat the exercise. This illustrates the importance of considering two-way directions of causation and complex interplay between risk factors in psychiatric research.

6. For the example(s) in question 5, discuss implications for prevention/treatment which arise out of each combination. Are there any differences? Does causation matter?

7. How might a research project disentangle some of these difficulties?

References

Haynes, R.B., Sackett, D.L., Guyatt, G.H., and Tugwell, P. (2006). *Clinical epidemiology: how to do clinical practice research*, 3rd edn. Philadelphia, PA: Lippincott Williams & Wilkins.

Hill, A.B. (1965). The environment and disease: association or causation? *Proceedings of the Royal Society of Medicine*, **58**, 295–300.

Mayeux, R. and Small, S.A. (2000). Finding the beginning or predicting the future? *Archives of Neurology*, 57, 783–784.

Rose, G. (1985). Sick individuals and sick populations. *International Journal of Epidemiology*, 14, 32–38.

Rothman, K.J. and Greenland, S. (1998). Causation and causal inference. In: Rothman, K.J. and Greenland, S. (eds.). *Modern epidemiology*, pp. 7–28. Philadelphia, PA: Lippincott Williams & Wilkins.

Chapter 17

Critical appraisal

Jo Thompson Coon and Rebecca Abbott

What is critical appraisal?

> A 21st century clinician who cannot critically read a study is as unprepared as one
> who cannot take a blood pressure or examine the cardiovascular system.[1]

In 'Evidence based medicine and the medical curriculum', Professor Paul Glasziou argues
that the medical curriculum needs to take into account the rapidly expanding and changing information that today's practitioners encounter, and that 'the necessary skills (for
doing so) must be taught and assessed with the same rigour as the physical examination'
(Glasziou, 2008). The concepts outlined in his paper are of importance to all health professionals and health-based researchers.

But what is meant by critical appraisal, or as some people term it, critical evaluation?
Critical appraisal is the process of carefully and systematically examining research to
judge its trustworthiness, and its value and relevance in a particular context (Burls, 2009).
In other words, critical appraisal means evaluating a piece of research in an objective and
structured way to assess its validity compared to other research and its applicability in
similar populations and/or settings. Critical appraisal aims to take account of both the
internal and external validity of the research. In this context, internal validity refers to the
extent to which the study methods and analysis allow for appropriate conclusions about
the study population being evaluated, and external validity refers to the extent to which a
study's results (regardless of whether the study is descriptive or experimental) can be gen-
eralized/applied to other people or settings. Table 17.1 shows the comparable appraisal
concepts, first proposed by Guba and Lincoln (1981), which are used in the assessment of
both quantitative and qualitative research.

General principles

First and foremost, critical appraisal demands a common-sense approach. Like any skill,
dedicated time and practice is needed to develop your appraisal skills. It is good practice
to read the whole research article a couple of times before attempting to undertake any

---

1 Reproduced with permission from Glasziou, P. et al. Evidence based medicine and the medical curriculum. *BMJ*, 2008;337:a1253. Copyright © 2008, British Medical Journal Publishing Group. doi: https://
doi.org/10.1136/bmj.a1253.

Table 17.1 Analogous concepts in critical appraisal of quantitative and qualitative research

Traditional criteria for judging quantitative research	Alternative criteria for judging qualitative research
Internal validity	Credibility
External validity	Transferability
Reliability	Dependability
Objectivity	Confirmability

appraisal, as aspects of the research method or findings may not be reported where you might expect to find them. It is not uncommon to find yourself reading a section of a research paper several times.

While the approach to critical appraisal will differ according to the type of research being assessed, there are some universal aspects of appraisal to consider when reading any research paper. This can be thought of as four key questions:

◆ Was the research design appropriate for the question?

◆ Were the methods used reliable/appropriate?

◆ Is/are the author/s interpretation valid?

◆ Are the findings relevant to the population more widely or other populations/settings that you are interested in?

One of the key components of appraisal is to consider whether there is any bias in the research. Bias can be defined as any systematic error in the study that leads to distortion of the results (Gerhard, 2008). Bias can occur at any stage of research, and can occur with all types of study designs. Bias is not a dichotomous variable, and interpretation of bias cannot be limited to simply asking: 'Is bias present or not?' Instead, when appraising research evidence the degree to which attempts were made to limit the bias by appropriate study design, methods, and implementation should be considered. As some degree of bias is nearly always present in a published study, readers must also consider how bias might influence a study's conclusions.

While several classification systems of bias have been proposed, they can broadly be described as 'confounding', 'selection', and 'information' bias (Gerhard, 2008). Bias can be introduced by factors that determine who is exposed to the intervention or phenomena of interest in the population (confounding bias), factors related to who is included in the study (selection bias), and errors of assessment and measurement (information bias). Sometimes, these classifications are broken down further; for example, as you will see later in the chapter, five specific types of bias are addressed in the appraisal of randomized controlled trials (RCTs). Irrespective of the terminology or classification used, it is important to understand that bias may result in estimates of effect that are either smaller or larger in magnitude than the true effect, or may even reverse an association/effect.

Critical appraisal of specific study designs follows this section, but with any scientific paper there are some key questions to consider, which help to assess the level of potential bias in the research (Box 17.1). Some questions may be more relevant to quantitative research than qualitative research, but largely the same questions can be asked of both.

Why is critical appraisal important in practice and research?

In order for practitioners and researchers to be able to use the best available evidence in clinical decision-making and programme design, skills in appraising research in an objective and structured way (critical appraisal skills) are essential. The methodological rigour of research studies varies considerably; almost all research is flawed in some way. Consideration of the reported findings of a piece of a research in the context of the study design and its associated methodological limitations is important to avoid drawing erroneous conclusions. The hierarchy of evidence, first proposed by the Canadian Task Force on the Periodic Health Examination in 1979 and now widely accepted in the medical literature, provides guidance as to the relative weight that can be attributed to a particular study design (Canadian Task Force, 1979). Systematic reviews with or without meta-analyses (the pooling of results from a number of similar RCTs) are considered to provide the most robust findings and observational studies such as single case reports the least robust (Centre for Evidence-Based Medicine, 2009). However, it is important to remember that the hierarchy provides guidance rather than absolute rules and in some situations, a well-designed observational study may provide more robust and relevant evidence than a poorly designed and conducted RCT. It is also important to consider that there are some circumstances in which randomization is not possible or indeed is unethical, and in such cases well-designed observational studies are the best evidence. Examples of such studies include those investigating the adverse effects of smoking or those assessing the benefits of breastfeeding.

Critical appraisal tools

There are a large number of tools, often referred to as checklists, to help with critical appraisal (see Table 17.2 for some of the most common ones). The majority guide the reader though a series of questions with a *yes/no/not sure* answer, and some have a summative appraisal based on the number of yes or no answers as an overall indication of study rigour. Others, like the Cochrane risk of bias tool involve a judgement about the degree of bias for each assessment item, which are not then combined (Higgins et al., 2011). Some checklists provide useful accompanying notes to help guide the reader with specific examples of what may be considered a low risk of bias, or a reasonable attempt to minimize bias; take time to read these as they will save time, and help with consistency in appraising studies.

In the next part of this chapter, we will address the appraisal issues to consider with the more common study designs within the epidemiology literature, and highlight the main questions to consider when appraising them.

Box 17.1 Generic appraisal questions to consider when reading any research study

Introduction

Is (are) the reason(s) for the study clearly stated? Is there a need for the study?
Is the review of the literature comprehensive?
Is there a clear research question?

Methods

Is the study design appropriate and does it link to the research objective?
Is the sample size appropriate/adequate and is there sufficient detail on population and setting?
For quantitative studies, is the primary outcome appropriate and is there sufficient length of follow-up?
Are the data collection methods and tools sufficiently described and are they appropriate and valid?
Is there a description of how data is to be analysed? Where appropriate are there sufficient details on the statistical methods to be used and are they appropriate?
Is there due consideration of ethical issues?

Results

Did the study proceed as planned? Are planned primary and secondary outcomes reported? Was there much attrition?
Are findings described adequately? Are data analyses correct?

Discussion/conclusion

What do the main findings mean?
Are the conclusions justified?
How do the findings compare with what others have found?
Are the findings generalizable?
What are the strengths and limitations of the research?

Critical appraisal of cross-sectional studies

A cross-sectional study measures the prevalence of health outcomes or determinants of health, or both, in a population at one point in time or over a short period. Bias may arise because of factors affecting a selection of the study population (inclusion/exclusion criteria). Furthermore, for studies assessing association, they can be limited by the fact that they are carried out at one time point and give no indication of the sequence of

Table 17.2 Common checklists and tools for critical appraisal

Checklist	Use	Website
Effective Public Health Practice Project: Quality Assessment Tool for Quantitative Studies	A global checklist which can be used across a range of study designs	http://www.ephpp.ca/tools.html
Critical Appraisal Skills Programme (CASP)	A range of checklists for common study designs	http://www.casp-uk.net/
Centre for Evidence-Based Medicine (CEBM)	A range of checklists for common study designs	http://www.cebm.net/critical-appraisal/
Scottish Intercollegiate Guidelines Network (SIGN)	A range of checklists for common study designs	http://www.sign.ac.uk/methodology/checklists.html
National Heart Lung and Blood Institute (NHLBI)	A range of checklists for common study designs	http://www.nhlbi.nih.gov/health-pro/guidelines/in-develop/cardiovascular-risk-reduction/tools
Cochrane risk of bias tool	A tool aimed at RCTs	http://handbook.cochrane.org/chapter_8/8_5_the_cochrane_collaborations_tool_for_assessing_risk_of_bias.htm
Downs and Black checklist	A tool for randomized and non-randomized studies	http://www.nccmt.ca/resources/search/9
Newcastle–Ottawa Scale (and adaptations of)	A checklist aimed at case–control studies, cohort studies, and cross-sectional studies	http://www.ohri.ca/programs/clinical_epidemiology/oxford.asp
ROBINS-I (Acrobat NRSI)	Non-randomized clinical controlled trials	https://sites.google.com/site/riskofbiastool/
AMSTAR 2	Tool for systematic reviews	http://amstar.ca/
ROBIS	Tool for systematic reviews	http://www.bristol.ac.uk/social-community-medicine/projects/robis/

events—whether exposure occurred before, after, or during the onset of the disease outcome. This being so, it is impossible to infer causality. Therefore, when appraising cross-sectional research it is important to assess how representative the study population was of the population of interest: for example, how were the participants recruited, how many were recruited from those that were eligible, and what was the attrition rate? See Box 17.2 for questions to consider when appraising cross-sectional studies.

Critical appraisal of case–control studies

The starting point of most case–control studies is the identification of cases. Once the outcome status is identified and participants are categorized as cases, controls (participants without the outcome but from the same source population) are then selected. Data about

Box 17.2 Questions to consider when appraising a cross-sectional study

Research question and design

Is the research question or objective in this paper clearly stated?
Can a cross-sectional study design answer the question?

Methods

How was the sample chosen—is it appropriate?
Is the sample size justified and is there an adequate power description?
What is the response rate into the study? (At least 50%?)
Is the study population representative of the source population?
How big is the loss to follow-up (>20%, >50%)?
For association studies, are key potential confounding variables measured and statistically adjusted for?

Findings and interpretation

Has the research question been answered?
Are the findings credible?
Can the results be applied to other relevant populations?

exposure to a risk factor or several risk factors are then collected retrospectively, typically by interview, from records, or survey. As information about exposure is typically collected by self-report, interview, or from recorded information, these types of studies are susceptible to recall bias and interviewer bias, and will rely on the completeness or accuracy of recorded information. These biases decrease the internal validity of the investigation and should be carefully assessed. Recall bias occurs when a differential response between cases and controls occurs. For example, a 'case' subject may unconsciously recall and report an exposure with better clarity due to the experience of illness. Interviewer bias occurs when the interviewer asks leading questions or has an inconsistent interview approach between cases and controls. Selection bias is important to consider in case–control studies with respect to how controls were selected: were controls selected from the same population as the cases? See Box 17.3 for questions to consider when appraising case–control studies.

Critical appraisal of cohort studies

The word 'cohort' has been adopted into epidemiology to define a set of people followed over a period of time. This has evolved to the modern epidemiological definition: 'a group of people with defined characteristics who are followed up to determine incidence of,

Box 17.3 Questions to consider when appraising a case–control study

Research question and design

Is the research question or objective in this paper clearly stated?
Is a case–control study an appropriate way of answering the question?

Methods

Are the cases and controls representative of the population of interest?
Is the exposure clearly defined and accurately measured?
Are the measurement methods similar in the cases and controls?
Is potential confounding taken into account?

Findings and interpretation

Has the research question been answered?
Are the findings credible?
Can the results be applied to the other relevant populations?

or mortality from, some specific disease, all causes of death, or some other outcome' (Morabia, 2004). Cohort studies can be prospective or retrospective. Prospective studies are carried out from the present time into the future. Because prospective studies are designed using specific data collection methods, they have the advantage of being tailored to collect specific exposure data and may be more complete. However, some studies may require lengthy follow-up while waiting for events to occur. Adequacy of follow-up time is an important appraisal question. Retrospective cohort studies, also known as historical cohort studies, are carried out in the present time and look to the past to examine medical events or outcomes. The primary disadvantage of this study design is the limited control the investigator has over data collection. The existing data may be incomplete, inaccurate, or inconsistently measured between subjects.

Cohort studies should be carefully assessed for both selection and attrition bias. The hallmark of a cohort study is defining the selected group of participants by exposure status at the start of the investigation. It is critical that both the exposed and unexposed groups should be selected from the same source population. Participants who are not at risk for developing the outcome should not have been included in the study. Because prospective cohort studies may require long follow-up periods, loss to follow-up should be assessed. Loss to follow-up is a situation in which the researcher loses contact with the participants, resulting in missing data. If too many are lost to follow-up, the internal validity of the study is reduced. See Box 17.4 for questions to consider when appraising cohort studies.

Box 17.4 Questions to consider when appraising a cohort study

Research question and design

Has the research question or objective in the paper been clearly stated?
Is the chosen study design appropriate?
Who has been studied, and are they clearly specified and defined?

Methods

Is potential confounding taken into account?
Is follow-up adequate? (Is the time frame sufficient enough to allow any effect of exposure and outcome to occur, if present)?
Are the measures of exposure valid and reliable (and independent from outcome measures)?
Are the measures of outcome valid and reliable (and independent from exposure measures)?
How big was the loss to follow-up (>20%, >50%)?

Findings and interpretation

Has the research question been answered?
Are the findings credible?
Can the results be applied to the other populations?

Critical appraisal of ecological studies

Ecological studies are observational studies which examine the evidence for associations by testing for correlations between average levels of an exposure and the prevalence or incidence of an outcome across different populations. Examples of the types of data reported in ecological studies include income inequality, area-level deprivation, and prescription rates which are reported at the population or group level (e.g. school, county, or country), rather than at the individual level.

As with all study types, the first step in critically appraising an ecological study is to consider whether you have sufficient information to assess whether the study has been properly conducted, analysed, and interpreted. The interpretation of ecological studies is prone to a specific type of confounding bias known as ecological fallacy. Ecological fallacy occurs when inferences and conclusions are drawn about individuals based only on the analyses of group data (Portnov et al., 2007). Additional considerations for ecological studies include whether the aims of the study take into account the limitations of the method; for example, ecological studies are not suitable to establish the causes of behaviours or to identify risk factors, whether the population has been clearly defined, and whether the data has been collected from a reliable source, is relevant and accurate, and any potential biases associated with the data source have been explored. See Box 17.5 for questions to consider when appraising ecological studies.

Critical appraisal of clinical trials

Randomized clinical trials

RCTs are probably the most simple research studies to critically appraise and interpret. The aim of randomization is to produce comparable treatment and control groups and to ensure that potential confounders are equally distributed between groups. Any difference in outcome may then be attributed to the intervention and, if conducted well, it is possible to be fairly confident that the results of RCTs are correct at least for the type of participants included. While flaws in the design, conduct, analysis, and reporting of

---

Box 17.5 Questions to consider when appraising an ecological study

Research question and design

Is the research question or objective in this paper clearly stated?
Who has been studied and are they clearly specified and defined?

Methods

Is exposure measured at the individual or ecological (aggregate) level?
Is the main outcome measured at the individual or ecological (aggregate) level?
Are the exposures clear, specific, and measurable?
Is there any likelihood of exposure misclassification?
Is the outcome clear, specific, and measurable?
Is there any likelihood of outcome misclassification?
Are confounders measured at the individual or ecological (aggregate) level?
Have the authors identified all potentially important confounders? Is the adjustment adequate? Is residual confounding likely?

Findings and interpretation

Is the unit of analysis clearly defined?
Is the type of inference intended clearly stated?
Have the authors considered ecological bias while interpreting their results?
Are the interpretations consistent with the ecological design used, unit of analyses, and unit of inference?

RCTs may influence the credibility of findings, the process of systematically critically appraising studies can highlight areas of concern. Potential sources of bias include *selection bias* (sequence generation and allocation concealment), *performance bias* (blinding of participants and personnel), *detection bias* (blinding of outcome assessors), *attrition bias* (incomplete outcome data), and *reporting bias* (selective reporting).

Selection bias is minimized by using appropriate methods of randomization such as computer-generated random numbers and by preventing researchers from influencing which participants are assigned to which treatment group (allocation concealment). Allocation concealment is possible in all trials even those which do not utilize blinding; methods of allocation concealment include the use of sequentially numbered, opaque, sealed envelopes; pharmacy controlled methods; central randomization using telephone or email; and sequentially numbered containers (Schulz and Grimes, 2002). *Performance and detection bias* can be minimized by blinding or masking which people receive which treatment. Any number of those involved in the conduct of a clinical trial may be blinded to the assigned intervention so that they are not influenced by that knowledge; for example, the trial participants, the investigators or healthcare providers, those collecting outcome data (the assessors), and/or the statisticians analysing the data. Well-reported studies will explicitly state who was blinded and how. Attrition or loss of participants during the follow-up of a trial leads to the collection of incomplete outcome data. Differences between randomized groups in the number or characteristics of participants lost to follow-up can introduce *attrition bias*. Selective reporting of a subset of the original recorded outcome variables on the basis of the results is an example of *reporting bias* (Kirkham et al., 2010). Covered in more detail within Chapter 12, the issue of how data were analysed is also an important consideration for critical appraisal. Ignoring everyone who has failed to complete a clinical trial will bias the results, usually in favour of the intervention. It is, therefore, standard practice to analyse the results of comparative studies on an intent-to-treat basis. Did the study include data from all participants as randomized in the analysis (intention to treat), or were data only from those who completed the intervention (per protocol) included? The key factors, therefore, to look for when appraising an RCT are the descriptions of allocation (randomization and allocation concealment), blinding, follow-up of participants, methods of data collection and analysis, sample size, presentation of results, and the applicability to the local population (Box 17.6).

Non-randomized clinical trials

In non-randomized clinical trials, participants are allocated to a comparison group using methods other than randomization; this means that groups are unlikely to be comparable at baseline. Differences in the characteristics of participants at baseline which are associated with the outcome of interest will result in confounding. An important part of the process of critically appraising a non-randomized clinical trial will therefore be in making judgements about imbalances in the groups at baseline and the appropriateness of efforts to account for these during analysis and interpretation.

Box 17.6 Questions to consider when appraising clinical trials

Research question and design

Did the trial address a clear and focused question?
Are the participants assigned to treatment groups by a randomized process?
Are the participants, healthcare providers, and outcome assessors blind to treatment allocation?
Do the authors provide statistical justification for the number of participants included in the trial?

Methods

Do all the participants complete the trial?
How did the authors deal with missing data?
How large is the treatment effect?
How precise is the estimate of the treatment effect?

Findings and interpretation

Can the results be applied to your context or population?
Were all clinically important outcomes considered?
Are the benefits worth the harms and costs?

Critical appraisal of qualitative research

With qualitative researchers hailing from a variety of disciplines and theoretical backgrounds, it is not surprising that there has been much debate as to whether and how quality appraisal should be applied to qualitative research (Dixon-Woods et al., 2004). Over one hundred sets of proposals on quality in qualitative research have been identified (Dixon-Woods et al., 2004). Some of the more commonly used critical appraisal tools for qualitative research include those by the Critical Appraisal Skills Programme (CASP; see 'Further reading'), Wallace et al. (2004), the Quality Framework (Spencer et al., 2003), and Walsh and Downe (2006).

For a general approach to appraisal of qualitative research, Greenhalgh (2010) recommends asking nine questions as you read the paper:

1. *Does the paper describe an important clinical problem addressed via a clearly formulated question?* As in any research paper, a statement of why the research was done and what specific question it addressed should be included. Qualitative papers are no exception to this rule.

2. *Is a qualitative approach appropriate?* Qualitative methods are ideal for exploring, interpreting, or obtaining a deeper understanding of a particular clinical issue. If,

however, the research aims to determine the incidence of a disease or the frequency of an adverse drug reaction, qualitative methods are clearly inappropriate.

3. *How were (a) the setting and (b) the subjects selected?* In qualitative research, the purpose is often to gain an in-depth understanding of the experience of particular individuals or groups, and therefore the research needs to involve individuals or groups who meet this requirement.

4. *What is the researcher's perspective, and has this been taken into account?* While qualitative research may be perceived to be more open to observer/researcher bias, this should not discredit the research. The role and influence of the researcher should be made explicit.

5. *What methods did the researcher use for collecting data and are these described in enough detail?* These need to be presented in sufficient detail to enable the reader to feel as though they have enough information about the methods to make a valued judgement about whether this was a sensible and adequate way of addressing the research question.

6. *What methods did the researcher use to analyse the data—and what quality control measures are implemented?* The author(s) should show how they have systematically analysed their data, and how they interpreted items of data that contradicted or challenged the theories derived from the majority, and how disagreements on subjective judgements were dealt with.

7. *Are the results credible, and if so, are they clinically important?* Ideally, the results should be independently and objectively verifiable (e.g. by including longer segments of text in an appendix or online resource), and all quotes and examples should be indexed so that they can be traced back to an identifiable interviewee and data source.

8. *What conclusions are drawn, and are they justified by the results?* It is necessary to ask whether the interpretation placed on the data accords with common sense and that the researcher's personal, professional, and cultural perspective is made explicit so the reader can assess the 'lens' through which the researcher has undertaken the fieldwork, analysis, and interpretation.

9. *Are the findings of the study transferable to other settings?* The more the research has been driven by progressive focusing (exploring new relationships and concepts) and iterative data analysis (revisiting the data and reshaping the research methods and hypothesis as you go along), the more its findings are likely to be transferable beyond the sample itself. For example, iterative adjustments to the sampling frame made during the research study may enable the researchers to develop a theoretical sample and test new theories as they emerge.

Critical appraisal of systematic reviews

In circumstances where there is more than one study addressing a question, a systematic review may be conducted to bring together the findings from the best available studies and to try and obtain an estimate of the combined effects. Systematic reviews are conducted using explicit and systematic methods to identify, synthesize, and evaluate the results of relevant research. Systematic reviews of RCTs are generally considered to be the most robust form of evidence on which to base decision-making. However, not all systematic reviews are methodologically sound. A protocol containing a clear, focused research question, corresponding inclusion and exclusion criteria, and detailed methods for how the review will be conducted should be published or registered before the review is undertaken. Given that systematic reviews aim to summarize the best available evidence, assessing the likelihood that the search has missed important studies is also an important step in the critical appraisal process. The quality of all the included studies in the review should be adequately assessed using a critical appraisal tool appropriate to the study design. There are many methods available with which to synthesize the results of individual studies within a review; the most commonly known statistical method is meta-analysis but this is not always appropriate due to clinical or statistical heterogeneity in the included studies. The methods for analysis should be pre-specified and justified in the protocol and described within the publication. See Box 17.7 for questions to consider when appraising systematic reviews.

Practical exercise

Read through the following journal article and answer the critical appraisal questions in Box 17.4. You could also try using one of the named checklists/tools referred to in the 'Further reading' section at the end of this chapter, such as those provided by CASP, or

---

Box 17.7 Questions to consider when appraising a systematic review

Research question and design

Did the review address a clear and focused question?

Methods

Were the best sorts of studies to address the question identified and included?
What is the likelihood that the authors have missed some important and relevant studies?
Were studies selected and data extracted using two independent reviewers?
If the results of individual studies were combined statistically, was it reasonable to do to?

Findings and interpretation

Can the results be applied to your context or population?
Were all clinically important outcomes considered?
Are the benefits worth the harms and costs?

the Scottish Intercollegiate Guidelines Network (SIGN). In the following sections you will find our interpretation of the study.

Kidger, J., Heron, J., Leon, D.A., Tilling, K., Lewis, G., and Gunnell, D. (2015). Self-reported school experience as a predictor of self-harm during adolescence: a prospective cohort study in the South West of England (ALSPAC). *Journal of Affective Disorder*, 173, 163–169.

Research question and design

Is the research question or objective in this paper clearly stated?

Yes—the research questions are stated clearly at the end of the introduction. Specifically the paper examines two questions: (1) is there an association between experiences of school at age 14 and self-reported self-harm at age 16? (2) Does the association between school experience and subsequent self-harm differ among those who self-harm with suicidal intent, compared to those who self-harm without suicidal intent? The authors are also clear to state that they are not able to examine temporal order, as they did not measure the 'outcome' at baseline.

Is the chosen study design appropriate?

Partly. The study from which the authors drew the data was a prospective cohort design which is suited to investigating the effect of an exposure over time for an outcome. However, it is clear that this particular analysis is not part of the original research question and is drawn out of a retrospective look at the data collected. While still appropriate, it does have implications, as variables which would have been of interest and given more rigour to the study (such as self-harm), were not collected. As stated earlier, the authors declare from the outset that there are some issues regarding the temporal order, however, they have tried to account for this by being explicit in their question. They have clearly stated that they are looking at the exposure of school experience at time A (age 14) and outcome of self-harm at time B (age 16).

Who has been studied, and are they clearly specified and defined (are they representative of a defined population)?

The cohort is well defined and described. They are appropriate for the research question being asked.

Methods

Is potential confounding taken into account?

Yes—a reasonable approach was used. The authors are clear in that they identified possible confounders from the literature a priori, and these are taken into account in the analyses. However, there are other measures of potential confounding that are not assessed (such as bullying).

Is follow-up adequate? (Is the time frame sufficient enough to allow any effect of exposure and outcome to occur, if present?)

The research question asked about a 2-year time frame. It seems reasonable, in this context, that this is a realistic time for the exposure to have an effect on the outcome. The authors are clear to state that there could have been a preceding/ongoing effect at baseline, but were not able to answer or address this.

Are there sufficient measures of exposure and are the measures valid and reliable (and independent from outcome measures)?

This is difficult to answer, and we would interpret this as 'not clear'. While considerable detail is provided about the process of choosing a few items from the original 39 items asked about school-related experiences, the validity and reliability of those few items is not known. The authors state that they chose not to look at the 'whole factors', which had come from the factor analysis, as the single items allowed them to compare to their own previous research. It is not clear whether these single items therefore were the most appropriate measure of school experience. With regards to being independent of self-harm, this is not known, as self-harm was not measured.

Are there sufficient measures of outcome and are the measures valid and reliable (and independent from exposure measures)?

Self-harm appeared to be assessed by asking one self-report question. No information is provided about the reliability of this question, whether it came from an established questionnaire, or whether it is the gold standard approach to assessing self-harm. As stated previously, it is difficult to establish whether this measure is independent from the measure of school experience, as there is a possibility that mood may affect one's response to a question about self-harm. The authors acknowledge these limitations in their discussion.

How big is the loss to follow-up (>20%, >50%)?

The authors achieved a 70% response rate at age 16 from those who had returned questionnaires at age 14. The group who returned data at age 16 (70%) were significantly different from those who did not (30%) in aspects related to perceptions of school. This is important. Bias already exists given that this is a select sample of less than 50% of the original cohort. The authors report that this select sample are more likely to be female, have higher educational qualifications, and come from a family with a higher wage and a mother in a non-manual social class.

Findings and interpretation

Is the research question answered?

Both research questions posed were answered.

Are the findings credible?

While the findings are credible, there remains a key uncertainty about whether perceptions of self-harm were already different at baseline. This is one of the issues with retrospective analyses alluded to earlier in this chapter; sometimes the measures relied on are incomplete. This study would have benefited from a measure of the outcome variable at age 14. Furthermore, while the measure of outcome and exposure are both self-report and their validity is not established, and they are not entirely independent from each other, there are few alternatives to measuring perception variables such as these.

Can the results be applied to the other populations?

Yes, it is reasonable to assume that the study findings may also apply to other UK school-age populations. However, the population of 4000 adolescents was biased in being those who were more likely to stay with a cohort study (selection bias), and in this particular case, were biased in terms of gender, education, and socioeconomic status.

Further reading

Greenhalgh, T. and Taylor, R. (1997). How to read a paper: Papers that go beyond numbers (qualitative research). *BMJ*, **315**, 740.

Guyatt, G.H. and Rennie, D. (1993). Users' guides to the medical literature. *JAMA*, **270**, 2096–2097. [Part of a JAMA series: 'Users guide to the medical literature'—for the whole series, see http://www.hopkinsmedicine.org/gim/training/osler/osler_jama_steps.html]

Websites

Centre for Evidence-Based Medicine (CEBM): http://www.cebm.net/critical-appraisal/

Cochrane: http://handbook.cochrane.org/

Critical Appraisal Skills Programme (CASP): http://www.casp-uk.net/#!appraising-the-evidence/c23r5

Effective Public Health Practice Project (EPHPP): http://ephpp.ca/

Enhancing the Quality and Transparency of Health Research (EQUATOR) Network: http://www.equator-network.org/

Joanna Briggs Institute (JBI): http://joannabriggs.org/index.html

Scottish Intercollegiate Guidelines Network (SIGN): http://www.sign.ac.uk/methodology/checklists.html

References

Burls, A. (2009). *What is critical appraisal?* London: Hayward Group. http://www.whatisseries.co.uk/what-is-critical-appraisal/.pdf

Canadian Task Force (1979). The periodic health examination. Canadian Task Force on the Periodic Health Examination. *Canadian Medical Association Journal*, **121**, 1193–1254.

Centre for Evidence-Based Medicine (2009). Oxford Centre for Evidence-based Medicine – levels of evidence (March 2009). http://www.cebm.net/oxford-centre-evidence-based-medicine-levels-evidence-march-2009/

Dixon-Woods, M., Shaw, R.L., Agarwal, S., and Smith, J.A. (2004). The problem of appraising qualitative research. *Quality and Safety in Healthcare*, **13**, 223–225.

Gerhard, T. (2008). Bias: considerations for research practice. *American Journal of Health-System Pharmacy*, **65**, 2159–2168.

Glasziou, P. (2008). Evidence based medicine and the medical curriculum. *BMJ*, **337**, a1253.

Greenhalgh, T. (2010). *How to read a paper: the basics of evidence-based medicine.* Hoboken, NJ: BMJ Books, Wiley-Blackwell.

Guba, E.G. and Lincoln, Y.S. (1981). *Effective evaluation: improving the usefulness of evaluation results through responsive and naturalistic approaches.* San Francisco, CA: Jossey-Bass.

Higgins, J.P., Altman, D.G., Gøtzsche, P.C., Jüni, P., Moher, D., Oxman, A.D., et al. (2011). The Cochrane Collaboration's tool for assessing risk of bias in randomised trials. *BMJ*, **343**, d5928.

Kirkham, J.J., Dwan, K.M., Altman, D.G., Gamble, C., Dodd, S., Smyth, R., and Williamson, P.R. (2010). The impact of outcome reporting bias in randomised controlled trials on a cohort of systematic reviews. *BMJ*, **340**, c365.

Morabia, A. (2004). *A history of epidemiologic methods and concepts.* Basel: Birkhaeuser Verlag.

Portnov, B.A., Dubnov, J., and Barchana, M. (2007). On ecological fallacy, assessment errors stemming from misguided variable selection, and the effect of aggregation on the outcome of epidemiological study. *Journal of Exposure Science and Environmental Epidemiology*, **17**, 106–121.

Schulz, K.F. and Grimes, D.A. (2002). Allocation concealment in randomised trials: defending against deciphering. *Lancet*, **359**, 614–618.

Spencer, L., Ritchie, J., Lewis, J., and Dillon, L. (2003). Quality in qualitative evaluation: a framework for assessing research evidence. Cabinet Office. https://www.gov.uk/government/publications/government-social-research-framework-for-assessing-research-evidence

Wallace, A.C., Quilagars, D., and Baldwin, S. (2004). Meeting the challenge: developing systematic reviewing in social policy. *Policy and Politics*, **32**, 455–470.

Walsh, D. and Downe, S. (2006). Appraising the quality of qualitative research. *Midwifery*, **22**, 108–119.

Chapter 18

Statistical techniques in psychiatric epidemiology

Lisa Aschan, Jayati Das-Munshi, Richard Hayes, Martin Prince, Marcus Richards, Peter Schofield, and Robert Stewart

Introduction

Epidemiology and medical statistics have been partner disciplines since the nineteenth century, despite disagreement between their founding fathers (William Farr took quite some time to accept John Snow's findings on cholera transmission). It is beyond the scope of this book to provide a comprehensive guide to medical statistics, and there is no shortage of excellent source material both in textbooks and online. However, it would also be inappropriate to gloss over the topic entirely, particularly as there are a number of new challenges, controversies, and techniques which are becoming increasingly relevant in psychiatric epidemiology. We begin with a summary of the discrete uses of statistical techniques in epidemiological research, followed by some guidance on constructing regression models—a common task, but one which it is important to think through carefully. This topic is developed further through a more detailed consideration of mediating and causation, which are particularly important in our specialty because of the long and complex pathways of causation, and lifelong interrelationships between exposure and outcome states characteristic of mental disorders and their risk factors. Finally, four key emerging themes are considered: the use of propensity scores, dealing with missing data, multilevel modelling, and latent class analyses.

The three uses of statistics

As described in Chapter 15, the purpose of carrying out a research project is to describe a property of a particular sample and then use this information to make an inference about the wider population from which that sample was drawn. If nothing can be inferred about the wider population, the findings from the sample are of little relevance to anyone beyond the investigators. The process of inference can be described as a series of steps, considering what the study seeks to contribute to the underlying scientific question and excluding alternative explanations for the observed findings: from data quality (i.e. the accuracy with which the original sample is described), through chance and bias (concerning the relationship between the sample and the source population), to confounding and other factors relating to causality. Statistical techniques are required in three respects: to describe the sample, to draw inferences about the source population, and to allow confounding influences to be evaluated.

Application 1: describing data

Quantitative data need to be communicated by researchers to their audience. While it would be possible to carry out this communication simply by publishing the research database (and a number of journals are exerting pressure on authors to do just this), it is more common practice to describe variables and their relationships numerically using statistical techniques. Proportions or percentages are therefore used to describe distributions of categorical covariates, or more complex parameters such as prevalences, risks, and rates. Continuously distributed variables might be described using a mean and standard deviation, moving on to more complex parameters such as alternative measures of central tendency and spread (median, interquartile range, etc.) when distributions differ from the normal.

Relationships between variables also have to be described numerically and these range likewise from simple parameters, such as the difference in the risk of an outcome between two groups, through to coefficients derived from regression analyses. All are still used as a means of communicating a property of the sample in a research study from the researcher to a wider audience. A difference between two mean values is described simply as one value minus another, and a prevalence ratio is one value divided by the other. Coefficients from regression analyses are more complex to derive and interpret, although at their heart are still simply properties of numeric data which can be communicated. The choice of regression analysis depends on the nature and distribution of the variable being modelled (most commonly the 'outcome variable' in an analysis), but all come down to the fact that a line on a graph can be described by an equation and the numbers (coefficients) in that equation can therefore be used to communicate the properties of that line. All regression analyses involve the statistical program plotting the values of one variable against another in the sample and attempting to find a line which 'best fits' the resulting points on the graph. Unless specified otherwise, a straight-line relationship is sought by the program and the coefficient for the slope of the line can be used as a way of communicating how much a variable on the y-axis can be expected to alter for each unit change in the x-axis variable. Linear regression analyses simply describe that unmodified relationship and require the residuals to be normally distributed (although often with some relaxation of the requirement possible where samples are large). Logistic regression analyses are used for binary dependent variables (e.g. case/control) and derive their coefficients by modelling the log odds of that dependent variable against the independent (x-axis) variable, back-transforming the slope coefficient through an anti-log function to generate an approximation of the odds ratio. Proportional hazard models are used for survival functions, and other outcomes require regression analyses which suit their distributions (e.g. counts are frequently modelled with Poisson regression). The mathematical models and assumptions behind regression analyses differ; however, all serve the same purpose to describe and communicate a relationship between variables.

Application 2: relating the sample to the population

Communicating findings in the sample is not enough; someone reading about the research study needs to know what can be said about the population that the sample is meant to represent. Statistical techniques here are used to describe a hypothetical construct called the 'sampling distribution'. This simply reflects the fact that if the study was carried out repeatedly under exactly the same conditions but in different samples, its findings would never be exactly the same. If it was repeated an infinite number of times, the observed values of any measured parameter would show a normal distribution. The standard deviation of this hypothetical distribution is called the 'standard error' and can be calculated from the properties of the sample and the measurement taken. Any statistic measured in the sample has a standard error, whether this is the prevalence or incidence of an outcome, the proportion or mean level of an exposure, or the regression coefficient reflecting the relationship between the two. As described in Chapter 15, these standard errors can be used to calculate confidence intervals for any parameter and determine p-values for associations. These in turn are used to extend what can be communicated between the person reporting research and the person reading or listening to this report. Importantly, the statistics here assume that the sample is representative of its source population and therefore are not able to take account of any bias in sampling or measurement. Minimizing bias is therefore the primary consideration in study *design* rather than *analysis*.

Application 3: investigating independence

Beyond describing a relationship between two parameters, and providing information on the likely precision of this relationship derived from the standard error of the sampling distribution, most researchers will wish to investigate and minimize potential confounding factors. Before the development of computers capable of running the standard statistical software we use today, the ability to assess the independence of associations was very limited and it is not surprising that early epidemiological research focused on defining major risk factors with strong effects. A major advantage of regression analyses is the ability to enter several variables simultaneously and generate coefficients which reflect the independent individual contribution of each one to variation in the outcome—that is, 'adjusted' for each other. This is therefore the third task of statistics in epidemiological research.

Strategies for model building in multivariable analysis

Regression analyses therefore provide the opportunity to investigate the independence of different predictors of a single outcome. This opportunity tends to be used in one of two approaches, depending on the objectives of a research project, and it is helpful for the researcher to be clear which approach is desired before constructing regression models. In either case it is important to act judiciously, and to justify carefully the inclusion and exclusion of variables in the model.

The first type of study has a particular hypothesized exposure–outcome association of interest. This association will have been described 'unadjusted' and the researcher will be using regression analyses to adjust that particular association for other potential confounding factors in order to investigate whether it remains independent. For example, in a study investigating the experience of migration as a risk factor for depression onset, a risk ratio may have been calculated in migrant compared to non-migrant participants and the next stage will be to adjust this risk ratio for other factors such as age, gender, pre-migration socioeconomic status, etc. The interest remains, however, on the coefficient for migration status and whether it changes following adjustment.

The second type of study is more exploratory and has an outcome of interest with a range of potential predictors. There are no predominating hypotheses and the objective is primarily to describe the most important of these potential predictors, using regression analyses to calculate their independent contributions and to filter out those factors which do not meaningfully contribute. So an example of this would be a study of incident depression in a population of interest where a number of exposures are under consideration (which might include migration status but not as a particular focus), where these are considered of equal interest and where the final report will describe the most parsimonious model—that is, limited to the exposures which are most independently predictive.

Approach 1: investigating a hypothesized association and controlling for confounding

So the aim in principle here is to include in the model all potential confounding variables in order to establish whether or not there is an independent association between the hypothesized exposure–outcome association, free of confounding. Potential confounding variables will be independently associated with both the exposure and the outcomes, so a useful first step is to carry out exploratory unadjusted analyses to discover which of the variables assessed in the study meet these criteria. For example, in an imaginary example of a case–control study testing the hypothesis that the experience of child sexual abuse (CSA) may be associated with major depression in young adulthood, you might detect the pattern of associations shown in Table 18.1.

In this instance, female gender, low education, lower parental social class, parental divorce, alcohol dependency, and deliberate self-harm are identified as potential confounders. However, caution must now be exercised:

1. In establishing whether or not there is an association between potential confounder and both exposure and outcome you should focus more on the size of the effect for the association rather than the p-value or statistical significance. Remember that the latter will be dependent upon the statistical power for the comparison, which may be

Table 18.1 Potential confounders associated with childhood sexual abuse (exposure) and depression (outcome)

Potential confounders associated with exposure (CSA)	Potential confounders associated with outcome (major depression)
Female gender	Female gender
Leaving school early	Leaving school early
No qualifications	No qualifications
Lower parental social class	Lower parental social class
Parental divorce	Parental divorce
Alcohol dependency	Alcohol dependency
Deliberate self-harm	Deliberate self-harm
	Recent adverse life events
	Family history of major depression
Learning difficulties	
Remote rural residence	Urban residence

limited for uncommon exposures that may nevertheless be important confounders. If in doubt, include it in the final model.

2. There may be a lot of missing values for certain potential confounding variables. The regression model will be derived from the subset of participants with *complete data for all variables included in the model*. Inclusion of such variables in the adjusted model will certainly lead to loss of power, and may also bias the estimate of the association under study. Strategies for dealing with missing data are discussed later in this chapter.

3. A confounder is *independently associated* with both exposure and outcome. Therefore the association with the outcome does not depend upon the association with the exposure and the 'confounder' is not *on the causal pathway* between exposure and outcome. Looking at the earlier examples, it seems highly likely that alcohol dependency, given our knowledge of likely mechanisms, is on the causal pathway between CSA and major depression, rather than a true confounder. The traumatic experience of CSA is likely to lead to alcohol dependency, which in turn increases the risk for major depression. It would be incorrect to adjust in the final model for such a causal pathway variable as it is likely to lead to an underestimate of the true association between CSA and major depression. Under these circumstances, a successful intervention targeted at alcohol dependency would reduce the prevalence of major depression, while an intervention targeted at the prevention of CSA would reduce the incidence both of alcohol dependency (the mediating variable) and of major depression (the ultimate outcome of interest). Rural/urban residence in this example illustrates what is sometimes called 'negative confounding'—where a factor is associated with the exposure and the outcome in different directions. If the potential confounding effect of area of residence is

not accounted for, then the true strength of the association between CSA and major depression may be underestimated.

4. Some true potential confounders may be highly correlated with each other. The obvious example in Table 18.1 is 'leaving school early' and having 'no qualifications'. Most of those in the first category would also be in the second category and there may be very few individuals who have left school early and have qualifications. Under these circumstances the correct approach is to include one or other of the variables in the final model, but not both. They are effectively measuring the same thing, so nothing is lost through this strategy in terms of control of confounding. If both variables are included then there is a high risk of *collinearity* in the resulting model. In practical terms, as a consequence of some cells in the model being empty or being represented by few participants, there is considerable imprecision in the estimation of the model coefficients. The results are likely to be capricious, with either both variables 'knocking themselves out' of the model or having very large standard errors.

Having finalized the list of potential confounders for which adjustment is to be made, inexperienced investigators are prone simply to enter the hypothesized exposure and all of the potential confounders simultaneously into the model in a single step. The correct approach is first to enter the hypothesized exposure, and then to enter, one by one, the potential confounding variables. At every stage, the effect of entering the new confounder upon the effect size for the main hypothesized exposure should be observed and recorded. In this way, the confounding effect of each and every variable can be elicited. To use the earlier example, with imaginary data, had all of the variables been entered simultaneously one might arrive at the model shown in Table 18.2.

The inference is that there is no association between CSA and major depression having adjusted for the potential confounding effects of female gender, leaving school early, lower parental social class, and parental divorce. However, we are none the wiser as to which of these variables is responsible for the confounding effect. Entering the same variables sequentially, we might observe the results as shown in Table 18.3.

From this data it is immediately apparent that the unadjusted association between CSA and major depression (odds ratio 2.4) is likely to be spurious, confounded by gender.

Table 18.2 Association between childhood sexual abuse (exposure) and depression (outcome); fully adjusted model

Variable	Odds ratio (95% confidence intervals)
CSA	1.0 (0.5–1.5)
Female gender	2.5 (1.6–3.7)
Leaving school early	2.1 (1.4–2.9)
Lower parental social class	1.4 (0.7–2.9)
Parental divorce	3.0 (0.8–9.9)

Table 18.3 Association between childhood sexual abuse (exposure) and depression (outcome); sequentially adjusted model

Variable	Step 1	Step 2	Step 3	Step 4	Step 5
CSA	2.4 (1.2–4.8)	1.3 (0.6–2.0)	1.3 (0.6–2.0)	1.2 (0.6–1.8)	1.0 (0.5–1.5)
Female gender		2.6 (1.7–3.6)	2.3 (1.4–3.2)	2.4 (1.5–3.5)	2.5 (1.6–3.4)
Leaving school early			1.9 (1.2–2.5)	1.9 (1.2–2.5)	2.1 (1.4–2.8)
Lower parental social class				1.6 (0.9–3.3)	1.4 (0.7–2.9)
Parental divorce					3.0 (0.8–9.9)

Step 1 CSA
Step 2 CSA + gender
Step 3 CSA + gender + leaving school early
Step 4 CSA + gender + leaving school early + parental social class
Step 5 CSA + gender + leaving school early + parental social class + parental divorce

Women are at increased risk for major depression, and independently are more vulnerable to CSA. This impression could be confirmed by repeating the sequential modelling process, entering first CSA, followed by leaving school early, parental social class, and parental divorce (likely to have a minimal effect on the association of interest), and then in a final step entering gender (likely to substantially reduce the odds ratio for the association between CSA and major depression). Alternatively, some researchers prefer to display a table with individual adjustments (e.g. CSA adjusted for gender, CSA adjusted for leaving school early, CSA adjusted for parental social class, etc.) before a sequential model is assembled.

The way we have looked at this example also illustrates the focus of this first approach. In evaluating the regression output, we are really only looking at the top row of coefficients—that is, those for CSA as the exposure of interest—and our interest is on how much the coefficients change with the addition of other covariates into the model. The fact that female gender and leaving school early happen to be independently associated with the outcome are only of secondary interest for this particular study. In communicating findings, particularly in journals with limited space for large tables, it would often be considered sufficient simply to display the coefficients relating to CSA as an exposure using separate, then sequential adjustments.

Approach 2: building a parsimonious predictive model

As described previously, the scenario here is a study which seeks to investigate and describe the most important predictors of an outcome without focusing on any one single exposure. The overriding objective is therefore to identify the best and most efficient prediction for the outcome measure, at the cost of the fewest degrees of freedom. This contrasts with the strategy for control of confounding where the aim is to saturate the model with inclusion of all plausible confounding variables, while concentrating upon the impact of these potential confounders upon a single hypothesized exposure–outcome association. The analysis now is by definition post hoc and exploratory, rather than hypothesis driven, but the findings on the apparent independent effects of multiple variables may be used to generate hypotheses for future study. Hence, in the case of the example of the case–control study described earlier, the parsimonious model might well include recent adverse life events and family history of depression, which were unadjusted risk factors for major depression, while not associated with CSA, as well as CSA and the potential confounders listed previously. The strategy for model building should still be judicious. For example, likely mediating variables on the pathway between CSA or other risk factors and major depression might still be excluded.

For the generation of such parsimonious models, forward or backward stepwise regressions are sometimes carried out. In forward stepwise regression, the statistical software first enters the most strongly associated variable according to a variety of possible criteria such as the likelihood ratio, which is the reduction in likelihood (essentially the improvement of fit of the model) divided by the number of degrees of freedom consumed. Next it tests whether model fit can be improved significantly by adding in another variable and/or by removing the first variable. This process is continued until the fit of the model cannot be improved by entering or removing any more variables. Backwards stepwise regression uses essentially the reverse process. All variables are entered and then variables are removed and/or re-entered sequentially until no further variables can be removed or re-entered without a significant deterioration in the fit of the model.

These stepwise regressions are superficially attractive, but can lead to capricious results and are probably best avoided. For example, they may fail to recover the 'true' model and it is often unclear what the criteria are for selection; therefore, it becomes difficult to others to draw inferences. While stepwise models are sometimes considered as an initial step to identify a subset of independent predictor variables of interest, it is preferable to build predictive models manually, to see if a more informative result can be achieved. There is no one correct approach; as with all exploratory techniques, the final results should be inferenced with due caution. In any exploratory regression, you can judge for yourself whether extension of an existing model to include an additional variable significantly improves upon the fit of the model, by carrying out a likelihood ratio test (in logistic regression) or an F-test (in multiple linear regression).

Mediation and causal inference

Mediation and causal inference are closely intertwined concepts in epidemiology. Indeed, the term mediation implies 'causal pathways along which changes are transmitted from causes to effects' (Pearl, 2014). This is distinct from true confounding, where known or unknown *competing* factors obscure causal inference. Two important points should be made. First, although mediation implies causality, as noted, causality is not exclusive to mediation, since an exposure and outcome can be linked through confounding by common cause processes (see later) that are independently connected to both. Second, the distinction between mediation and confounding is fundamentally theoretical, since mediators and confounders can have similar empirical effects when adjusted out of an exposure–outcome association. In the example provided earlier in this chapter, adjusting for female gender and no qualifications may result in similar magnitudes of attenuation of the association between CSA and major depression. However, while females may be at greater risk of exposure to CSA, and also of adult affective disorder, this is confounding by common cause rather than a mediational chain linking exposure and outcome. On the other hand having no qualifications may indeed act as a mediator; CSA can result in psychiatric problems which, in addition to themselves increasing the risk of major depression through the life course continuity, may interfere with school performance, with long-term consequences for this outcome via low socioeconomic attainment. Similarly, revelation of CSA may lead to parental divorce, which can also exacerbate risk of major depression (particularly in females; Rodgers, 1994).

In both examples it can be seen that the concept of mediation implies temporal sequence, with the mediator necessarily occurring between the exposure and outcome to play a role in the causal chain. Referring back to the CSA example, this again is in contrast to female gender, which cannot be altered by CSA (unless, plausibly if rarely, the latter leads to medical sex reassignment). Modelling a temporal sequence has its historical roots in path analysis, which is a form of multivariable regression analysis that can estimate indirect as well as direct associations between a set of variables. It is also a form of structural equation modelling, except that single indicators are used rather than latent variables (see later in this chapter). Figure 18.1 is a simple illustration, based on models estimated by Richards and Sacker (2003). All paths are mutually independent.

Here, the conceptual framework is that father's occupational social class is associated with adult cognitive function via a causal path through childhood cognitive development and educational attainment; the direct path between father's social class and adult cognition was not statistically significant and is not shown. On the other hand, direct as well as indirect paths occur between father's social class and educational attainment, and between childhood and adult cognition. It can also be seen that education is associated with adult cognition independently of childhood cognition and father's social class. Note that, depending on their exact timing, the temporal sequence of these variables cannot be meaningfully rearranged. For example, although there is a dynamic bidirectional association between cognition and educational attainment, it is impossible for the latter to cause a change in cognition prior to school age. However, careful thinking about causality is required beyond such strict timing; for example, childhood cognition cannot influence

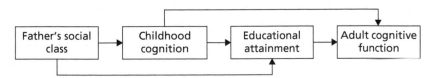

Figure 18.1 Association between father's social class and adult cognitive function: possible causal pathways.

father's social class classified before birth, but it is possible that childhood cognitive development and educational progress could be a cause of father's occupational mobility through pathways involving geographical relocation and school selection.

The limitations of randomized controlled trials and addressing confounding using propensity scores

As discussed in earlier chapters, randomized controlled trials (RCTs) are considered the 'gold standard' research design for inferring causality. However, obtaining evidence of this quality is not feasible or ethical for every research question, and randomized trials themselves may have limited generalizability because of overly restrictive inclusion and exclusion criteria. There has therefore been increasing interest in improving causal inference from observational study designs. In this respect, propensity scores are becoming increasingly popular, particularly in observational studies of medication-related exposures. RCTs are clearly the gold standard for establishing medication efficacy, primarily because randomization essentially negates the influence of both known and unknown confounding factors, removing these as alternative explanations for an observed difference in outcome. However, observational data from 'real-world' clinical settings can provide useful complementary information on the risks and benefits of medications, although 'confounding by indication' is an important issue which can distort results.

Confounding by indication arises because the assignment of treatment to patients in routine clinical practice is not random. In particular, medications are prescribed to address particular illnesses or symptoms, the characteristics of patients who receive a given treatment may be systematically different from those who do not, and the illness or symptoms for which a medication was prescribed may be the cause of the outcome under investigation rather than the medication itself. For example, people taking clozapine, a third-line antipsychotic for treatment-resistant psychosis, may well have more severe psychopathology than those who have not been prescribed this antipsychotic (Hayes et al., 2015). This does not necessarily mean that clozapine causes these severe symptoms; instead, it is more likely that clozapine was prescribed to treat these symptoms.

Given the effectiveness of RCTs, in removing the influence of confounding by indication, why is there a need for observational medication studies at all? Despite their utility, RCTs have important limitations, particularly their tendency to be conducted under idealized circumstances, in restricted populations, and over limited time spans (Booth et al., 2014). Patients who participate in RCTs are often more homogeneous than those who will ultimately be prescribed the treatments under investigation, and people may be excluded who have particular comorbidities or who take additional medications. Due to the expense of maintaining RCTs, participants are often followed up for limited time spans, which can mean that longer-term medication effects are not recorded or investigated. Furthermore, the treatment regimens in RCTs may be an idealized version of how these medications are delivered clinically, and medications in practice may be used in a variety of ways that are beyond the scope of most RCTs. For example, in the treatment of people with schizophrenia, multiple antipsychotics may be prescribed (Kadra et al., 2016) despite potential adverse effects. Additional medications may be prescribed for a range of reasons including treating specific symptom domains, as an alternative to increasing the dose of the current medication (Barnes et al., 2011), or to counteract specific side effects (Fleischhacker et al., 2010). Moreover, clinicians may increase the dose or switch medications in pursuit of an optimal therapeutic effect (Barnes et al., 2011). Observational studies embedded in real-world clinical practice can address many of these issues. In addition, observational studies can examine risk factors which would be unethical to randomize: for example, the association between maternal alcohol consumption during pregnancy and adverse outcomes in the child (Lundsberg et al., 1997).

Propensity score methods provide an alternative to conventional multivariable models which may have advantages in some settings, and there has been an increase in the use of this technique in published research (Sturmer et al., 2006). A propensity score is the probability for treatment assignment based on a set of patient characteristics, including severity of illness and other clinical factors (Rosenbaum and Rubin, 1983); in other words, it is the likelihood that a patient will be prescribed a particular treatment. By attempting to balance treated and non-treated groups more robustly on observed characteristics, the aim is to obtain more genuine estimates of treatment effects (Okoli et al., 2014). In practice, the propensity score is most often estimated using a logistic regression model in which treatment status is regressed on observed patient characteristics. There are a number of approaches to selecting which characteristic to include when calculating propensity scores. These include: (1) including all factors which might impact treatment; (2) starting with factors which may impact treatment then using stepwise procedures to reduce the number of variables included in the model (Patrick et al., 2011); and (3) selecting factors which are associated with both treatment and outcome.

Ultimately these initial regression analyses end up assigning each individual a single propensity score which can be used in a number of ways to address confounding by indication: as a covariate to be adjusted for in the main regression analysis, or as a factor for stratification, matching, or restriction (Glynn et al., 2006; Okoli et al., 2014). Stratification or matching on propensity scores generally involves removing those individuals without comparable controls and can therefore lead to reduced precision because of a smaller sample size. Adjusting for a propensity score by including it as a covariate in a multivariable model will permit the inclusion of treated and untreated participants who would have been dropped due to the lack of appropriate matches; however, the inclusion of these individuals in the analysis may increase bias. Another approach is to trim the tails of the propensity score distribution. In this case, one can graphically represent two distributions of propensity scores comparing those who did and did not receive the given treatment. The lowest and highest ends of this range may well correspond to regions where there is no overlap between the two distributions. For example, the lowest propensity scores may be generated by individuals for whom the treatment is contraindicated or whose symptoms are not sufficiently severe to warrant treatment, while the highest propensity scores may be generated by people who definitely require the treatment. By trimming these tails we are left with the region of overlap between the two distributions corresponding to a group of patients who would all stand a chance of being treated or not treated.

Despite the attractiveness of the approach, it should be borne in mind that most studies which have applied both conventional multivariable and propensity score approaches in their analyses have obtained similar results for both methods; however, there is some evidence that propensity score methods may produce estimates closer to the null (Shah et al., 2005). Also, where relevant confounders have not been measured, propensity score methods display similar bias to conventional approaches (Drake, 1993). Nevertheless, regression analyses using propensity scores do have advantages in some circumstances. Examining propensity scores distributions for treated and untreated groups can make it possible to identify and remove individuals who have contraindications or absolute indications and hence are not reasonable to include in comparisons. Also, in situations where there are seven or fewer events per confounding factor included in the model, propensity score adjustment may produce more precise and less biased estimates than logistic regression (Cepeda et al., 2003). Finally, there is evidence that matching on the propensity scores will allow a better balance of measured covariates between treatment and control groups than conventional matching (Glynn et al., 2006).

Dealing with missing data

All epidemiological studies at some point will be affected by missing data, and as mentioned earlier, this can present major challenges for interpreting statistical analysis output. Data may be missing for whole variables or for parts of a variable: for example, if part of a question was not understood by respondents, or if sensitive questions were asked which participants opted not to answer. Errors in inputting data at the data collection phase may lead to missing data, especially if it is not possible to later retrieve correct values. In longitudinal studies such as RCTs or cohort studies, missing data may arise when participants are lost to follow-up, referred to as 'attrition'.

Missing data have the potential to introduce bias into a study and may also impact the precision and power of a study to detect differences. In the past, missing data may have been unreported in research reports; however, ignoring or not reporting missing data is now less acceptable and reporting guidelines such as Strengthening the Reporting of Observational Studies in Epidemiology (STROBE), now explicitly recommend that proportions of missing data are reported in all studies, alongside the statistical methods used to deal with missing data. What follows is a brief overview of missing data and some of the approaches which may be taken to deal with this. Interested readers considering statistical procedures to handle missing data, such as multiple imputation, are recommended to read about this topic in more detail (some suggestions are provided at the end of this chapter in 'Further reading') and to consider attending one of the growing number of courses on handling missing data and/or consult an expert before attempting these procedures.

Types of missing data

Data 'missingness' is commonly classified into one of three groups: missing completely at random (MCAR), missing at random (MAR), and missing not at random (MNAR). Definitions and examples of these scenarios are provided in Box 18.1. The distinctions are important because they have implications for the analysis strategy, particularly on whether any strategy is required at all, or whether it is likely to be justifiable. For example, if assumptions for MCAR are satisfied, complete case analyses may be used although power and precision in the study may be affected. Distinguishing between MAR and MNAR scenarios may be difficult and cannot be based simply on analyses of observed data. Instead, plausible mechanisms which could underlie the missingness should be considered. For example, MNAR mechanisms may be suspected if currently depressed

---

Box 18.1 Missing data mechanisms and examples

Missing completely at random (MCAR)

Missing values in the dataset are not predicted by observed or unobserved values within the dataset.

Example: in a study of cortisol levels in depression the lab worker drops a tray of test tubes. In this scenario, a random batch of blood tests has been lost. The probability of participants missing data on cortisol levels in this study is not predicted by other observed or unobserved values within the dataset and is completely random. Under these conditions, analyses utilizing complete case methods will not introduce bias into the study, although resultant missing data could have a detrimental impact on sample size, resulting in loss of precision.

Missing at random (MAR)

Missing values within the dataset can be explained by other observed variables in the dataset and do not depend on unobserved data.

Example: in a study, only older women had an assessment of mental state. This is an example of MAR since age and sex (fully observed within the dataset and included in the analyses) predict missingness for the 'mental state' variable.

Missing not at random (MNAR)

In this scenario, missing data is dependent on unobserved variables.

Example: in a study of dementia in primary care, only people with suspected cognitive impairment have a Mini-Mental State Exam (MMSE). This is an example of MNAR since measurement of the outcome (cognitive impairment) predicts missingness on MMSE score.

participants are thought to be less likely to be followed up in a longitudinal study. MAR assumptions can be made more plausible if there are many observed variables within the dataset which predict missingness, and if these are used in the final analyses to account for missing data mechanisms. MAR assumptions underlie statistical approaches such as multiple imputation (see 'Handling missing data') which attempt to deal with missing data.

Handling missing data

Most statistical packages will perform complete case analyses by default—that is, the analyses will be restricted to participants with complete data on all variables in a given regression model. The inclusion of many variables in a model with varying proportions of missing responses may have important consequences for the final model in terms of the sample size, since any participant providing incomplete data will be dropped. In addition, unless the missing data mechanism is MCAR, such models will be subject to bias. Clearly the situation can potentially be solved by re-contacting participants to retrieve any missing data, although in reality this is usually not feasible. A pragmatic approach might be to restrict regression models to variables which have relatively complete information, in order to minimize the loss of participants with missing data, although this may not be possible if the analysis is dependent on the inclusion of such variables in models. For missing outcome data in RCTs, investigators may opt to use methods such as 'last observation carried forward', whereby the last measurement on a subject who is lost to follow-up is used for analysis instead; however, this approach introduces bias if people are discontinuing follow-up because of an adverse outcome (or because they are feeling better), and it may be more parsimonious to assume treatment failure in those who fail to complete. Investigators may consider dealing with missing data by substituting values—for example, replacing a missing data point with the mean value for the variable in question (single imputation); however, this can have adverse consequences, as variability in the estimates will be artificially reduced. In general, these approaches have been heavily criticized as introducing bias and are not recommended.

It is also worth bearing in mind that not all statistical models are restricted to complete case analyses. Mixed models used for the analysis of repeated measures will include all cases regardless of whether they have missing measurement points and will estimate the trajectory of the measure from those points which are available. So for example, in a RCT estimating changes in depressive symptoms over the course of seven successive examinations, it would be conventional to use a statistical procedure which calculated these trajectories using the data available, regardless of whether a participant had participated at all seven time points. Clearly there would still be a potential for bias if attrition during the study was influenced by poor outcome (because the measurement points prior to attrition might give an over-optimistic trajectory) and clearly there need to be sufficient numbers of measurement points to calculate an overall trajectory (e.g. people who are only present at the baseline interview are not going to contribute to the output); however, this approach does at least provide information which is more complete, and therefore less biased, than an analysis that only considered baseline and final measurement points.

If missing data are thought to be MAR then a number of statistical procedures exist which can help to estimate missing values within the dataset, thus improving statistical power without introducing bias into the analyses. There are a number of approaches to handling missing data, which include inverse probability weighting, maximum likelihood approaches, and imputation procedures. Imputation procedures have already been mentioned and may involve substituting missing values for another value (e.g. a mean). We have previously described such approaches as highly problematic. However, approaches which deal with missing data using *multiple* imputation differ from this, and are widely utilized. As multiple imputation is widely used and readily implemented through a range of statistical packages, a brief overview is provided in Box 18.2.

In conclusion, missing data are a common problem in epidemiology. Aside from attempting to minimize the loss of data, researchers should ensure that, when it occurs, they report proportions of missing data and consider whether this could have impacted the study's findings, through bias or loss of precision. Statistical methods to deal with missing data, such as multiple imputation, are becoming increasingly considered as the required computational power is increasingly available to run these. However, they remain relatively specialized techniques and expert advice is recommended.

Multilevel modelling approaches to clustered data

As described earlier, regression analyses are used as one way to describe relationships between variables in a dataset. In its simplest form, this is achieved by the statistical program plotting out the individual exposure–outcome combinations on a graph and finding a line which 'best fits' the result. The two coefficients derived from that line are the number which defines the slope—usually the most important for communication because it describes the relationship between the two variables—and the number which defines the 'intercept', the value of the outcome when the exposure is zero. Mathematically this is expressed as:

$$y = \beta_0 + \beta_1 x$$

where β_0 is the intercept, and β_1 the slope (the change in the outcome y for each unit change in the exposure x). When multiple exposures (independent variables) are entered into the regression, the hypothetical graph becomes complex and multidimensional, but the equation remains relatively straightforward with the addition of more slope coefficients. So for four independent variables, this would be:

$$y = \beta_0 + \beta_1 x_1 + \beta_2 x_2 + \beta_3 x_3 + \beta_4 x_4$$

However, this equation only describes the properties of the best fit line itself. The actual y values for each individual are never going to lie exactly on the line predicting them from the x values and the coefficients; instead, they will each exist some distance away from that predictive line. The sum of these distances for each individual represents an 'error'

Box 18.2 Multiple imputation

Under assumptions of MAR, multiple imputation deals with the problem of missing data by using observed variables within the dataset to estimate missing values. The procedure is based on the probability distribution of variables within the observed dataset and as such uses a Bayesian framework, to 'fill in' or impute missing data. There are a number of steps which need to be followed:

1. *Assess the data to understand patterns of missingness.* Before commencing multiple imputation, researchers usually spend some time trying to understand patterns of missingness within their dataset, particularly proportions missing and distributions of variables. The researcher may at this stage identify a number of observed variables within the dataset which predict missingness. These will be used to inform the imputation regression equation which will be used to create imputed datasets as outlined in step 2. The variables which will be used in the imputation regression to produce imputed datasets do not necessarily need to be those used for final analyses; however, any variables or outcomes which are planned for analyses must be included in the imputation regression.

2. *Create multiple copies of the original dataset, where missing values are 'filled in' using imputation.* The full probability distribution of the dataset is used to fill in plausible values for missing data, and multiple copies of the dataset (each with slightly different values, which reflect the uncertainty) are created. The imputation regression equation, developed in step 1 is used to create imputed datasets. The total number of imputed datasets derived in this step should reflect the proportion of missing data (White et al., 2011), although previously investigators tended to impute between five and ten datasets. As computational power has improved, it is more common these days to impute a much larger number of datasets.

3. *Estimates from multiply imputed datasets are brought together for final analyses.* In the final step, associations are estimated across each of the datasets. Finally, imputed estimates are brought together to provide a final combined estimate, in which the coefficient and standard error should reflect the variability between imputed datasets as well as uncertainty due to missing data.

There are a number of potential errors which may occur when carrying out these procedures (see White et al. (2010) and Sterne et al. (2009) for more detail). In particular, the analytic model should reflect the imputation regression; for example, any anticipated interactions in the analysis phase should be included in the imputation regression equation. The outcome variable must be included in the imputation regression also. If this is not done, then the resulting analyses will be biased.

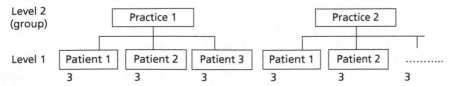

Figure 18.2 Multilevel hierarchy example—GP practices.

variable which can simply be added on to the end of the regression equation so that it now expresses all data points for that individual rather than just the best fit line.

Whenever we apply regression methods in conventional samples we assume that what is unexplained by our model, the error variables described previously, can be treated simply as random variation. This implies that errors are independent because the participants in the study are a simple random sample of their source population. However, we are often faced with data that is clustered in some way so that this no longer applies. For example, antidepressant use among patients may be clustered by general practitioner (GP) practice due to prescribing differences between practices. Some practices may be more likely to concentrate on treating depression using medication while others may favour talking treatments such as cognitive behavioural therapy. Furthermore, practices themselves are situated within regions and there are likely to be regional differences in the availability of cognitive behavioural therapy. We may approach clustering as simply a nuisance factor to adjust for in order to ensure the accuracy of our estimates. Alternatively, we may be interested in exploring the effect of these different groupings and choose to model processes occurring both at individual (patient) level and group (GP practice or region) level(s). Multilevel models allow us to do this within the same statistical model (Figure 18.2).

How does this work?

As described previously, with any regression we aim for a model that best fits the data, given outcome y and a set of predictor variables $x_1 \ldots x_k$:

$$yi = \beta_0 + \beta_1 x_1 1i + \cdots + \beta_k x_{ki} + e_i$$

where e_i is the error or unexplained difference between predicted y and observed y_i for each individual i. With a multilevel model we split this unexplained component into separate components for each level of analysis. So for a two-level model we would have:

$$y_{ij} = \beta_0 + \beta_1 x_{1ij} + \cdots + \beta_k x_{ki} j + u_j + e_i j$$

where j represents each group (e.g. GP practice) and i represents each individual (patient) within the Jth group. We now have an extra component u_j that represents unexplained

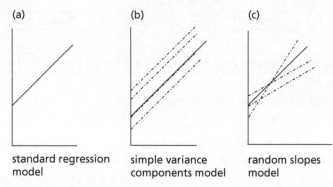

Figure 18.3 Regression models compared.

variation at the group level (GP practice in our example) and another, e_{ij}, the remaining unexplained variation at the lower (patient) level. The group level variation u_j is assumed to be random, that is, covering a random sample of practices, with a normal distribution with variance var_u. The remaining variation e_{ij} is also assumed random, that is, a random sample of patients within practices. Both are therefore termed 'random effects', while the rest of the model comprises 'fixed effects'. For this reason we sometimes refer to these as mixed (fixed and random) effects models.

In graphical terms we now have a model where, instead of specifying a straight line, we have a series of possible parallel regression lines corresponding to a variable intercept. This is known as a 'simple variance components model' (Figure 18.3). We can then extend this further to include also a random effect for the β coefficients—allowing the slope of the regression line to vary. For example, say we were interested in the effect of age on antidepressant use. The relation between age and antidepressant use may take a different shape depending on the type of GP practice, that is, the slope of our regression line is therefore no longer fixed (β_1) but random (β_{1j}).

Multilevel modelling in practice

Having specified the form that our model should take, we then use statistical software to estimate the coefficients to arrive at a model that best fits the data. A typical modelling approach will start with the simplest model—a variance components model with no predictors. At this stage it is useful to look at the proportion of unexplained variation attributed to the group level(s)—known as the intra-class correlation (ICC):

$$ICC = var_u / (var_u + var_e)$$

Then we enter variables to try to explain the variation at different levels. For example, at level 1 we might adjust for the patient's age while at level 2 we could adjust for practice size. We may further develop the model allowing for random slopes in our regression coefficients.

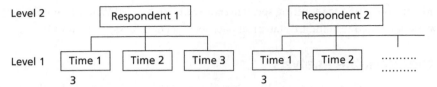

Figure 18.4 Multilevel hierarchy example—repeated survey measures.

Longitudinal data—repeated measures as level 1

Multilevel models can be extended to fit any kind of clustering so that, for example, we could look at the way that depression scores are clustered according to the interviewer administering the survey. We could extend this to look at how scores vary by neighbourhood and then by region. We could also extend this, in the other direction, to cover repeated observations made on the same individual—say, if we administered the survey at monthly intervals. This would allow us to investigate the extent to which depression scores change over time. We would then treat observations as the lowest level (level 1) and individuals at the group level (level 2)[1] (e.g. Figure 18.4).

This is necessary because repeated observations made on the same individual are almost always clustered. Often when we use a multilevel model to look at longitudinal data we are interested in how changes over time vary between individuals. We would therefore use a random slope model to look at this. It is important to note that repeated measures data require that particular attention is paid to how observations within individuals are inter-related. For example, observations occurring around the same time point are likely to be similar compared to observations occurring much earlier or later. This is known as auto-correlation and is something we would usually need to account for when specifying a longitudinal model.

Assumptions

We make much the same assumptions for multilevel regression as with any other type of regression. Essentially we treat each level as if it were a separate (but simultaneous) regression; therefore we make the same assumptions as we would for each regression in turn. Sample size limitations also apply in much the same way. The main drawback with studies underpowered at a group level is that a multilevel analysis will tell us no more than if we had used classical regression.

Software for multilevel modelling

Multilevel modelling approaches are now routinely used when analysing clustered data, and in the past two decades their use has grown rapidly. They have developed from being

---

1 This and the earlier diagram are clearly similar because they are demonstrating clustering as a common statistical challenge – the first indicating clustering by practice, the second indicating clustering by individual

an advanced technique requiring specialist software, such as MLWin, to something that is now incorporated in standard statistical packages, such as SPSS, Stata, and R.

Latent variable analysis

If the purpose of statistics is to allow the communication of numeric data between researchers, it is clear that the ability to communicate depends strongly on the meaning of the variables in the analysis. As described elsewhere in this book, mental health research faces particular challenges because of the nature of the disorders and health states being evaluated as outcomes, and the complexity of many of the constructs being evaluated as exposures. This has led to particular interest and experience in statistical techniques which help to refine the measurements used in research and those which can be derived from pre-existing data.

Specifically, a longstanding area of interest in mental health research has been the examination and quantification of unobservable constructs such as socioeconomic status or intelligence. These may be described as *latent variables*, because it is not possible to measure them directly. Latent variable analysis is a statistical method which makes it possible to estimate latent variables from *observed variables*, which are thought to be associated with the latent variable. The basic principle is that the responses on the observed measures are patterned according to their association with latent variable, which makes it possible to infer the latent variable of interest. Researchers may use latent variable analysis for several purposes, including understanding complex relationships, reducing data for practical reasons, revealing unknown underlying constructs, or testing theoretical underlying constructs.

Table 18.4 shows a traditional classification of latent variable analyses. This is based on the nature of the observed and latent variables—specifically, whether they are continuously distributed (e.g. age) or categorical (e.g. gender). However, recent developments in statistical software such as MPlus have made it possible to use a combination of continuous and categorical observed variables in latent variable analyses. As a result, the distinctions outlined in Table 18.4 have become less clear cut, and the terms 'latent profile analysis' and 'latent class analysis' are sometimes used interchangeably. This also applies to 'factor analysis' and 'latent trait analysis'.

Examples of latent variable analyses

Factor analysis involves examining the covariation between a number of observed variables in order to identify a smaller number of latent constructs—or *factors*. For example,

Table 18.4 Basic categorizations of latent variable analyses

Latent variable	Observed	
	Continuous	Categorical
Continuous	Factor analysis	Latent trait analysis
Categorical	Latent profile analysis	Latent class analysis

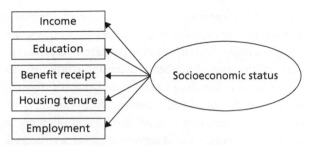

Figure 18.5 Factor analysis estimating a latent variable of socioeconomic status.
Adapted with permission from Aschan, L. et al. Suicidal behaviours in South East London: prevalence, risk factors and the role of socio-economic status. *Journal of Affective Disorders,* 150(2), 441–9. Copyright © 2013 Elsevier B.V. All rights reserved. DOI: https://doi.org/10.1016/j.jad.2013.04.037.

Aschan and colleagues (2013) estimated a latent variable of socioeconomic status from several continuous and categorical socioeconomic measures in a community sample in South East London (N = 1698). Informed by responses to the observed socioeconomic measures, a single continuous latent variable was identified ranging from low to high socioeconomic status. Figure 18.5 shows this in an ellipse and the observed socioeconomic variables in rectangles, which is the conventional way of depicting latent and observed variables. There are numerous examples of factor analysis in mental health research, including investigations of disorder states (e.g. dimensions underlying the Euro-D measure of late-life depressive symptoms reported by Prince et al. (1999)) and exposures (e.g. dimensions underlying the Parental Bonding Inventory and their cross-cultural applicability reported by Qadir et al. (2005)).

Latent class analysis is often described as the categorical equivalent to factor analysis. Instead of producing continuous measures, it classifies individuals into groups based on their responses to multiple observed variables. Thus, individuals within a latent class will have a similar pattern of responses to the observed variables used in the model. Latent class analysis is often used to identify subgroups within a specified population. For example, in a study of 818 persons with depressive disorder, Lamers and colleagues (2010) examined 16 depressive symptoms and identified three distinct latent classes: a severe melancholic class, a severe atypical class, and a class of moderate severity. The authors then examined these subtypes by risk factors of depression, indicating which specific risk factors may be part of their aetiology.

Exploratory versus confirmatory approaches to latent variable modelling

A researcher may either take a *confirmatory* or *exploratory* approach to their latent variable analysis. The confirmatory approach is theory driven and tests a predefined hypothesis or theory. This approach was applied in the factor analysis estimating socioeconomic status, described earlier (Aschan et al., 2013). Given that the researchers sought to identify a single theoretically defined construct of socioeconomic status, the analysis was restricted to models that only allowed one factor to be identified.

In contrast, the exploratory approach aims to identify an unknown number of latent constructs. Multiple models are typically run, and statistical criteria are used to inform which number of latent variables best captures the patterns of the observed variables. This approach was applied in the study described previously identifying subtypes of depression; models allowing for one to five classes were tested before the researchers determined that the three-class solution best fitted their observed data (Lamers et al., 2010).

Even when an exploratory approach is used, theory still plays an important part. It is, for example, important to ensure the observed variables are theoretically relevant to the latent construct of interest. Particularly when dealing with large datasets, it can be tempting to include more variables in attempts to improve the model; however, too many observed variables may in fact overwhelm the model and produce less meaningful results (Wurpts and Geiser, 2014). Theory also plays an important role in model selection. If the researcher relies too heavily on the statistical criteria, they may overlook model solutions which may have a slightly poorer model fit, but which generate more theoretically or clinically meaningful results.

Examples of advanced latent variable analyses

Often researchers want to test the associations between latent variables in statistical models as exposures or outcome variables. In the study described previously, Aschan and colleagues (2013) used socioeconomic status to examine the association with suicidal behaviours as an outcome. When a latent variable is used this way to test associations with observed variables, it is called *structural equation modelling*. Latent variable analyses may also consider changes in time, using *latent curve modelling*. Here, the researcher is interested in examining how observed variables cluster together over time. For example, if depressive symptoms were measured over multiple time points within the same people, it would be possible to identify specific trajectories of illness and recovery among persons with depression.

References

Aschan, L., Goodwin, L., Cross, S., Moran, P., Hotopf, M., and Hatch, S.L. (2013). Suicidal behaviours in South East London: prevalence, risk factors and the role of socio-economic status. *Journal of Affective Disorders*, **150**, 441–449.

Barnes, T.R. and Paton, C. (2011). Antipsychotic polypharmacy in schizophrenia: benefits and risks. *CNS Drugs*, **25**, 383–399.

Booth, C.M. and Tannock, I.F. (2014). Randomised controlled trials and population-based observational research: partners in the evolution of medical evidence. *British Journal of Cancer*, **110**, 551–555.

Cepeda, M.S., Boston, R., Farrar, J.T., and Strom, B.L. (2003). Comparison of logistic regression versus propensity score when the number of events is low and there are multiple confounders. *American Journal of Epidemiology*, **158**, 280–287.

Drake, C. (1993). Effects of misspecification of the propensity score on estimators of treatment effect. *Biometrics*, **49**, 1231–1236.

Fleischhacker, W.W., Heikkinen, M.E., Olié, J.P., Landsberg, W., Dewaele, P., McQuade, R.D., et al. (2010). Effects of adjunctive treatment with aripiprazole on body weight and clinical efficacy in schizophrenia patients treated with clozapine: a randomized, double-blind, placebo-controlled trial. *International Journal of Neuropsychopharmacology*, **13**, 1115–1125.

Glynn, R.J., Schneeweiss, S., and Sturmer, T. (2006). Indications for propensity scores and review of their use in pharmacoepidemiology. *Basic & Clinical Pharmacology & Toxicology*, **98**, 253–259.

Hayes, R.D., Downs, J., Chang, C.K., Jackson, R.G., Shetty, H., Broadbent, M., et al. (2015). The effect of clozapine on premature mortality: an assessment of clinical monitoring and other potential confounders. *Schizophrenia Bulletin*, **41**, 644–655.

Kadra, G., Stewart, R., Shetty, H., Downs, J., MacCabe, J.H., Taylor, D., and Hayes, R.D. (2016). Predictors of long-term (≥6months) antipsychotic polypharmacy prescribing in secondary mental healthcare. *Schizophrenia Research*, **174**, 106–112.

Lamers, F., De Jonge, P., Nolen, W.A., Smit, J.H., Zitman, F.G., Beekman, A.T., and Penninx, B.W. (2010). Identifying depressive subtypes in a large cohort study: results from the Netherlands Study of Depression and Anxiety (NESDA). *Journal of Clinical Psychiatry*, **71**, 1582–1589.

Lundsberg, L.S., Bracken, M.B., and Saftlas, A.F. (1997). Low-to-moderate gestational alcohol use and intrauterine growth retardation, low birthweight, and preterm delivery. *Annals of Epidemiology*, **7**, 498–508.

Okoli, G.N., Sanders, R.D., and Myles, P. (2014). Demystifying propensity scores. *British Journal of Anaesthesia*, **112**, 13–15.

Patrick, A.R., Schneeweiss, S., Brookhart, M.A., Glynn, R.J., Rothman, K.J., Avorn, J., and Stürmer, T. (2011). The implications of propensity score variable selection strategies in pharmacoepidemiology: an empirical illustration. *Pharmacoepidemiology and Drug Safety*, **20**, 551–559.

Pearl, J. (2014). Interpretation and identification of causal mediation. *Psychological Methods*, **19**, 459–481.

Prince, M.J., Beekman, A.T.F., Deeg, D.J.H., Fuhrer, R., Kivela, S.L., Lawlor, B.A., et al. (1999). Depression symptoms in late-life assessed using the EURO-D scale. *British Journal of Psychiatry*, **174**, 339–345.

Qadir, F., Stewart, R., Khan, M., and Prince, M. (2005). The validity of the Parental Bonding Instrument as a measure of maternal bonding among young Pakistani women. *Social Psychiatry and Psychiatric Epidemiology*, **40**, 276–282.

Richards, M. and Sacker, A. (2003). Lifetime antecedents of cognitive reserve. *Journal of Clinical and Experimental Neuropsychology*, **25**, 614–624.

Rodgers, B. (1994). Pathways between parental divorce and adult depression. *Journal of Child Psychology and Psychiatry*, **35**, 1289–1308.

Rosenbaum, P.R. and Rubin, D.B. (1983). The central role of the propensity score in observational studies for causal effects. *Biometrika*, **70**, 41–55.

Shah, B.R., Laupacis, A., Hux, J.E., and Austin, P.C. (2005). Propensity score methods gave similar results to traditional regression modeling in observational studies: a systematic review. *Journal of Clinical Epidemiology*, **58**, 550–559.

Sterne, J.A.C., White, I.R., Carlin, J.B., Spratt, M., Royston, P., Kenward, M.G., et al. (2009). Multiple imputation for missing data in epidemiological and clinical research: potential and pitfalls. *BMJ*, **338**, b2393.

Sturmer, T., Joshi, M., Glynn, R.J., Avorn, J., Rothman, K.J., and Schneeweiss, S. (2006). A review of the application of propensity score methods yielded increasing use, advantages in specific settings, but not substantially different estimates compared with conventional multivariable methods. *Journal of Clinical Epidemiology*, **59**, 437–447.

White, I.R., Royston, P., and Wood, A.M. (2011). Multiple imputation using chained equations: issues and guidance for practice. *Statistics in Medicine*, **30**, 377–399.

Wurpts I.C. and Geiser C. (2014). Is adding more indicators to a latent class analysis beneficial or detrimental? Results of a Monte-Carlo study. *Frontiers in Psychology*, **5**, 1–15.

Chapter 19

Genetic epidemiology: Overview

Frühling Rijsdijk and Paul F. O'Reilly

Introduction

The aim of this chapter is to demonstrate the principles behind some of the major genetic study designs used in psychiatry research (and complex disorder research more broadly). The first part of this chapter focuses on behavioural genetic designs, while the second part describes designs for 'gene mapping'. Behavioural genetics examines the genetic basis of behavioural phenotypes, including both disorders and 'normal' dimensional traits. The theoretical basis is derived from population genetics, including properties such as segregation ratios, random mating, genetic variance, and genetic correlation between relatives. The second part of the chapter deals with gene mapping designs, in which specific genetic variants or genomic regions associated with a disorder or trait are identified. Practical methods for the efficient analysis of the human genome have only recently emerged, but their development and that of the technologies that obtain genetic information is moving at a rapid pace. A brief outline of the most popular current approaches to the analysis of the genetics of complex human disorders will be provided.

Behavioural genetic designs

Genetic factors have neither an isolated nor static effect. Therefore, important considerations in behavioural genetics are (1) the relative contributions of genetic and environmental factors, (2) the interplay between genetic and environmental factors, and (3) the changing role of genetic factors in different stages of development. The major study designs are discussed here in the context of *categorical* and *dimensional traits*. Behavioural genetics is rooted in both psychiatry and psychology. Psychiatrists traditionally adopt a medical model where diseases are defined as categorical entities and diagnoses are either present or absent. Psychologists, on the other hand, prefer quantitative measures of, for example, cognitive ability and personality traits. The methodology of behavioural genetics research reflects this duality, although there is a trend to integrate the two approaches, especially for traits such as anxiety and depression where diagnostic categories can be seen as the extremes of a continuum of symptom severity.

Family studies

The aim is primarily to demonstrate familial aggregation of a disease or trait and to use this pattern to infer its likely mode of inheritance. Systematic ascertainment of affected individuals is important since over-inclusion of families with several affected individuals could lead to biased estimates of familial aggregation. To prevent such biases, a two-stage sampling scheme is adopted: a random sample of individuals with the disease is obtained (index cases or 'probands'); and the relatives of the probands are assessed for the presence or absence of the disease. The risk of disease in a relative of a proband is called 'morbid risk' or 'recurrence risk'. For a disease with variable age at onset, there is the problem of 'censoring'—namely that some unaffected individuals of a relatively young age may yet develop the disease in later life. Age adjustments in the calculation of morbid risk are made using, for example, the Weinberg (modified by Strömgren) method and survival analysis-based methods (lifetable or Kaplan–Meier estimators). A measure of *familial aggregation* is the 'relative risk ratio', which is the ratio of morbid risk among the relatives of cases to the relatives of controls, for a specific class of relatives (e.g. parent, sibling, and offspring). Schizophrenia, for example, has relative risk ratios of about 10 for siblings and offspring, and about 3 for second-degree relatives.

Ascertainment types

The systematic ascertainment of families through probands can lead to the complication that some families may have two or more probands. In the extreme case, if sampling is exhaustive and all affected individuals in the population are included as probands, then a family will have as many probands as affected members (*complete ascertainment*). At the other extreme, only a small proportion of the affected individuals in the population are included as probands, and almost all ascertained families will have only one proband (*single ascertainment*). In between these two scenarios, there is *multiple incomplete* ascertainment. Estimating morbid risk under multiple ascertainment is worked out by Weinberg using the '*proband method*' (Cavalli-Sforza and Bodmer, 1999, p. 857).

Inferring mode of inheritance

Simple Mendelian modes of inheritance such as autosomal dominant and recessive have predictable patterns of relative risk ratios. For a rare autosomal dominant disease, the ratios are 0.5 for parents, siblings, and offspring, 0.25 for second-degree relatives, and so on. For a rare recessive condition, the ratio is 0.25 for siblings, and other classes of relatives are rarely affected. However, most behavioural traits do not show such ratios because of the likely involvement of multiple genes and environmental factors in their cause. A popular model to explain the complexity of behavioural traits is the *polygenic model*, which posits a very large number of genes each of small effect (Neale and Cardon, 1992; Plomin et al., 2001). The cumulative effects of multiple genes lead to a continuous (normal) distribution, which fits well with quantitative characteristics, but is not directly applicable to categorical traits. The *liability-threshold model* proposes that many genes of small effect exert their influence on an unobserved normally distributed variable—known as a liability—and that the disease develops if this liability exceeds a certain threshold value

Adoption studies

A limitation of family studies is the inability to discriminate genetic from shared environmental factors (i.e. non-genetic factors that make family members more alike). There are several varieties of adoption studies. The *adoptees design* compares the adopted-away children of affected and unaffected biological parents, controlling for the affection status of the adoptive parents if known. If the affection status of the biological parents is related to morbid risk in the adoptee, after adjusting for the affection status of the adoptive parents, then genetic factors are implicated. The *adoptees' family design* compares morbid risk in the biological and adoptive families of affected adoptees, also considering information on the biological and adoptive families of unaffected adoptees if available. A greater morbid risk among biological than adoptive family members of affected adoptees would implicate genetic factors if not also observed for unaffected adoptees. Adoption studies are essentially family studies with the 'convenient' ability to interpret family resemblance as genetic rather than some combination of genetic and 'familial'.

Twin studies

The classical twin method is the most popular design in behavioural genetics. The existence of two types of twin pairs, monozygotic (MZ) and dizygotic (DZ), provides a natural experiment for untangling genetic from environmental factors. MZ twins are developed from the same fertilized ovum and are therefore genetically identical; DZ twins are developed from two separate fertilized ova and share on average 50% of their segregating genes. There are two main types of twin study: (1) those based on twin pairs ascertained through affected probands, and (2) those based on population twin registers. The former is appropriate for investigating relatively rare diseases, whereas the latter is better suited for studying common traits and quantitative dimensions. The inference of a genetic component from proband-ascertained twin pairs is usually based on a difference between MZ and DZ concordance rates. The most informative index is the proband-wise concordance rate, which is defined as the number of probands whose co-twins are affected divided by the total number of probands.

There are a number of assumptions made in the classical twin study. It is important to be aware of the implications of these and consider whether they are realistic in relation to the trait under study. The assumptions are that (1) MZ and DZ twin pairs share their environments to the same extent; (2) gene–environment correlations and interactions are minimal for the trait in question (if not, they get incorporated into the other variance components); and (3) twins are no different from the general population in terms of the trait in question. Procedures for testing these assumptions are discussed in detail elsewhere (Rijsdijk and Sham, 1992). When the assumptions are met, the classical twin design is the most powerful tool for investigating the relative contribution of genetic and environmental influences to individual differences in traits. The latent genetic and environmental influences can be categorized into several major sources. The relative importance of these can be inferred by comparing the observed correlations between MZ and DZ twins, with predicted correlations based on different sources of genetic and environmental factors playing a role. The sources of genetic and environmental variation considered in behavioural genetics are as follows:

♦ Additive genetic influences, A, represent the sum of the effects of the individual alleles at all loci that influence the trait.

♦ Non-additive genetic influences, D, which represent interactions between alleles of the same marker (dominance genetic variation) or different markers (epistasis).

♦ Environmental influences, C, that make family members more alike (common environmental variation) (e.g. socioeconomic status, parenting style, and diet).

♦ Unique environmental influences, E, that result in differences among members of one family (e.g. accidents, differential parental treatment, as well as measurement error).

The total phenotypic variance (P) of a trait is the sum of these variance components ($P = A + D + C + E$). To unravel the sources of variance and estimate their contribution, information from genetically informative subjects is essential.

Biometrical genetics and the twin method

MZ and DZ twins have different degrees of correlation for the genetic components A (1 vs 0.50) and D (1 vs 0.25) but the same degrees of correlation for the environmental components C (1 in both MZ and DZ pairs) and E (0 in both MZ and DZ pairs). Since D involves the interaction effects between alleles, for this source of variance to explain the correlation between relatives, they would need to have the same alleles identical by decent (alleles from same parental origin), which is 100% the case for MZ pairs, only 25% for siblings/DZ twins, and 0% for any other relative pair. Assuming that MZ and DZ twins experience the same degree of similarity in their environments, then any excess of similarity between MZ (compared to DZ) twins can be interpreted as due to the greater proportion of genes shared by MZ twins, and thus, gives us an estimate for A; an estimate for C is given by the difference in MZ correlation and the estimated effect of A. Differences in MZ twins can only be due to unique environmental influences and, thus, gives us an estimate for E.

Heritability (h^2), an index for the relative contribution of genetic effects to the total phenotypic variance is derived by using the simple Falconer's formula: h^2 is $2(r_{mz} - r_{dz})$, where r is the correlation coefficient. The relative contribution of the shared and non-shared environmental effects are given by: $c^2 = r_{mz} - h^2$; and $e^2 = 1 - h^2 + c^2$. More advanced covariance structure analysis is accomplished by structural equation modelling (SEM) software in which (multivariate) data from a range of different family groupings is analysed simultaneously by means of maximum likelihood estimation techniques (Neale and Cardon, 1992; Plomin et al., 2001).

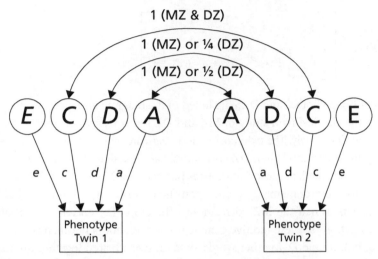

Figure 19.1 Path diagram for the basic univariate twin model. The additive (*A*) and dominance (*D*) factors are correlated 1 between MZ twins and 0.5 and 0.25 for DZ twins, respectively. Shared family environment (*C*) is correlated 1 for both MZ and DZ twins that are reared together in the same home. Unique environment (*E*) is the source of variance that results in differences among members of one family and is, thus, uncorrelated between members of MZ and DZ pairs. *a, d, c,* and *e* are the path coefficients for the *A, D, C,* and *E* effects, respectively.

Path diagram and structural equation modelling

The full twin model (for a single trait) is depicted in a path diagram (Figure 19.1) in which the observed trait for twin 1 and twin 2 is represented in rectangles and the unobserved (latent) genetic and environmental variables in circles. The single-headed arrows pointing from the latent variables to the observed traits represent causal paths. The path estimates (or regression coefficients) indicated by *a, c, d,* and *e* represent the effects of the latent variables on the trait in question. The square of these estimates represents the variance of the trait accounted for by the corresponding latent factor (Neale and Cardon, 1992).

The curved double-headed arrows represent correlations among the latent factors (i.e. for MZ pairs $r = 1$ for *A, D,* and *C*; for DZ pairs $r = 0.50$ for *A*, 0.25 for *D*, and 1 for *C*). The *genetic* covariance between twin 1 and twin 2 is the product of the paths linking the trait scores via *A* (for MZ: $a \times 1 \times a = a^2$; for DZ: $a \times \frac{1}{2} \times a = \frac{1}{2}a^2$). The covariance due to *C* and *D* can be derived in similar way. The total covariance is the sum of these chains via *A* and *C*. The expected variances and covariance of the traits within MZ and DZ pairs can then be written in terms of the different variance components:

$$\text{Cov}_{\text{MZ}} = \begin{bmatrix} a^2 + d^2 + c^2 + e^2 & a^2 + d^2 + c^2 \\ a^2 + d^2 + c^2 & a^2 + d^2 + c^2 + e^2 \end{bmatrix}$$

$$\mathrm{Cov}_{\mathrm{DZ}} = \begin{bmatrix} a^2 + d^2 + c^2 + e^2 & \dfrac{1}{2}a^2 + \dfrac{1}{4}d^2 + c^2 \\ \dfrac{1}{2}a^2 + \dfrac{1}{4}d^2 + c^2 & a^2 + d^2 + c^2 + e^2 \end{bmatrix}$$

Note that, although both C and D are included in the diagram and matrices, they are confounded in the classical twin study of MZ and DZ twins reared together and cannot be estimated simultaneously. The twin correlations indicate which of the two components is more likely to be present. When DZ correlations are less than half the MZ correlations, dominance is indicated, because D correlates perfectly for MZ but only 25% for DZ twin pairs. Common environmental influences, on the other hand, will make the DZ correlations greater than half the MZ correlations. Therefore, DZ correlations of about half the MZ correlations suggest additive genetic influences, but is not inconsistent with the presence of both C and D. In other words, data on twins reared together do not contain enough information to tease out the contrasting effects of C and D. If data of adoptive siblings are included (giving us an independent estimate of C), we can estimate the effects of both components. While path diagrams allow models to be presented in schematic form, they can also be represented as structural equations and covariance matrices and, since all three forms are mathematically complete, it is possible to translate from one to the other (Neale and Cardon, 1992). SEM represents a unified platform for path analytic and variance components models and is the current method that is used to analyse twin data. SEM is a statistical technique that tests hypotheses about relations among observed and latent variables. Many SEM programs are available, but packages like Mx (Neale, 1997) and more recently, OpenMx (Boker et al., 2011), were developed to model genetically sensitive data in a more flexible way.

Twin analysis of multiple traits

If multiple measures have been assessed in twin pairs, the model-fitting approach easily extends to analyse the genetic–environmental architecture of the covariance between the traits. With multivariate models we can investigate the genetic overlap between different disorders, the continuity of genetic factors at different stages of the illness, and the relationship between genetic factors and mediating or environmental variables (e.g. personality and stressful life events) in the development of illness. For depression and anxiety, two very common and commonly comorbid disorders, it was found that the substantial genetic component of both disorders is shared. Environmental factors, however, were different, and therefore important in shaping different outcomes (Kendler et al., 1992).

Categorical data for twins

Variance components models can also be applied to categorical twin data by assuming that the ordered categories reflect an imprecise measurement of an underlying *normal distribution of liability* with one or more *thresholds* (cut-offs) to discriminate between the ordered classes. The joint distribution of two categorical traits (twin 1 and twin 2 variables) is assumed to have a *bivariate normal distribution*, whose shape is determined by the relative proportions of twin pairs concordant and discordant for the observed categories (estimating tetrachoric correlations). The relative difference in derived MZ and DZ correlations will further inform on the usual twin method of variance decomposition, leading to an estimate of the heritability of the liability. The often-cited heritability estimates for psychiatric disorders are, strictly speaking, estimates of the *heritability of the liabilities* to the disorder.

Gene mapping designs

Linkage studies

The term linkage refers to the tendency for alleles from physically close genetic loci, on the same strand of DNA, to segregate together. The mechanism that explains this is genetic recombination. Recombination occurs infrequently along each chromosome per meiosis (once or twice on average) and therefore long stretches of sequence are passed on to the next generation intact, although these are broken down over many generations. The closer that two loci are together, the stronger their observed linkage, since the chance of being separated by a recombination event during meiosis reduces with physical distance. Nearby genetic loci are said to be 'linked'. This phenomenon is exploited to detect loci influencing genetic diseases, where alleles of a genetic marker close to a disease causing gene will tend to co-segregate with the disease and be shared among affected relatives. There are two main linkage methods: (1) analysis of the pattern of allele transmission in families relative to the pattern of disease transmission, and (2) analysis of the extent of allele sharing between affected family members (Sham, 1998). The former is commonly referred to as *linkage analysis*, performed as part of linkage studies. Statistical significance in linkage analysis is derived from likelihood ratios that compare the odds of segregation between the marker and the disease being the result of linkage, with the odds of it being the result of chance. It is customary to use the *logarithm of odds* or *LOD score*, with a score of 3 or higher indicating significance (a LOD of 3 is roughly equivalent to a p-value of 0.0001). The primary limitation of the linkage analysis method is that its power relies on the specification of the disease model in terms of a single gene frequency and a mode of inheritance, specifically in relation to a single dominant or recessive putative disease gene. This is a poor representation of the causal system for complex disorders, so while linkage studies have been extremely successful in identifying genetic susceptibility loci for rare or Mendelian disorders, aided by collecting family data enriched for cases, the method is not well designed for complex disease. This disadvantage has given rise to the development of 'non-parametric' *allele-sharing methods*.

The 'sibling pair analysis' relies on the relationship between the disease status and genetic markers of pairs of siblings (Sham, 1998). If a marker is linked to the disorder, then siblings with the same disease status will be more alike than those discordant for the disease. A more specialized form of this method is the *affected sibling method*, which considers only pairs of affected siblings and uses *identity by descent* rather than *identity by state.* Identity by state is measured when a sibling pair is simply alike for two marker alleles; identity by descent occurs when the two alleles are shown to come from the same chromosome in the previous generation (i.e. they are replicates of each other). The underlying intuition is that affected siblings will have received the same disease-causing allele from the same grandparental sequence of DNA, but that this allele will not be one of the genetic markers assayed as part of the study. The logic of the allele-sharing method can be extended to using affected relative pairs, which is more convenient when affected sibling pairs are rare (see, for example Curtis and Sham, 1994).

Association studies

While linkage studies test for association between marker alleles and the segregation of disease in families, association studies test for the association between alleles and disease in population samples. The principle of the study design is that a disease-causing allele should be more common in the disease population than in the control population, and thus the corresponding genetic variant(s) should be associated with disease status. It is this reliance on the association only, without exploiting known relatedness (as in linkage studies), that gives association studies their name. However, like linkage studies, association studies exploit linkage between genotyped markers and disease-causing variants, which over many generations in population samples is observed as correlation between nearby variants, known as linkage disequilibrium (LD). This LD is the key phenomenon that makes association studies possible (Figure 19.2), usually ensuring that a signal of association is observed at many variants across a susceptibility locus, even when the causal variant(s) is not included in the set of markers genotyped (Balding, 2006).

The application of association studies to population-based data is far more cost-effective than collecting family data, and thus allows them to exploit the large resources of existing cohort and case–control data sets. Consequently, association studies can be performed

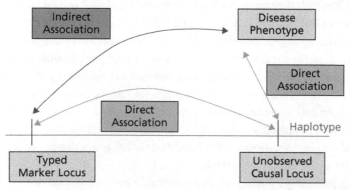

Figure 19.2 Testing of markers in genetic association studies. The association between the causal variant and the phenotype under study is implicitly highlighted by the association observed between a correlated genotyped variant and the phenotype.

Reproduced with permission from Balding, D. J. A tutorial on statistical methods for population association studies. *Nature Reviews Genetics* 7(10), 781–791. Copyright © 2006, Springer Nature. DOI: https://doi.org/10.1038/nrg1916.

on very large sample sizes, often via meta-analysis of different studies, making them highly powerful and thus able to detect the alleles of small effect expected to be associated with complex disorders. This explains their huge popularity in recent years. Association studies are typically performed either on a candidate gene list or across the entire genome in *genome-wide association studies* (GWASs). Each type of study is described in the following sections.

Candidate gene studies

One strategy for identifying genomic regions associated with a disorder is to test variants in genes that have a plausible biological link to the disorder. This link may derive from knowledge on relevant biological pathways, clinical evidence, or from the results of linkage studies. Prior to around 2007, testing such candidate genes was the only feasible way to perform association testing in large samples, given the cost of genotyping at the time. Depending on available funding and the disorder being investigated, a candidate gene study typically involves compiling a list of approximately 30 candidate genes considered most likely to harbour disease-causing variants, and 20–50 genetic variants are then genotyped across each gene and tested for association with the outcome (Tabor et al., 2002). While this approach was popular prior to the onset of GWASs, and is still sometimes applied now, many results from candidate gene studies that claimed statistical significance were underpowered and have since failed to replicate in larger studies (Munafò, 2006). Together with rapidly reducing genotyping costs, this motivated a transition in the field from the candidate gene design to the hypothesis-free approach of GWAS, which has come to dominate the field of gene mapping, and even to some degree genetics more broadly, over the last decade.

Genome-wide association studies

The turn of the century saw the completion of two landmark human genetic studies that paved the way for a new approach to gene mapping. In 2001, the Human Genome Project was completed, in which a full human genome sequence was deciphered for the first time (Lander et al., 2001). During 2003–2010 the three stages of the International HapMap Project were performed, in which a large portion of common genetic variation was assayed in samples of hundreds of individuals from the major worldwide populations (International HapMap Consortium, 2003; International HapMap 3 Consortium, 2010). Common genetic variation was captured by the HapMap project in the form of single nucleotide polymorphisms (SNPs) because these are by far the most abundant polymorphism in the human genome and the variant type that are most easily assayed. This comprehensive characterization of the human genome and of common genetic variation, in which the less frequent (minor) allele of a SNP is present in more than 1% of human chromosomes, motivated intense competition to devise affordable genotyping chips for assaying hundreds of thousands of SNPs across the genome. The subsequent drop in the cost of genotyping allowed genetic association studies to be performed across the entire human genome in large population samples for the first time (Sladek et al., 2007; Wellcome Trust Case Control Consortium, 2007).

The early genome-wide genotyping chips typically assayed around 500,000 SNPs, corresponding to around 1 SNP in every 5000 nucleotide bases of DNA sequence. The HapMap project showed that while this only captures a fraction of SNPs in genomic regions, the correlation among SNPs in most genomic regions is sufficient to ensure with high probability that a genotyped SNP will be in LD with, or 'tag', a causal variant (Figure 19.2). The key intuition underlying the GWAS design is that with a sufficiently large study sample, a statistically significant association will be observed by testing a genotyped SNP in LD with the causal variant, even when that causal variant has a small effect on the outcome, as is expected for complex diseases and psychiatric disorders (Stranger et al., 2011). The association tests themselves assess evidence of association between SNP genotypes and the trait or disorder, at each SNP independently, using statistical tests commonly applied in observational epidemiology: the chi-squared test, Fisher's exact test, the Cochran–Armitage trend test, and linear or logistic regression which allow covariates to be adjusted for (Balding, 2006). Prior to selecting which test to perform, the expected mode of inheritance given a causal effect should be considered; that is, whether the genotypes have a dominant, recessive, or additive effect on the outcome. The general assumption made in GWASs is that effects are additive, or more specifically that assuming additivity will have greatest statistical power (Iles, 2010), and so either the Cochran–Armitage trend test, regression models, or equivalent tests are typically applied.

While GWASs are relatively straightforward to perform, there are problems specific to genetic association testing that must be addressed in order to minimize false-positive findings and optimize statistical power.

Problems with genetic association testing

A distinct advantage of association testing in genetic studies over that in standard epidemiological studies is the limited opportunity for confounding factors to induce associations that do not reflect causality between the tested variables. The only true confounder in genetic association studies is population structure, whereby allele frequencies vary by geographical location and are thus indirectly associated with environmental risk factors that also vary by location, but statistical genetic methods can be applied that control for this extremely well (Price et al., 2010). However, other problems exist that require consideration. For example, given that only a fraction of genetic variants are typically genotyped or imputed, and then tested, it cannot be known whether a significant finding pertains to a causal variant or whether it is merely in LD with the causal variant. This makes it difficult to establish the precise biological mechanism responsible for the effect on the phenotype and can only be resolved through sequencing of the susceptibility locus. In GWASs, usually millions of SNPs are tested, producing a 'multiple testing problem'. In order to avoid a large number of false-positive findings that arise only due to this multiplicity of testing, GWASs impose a stringent significance threshold of $p = 5 \times 10^{-8}$, which maintains a family-wise error rate of 0.05. However, it has become clear that most complex diseases are highly polygenic in nature, with hundreds or thousands of genetic variants of small effect, which means that extremely large sample sizes are required to obtain statistical

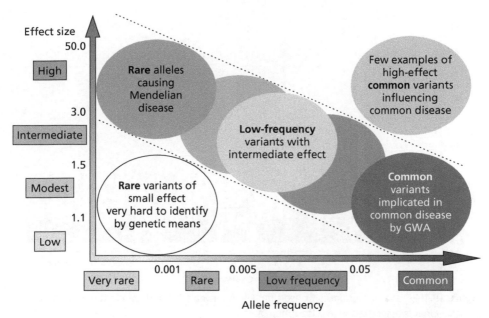

Figure 19.3 The challenge in detecting genetic variants as risk allele frequencies and effect sizes vary.

Reproduced with permission from Manolio, T. A. et al. Finding the missing heritability of complex diseases. *Nature*, 461, 747–53. Copyright © 2009, Springer Nature. https://doi.org/10.1038/nature08494.

significance for the majority of causal variants, given the stringent genome-wide significance threshold. With sample sizes in the tens of thousands, it may be possible to detect common variants of moderate effect or rare variants of large effect; however, detecting rare variants of intermediate or weak effect remains extremely challenging with present sample sizes (Figure 19.3).

Results from GWAS

The Wellcome Trust Case Control Consortium performed the first major GWAS study in 2007, conducting separate analyses in seven common diseases, including bipolar disorder (Wellcome Trust Case Control Consortium, 2007). In the years that followed, hundreds of GWAS were performed in search of common variants affecting a multitude of different traits, diseases, and disorders (Visscher et al., 2012). While this yielded thousands of genetic variants associated with hundreds of phenotypes affecting humans, there was a distinct paucity of findings for psychiatric disorders, leading to questions over the value of searching for common genetic determinants in psychiatry (Cirulli et al., 2010). However, many of these concerns were allayed in 2014 when the Psychiatric Genomics Consortium published their latest GWAS into schizophrenia (Ripke et al., 2014), finding 108 independent genes harbouring genome-wide significant associations (Figure 19.4). While the prevalence and heterogeneity of disorders such as major depressive disorder make finding their genetic determinants even more challenging, the latest findings (Wray

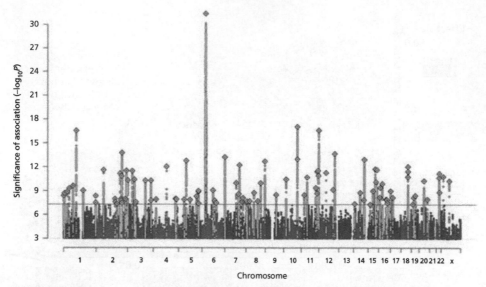

Figure 19.4 Psychiatric Genomics Consortium GWAS reveals 108 independent genes harbouring genetic variants associated with schizophrenia.

Reproduced with permission from Ripke, S. et al. Biological insights from 108 schizophrenia-associated genetic loci. *Nature,* 511(7510), 42–7. Copyright © 2014, Springer Nature. DOI: https://doi.org/10.1038/nature13595.

et al., 2018) suggest that further sample size increases will bring about a similar bounty of significant results (Hyman, 2014).

Downstream analyses and alternative approaches

In addition to standard genetic association testing, there are a number of downstream and alternative analyses performed that exploit genome-wide genetic data. One of the most frequently applied downstream analyses is pathway analysis. The standard approach involves assessing GWAS results for enrichment of small *p*-values among all gene sets that correspond to a known biological pathway. The top-ranked pathways highlighted are then usually interrogated for their biological link with the phenotype under study. Given marked differences in the performance of pathway analysis methods, a strategy of combining methods may be preferred and was used recently to highlight pathways shared among different psychiatric disorders (Network and Pathway Analysis Subgroup of Psychiatric Genomics Consortium, 2015). In addition to testing for the main effects of genetic variants, researchers may be interested in searching for interaction effects between variants and environmental factors. The most notable interaction effect identified to date is that between a variant of the serotonin transporter gene and stress life events on depression (Caspi et al., 2003), though replication studies into this have produced conflicting results.

Genetic association testing is generally performed on one SNP at a time and one phenotype at a time. However, methods have been developed that take a multivariate approach in order to increase the statistical power of discovery. These either perform joint testing across SNPs (Hoggart et al., 2007), across multiple phenotypes (O'Reilly et al., 2012), or both simultaneously (Zhou and Stephens, 2014). Recent major advances in the field have been the development of statistical genetic methods to estimate the heritability, co-heritability, and genetic correlation among phenotypes, as well as to perform risk prediction, from genome-wide SNP data (described in the following section).

Estimating heritability from SNP data and polygenic risk scores

Estimation of the variance in a trait explained by genome-wide SNP data in unrelated individuals is commonly referred to as genome-wide complex trait analysis (GCTA), though this is in fact the name of the software that performs this and other analyses (Yang et al., 2011). The method, introduced by Yang and colleagues (2010), exploits the so-called genomic relationship matrix between nominally unrelated individuals estimated from genome-wide SNPs, to estimate the variance explained by the SNPs in a linear mixed model. The proportion of genetic variation estimated by GCTA is in general substantially larger than that based on only the genome-wide significant SNPs, since it infers the total effect of all SNPs, accounting for much of the so-called missing heritability (Manolio et al., 2009). For human height, the genetic variance based on around 300,000 SNPS was estimated at 45% compared to 5% using around 50 GWAS-detected variants (Yang et al., 2010). The method has been further developed for analysing complex diseases in case–control studies (Lee et al., 2011) and extended to estimate genetic correlations between complex diseases (Lee et al., 2012). GCTA estimates confirm around two-thirds of twin-study estimates of heritability for traits such as cognitive ability (Plomin et al., 2013), but not for others, for example, childhood anxiety and behaviour problems (Trzaskowski et al., 2013). For the variation in liability to psychiatric disorders this method estimated the contribution of common variants to be between 17% and 29% (Cross-Disorder Group of the Psychiatric Genomics Consortium, 2013), with a high genetic overlap reported for schizophrenia and bipolar disorder and a moderate correlation between major depression and schizophrenia/bipolar disorder. An interesting possibility of this method is to derive heritability estimates for variables which do not show any variation among individuals in the same family (e.g. SES) and thus cannot be analysed using twin models.

The development of polygenic methods of inference, such as GCTA, is an active area of statistical genetics research, with LD score regression (Bulik-Sullivan et al., 2015) and polygenic risk score analyses (Dudbridge, 2013; Euesden et al., 2015) offering attractive alternatives and their own applications. For example, a review of schizophrenia polygenic risk score studies (Mistry et al., 2018) reported associations with a range of phenotypic measures, including depression, bipolar disorder, lower performance IQ, and negative symptoms. In addition, there was some evidence of associations with non-psychiatric disorders such as diabetes, rheumatoid arthritis, and Crohn's disease, supporting a hypothesis of common inflammatory pathways. A framework and checklist for future studies was proposed by the authors. While the most popular use of polygenic risk scores to date has been to test for shared aetiology among different phenotypes, there are a rapidly growing number of applications of the approach. For instance, polygenic risk scores have been in Mendelian randomization studies investigating associations between the genetic propensity to a hypothesized exposure and the mental health outcome of interest—for example, investigating polygenic scores for type 2 diabetes mellitus as putative risk factors for Alzheimer's disease (Walter et al., 2016). Developments in the genetic epidemiology of physical traits are therefore likely to have important applications in mental health research, an advantage of Mendelian randomization approaches being the ability to investigate more explicitly the relative likelihoods of causation, reverse causation, and confounding as explanations for an observed association.

References

Balding, D.J. (2006). A tutorial on statistical methods for population association studies. *Nature Reviews Genetics*, 7, 781–791.

Boker, S., Neale, M., Maes, H., Wilde, M., Spiegel, M., Brick, T., et al. (2011). OpenMx: an open source extended structural equation modeling framework. *Psychometrika*, 76, 306–317.

Bulik-Sullivan, B.K., Loh, P.R., Finucane, H.K., Ripke, S., Yang, J., Schizophrenia Working Group of the Psychiatric Genomics Consortium, et al. (2015). LD score regression distinguishes confounding from polygenicity in genome-wide association studies. *Nature Genetics*, 47, 291–295.

Caspi, A., Sugden, K., Moffitt, T.E., Taylor, A., Craig, I.W., Harrington, H., et al. (2003). Influence of life stress on depression: moderation by a polymorphism in the 5-HTT gene. *Science*, 301, 386–389.

Cavalli-Sforza, L.L. and Bodmer, W.F. (1999). *The genetics of human populations*. New York: Unabridged Dover.

Cirulli, E.T., Kasperaviciūtė, D., Attix, D.K., Need, A.C., Ge, D., Gibson, G., and Goldstein, D.B. (2010). Common genetic variation and performance on standardized cognitive tests. *European Journal of Human Genetics*, 18, 815–820.

Cross-Disorder Group of the Psychiatric Genomics Consortium, Lee, S.H., Ripke, S., Neale, B.M., Faraone, S.V., Purcell, S.M., et al. (2013). Genetic relationship between five psychiatric disorders estimated from genome-wide SNPs. *Nature Genetics*, 45, 984–994.

Curtis, D. and Sham, P.C. (1994). Using risk calculation to implement an extended relative pair analysis. *Annals Human Genetics*, 58, 151–162.

Dudbridge, F. (2013). Power and predictive accuracy of polygenic risk scores. *PLoS Genetics*, 9, e1003348.

Euesden, J., Lewis, C.M., and O'Reilly, P.F. (2015). PRSice: polygenic risk score software. *Bioinformatics*, 31, 1466–1468.

Hoggart, C.J., Chadeau-Hyam, M., Clark, T.G., Lampariello, R., Whittaker, J.C., De Iorio, M., and Balding, D.J. (2007). Sequence-level population simulations over large genomic regions. *Genetics*, 177, 1725–1731.

Hyman, S. (2014). Mental health: depression needs large human-genetic studies. *Nature*, 515, 189–191.

Iles, M.M. (2010). The impact of incomplete linkage disequilibrium and genetic model choice on the analysis and interpretation of genome-wide association studies. *Annals of Human Genetics*, 74, 375–379.

International HapMap Consortium (2003). The International HapMap Project. *Nature*, 426, 789–796.

International HapMap 3 Consortium (2010). Integrating common and rare genetic variation in diverse human populations. *Nature*, 467, 52–58.

Kendler, K.S., Neale, M.C., Kessler, R.C., Heath, A.C., and Eaves, L.J. (1992). Major depression and generalized anxiety disorder: same genes, (partly) different environments? *Archives of General Psychiatry*, 49, 716–722.

Lander, E.S., Linton, L.M., Birren, B., Nusbaum, C., Zody, M.C., Baldwin, J., et al. (2001). Initial sequencing and analysis of the human genome. *Nature*, 409, 860–921.

Lee, S.H., Wray, N.R., Goddard, M.E., and Visscher, P.M. (2011). Estimating missing heritability for disease from genome-wide association studies. *American Journal of Human Genetics*, 88, 294–305.

Lee, S.H., Yang, J., Goddard, M.E., Visscher, P.M., and Wray, N.R. (2012). Estimation of pleiotropy between complex diseases using single-nucleotide polymorphism-derived genomic relationships and restricted maximum likelihood. *Bioinformatics Application Notes*, 28, 2540–2542.

Manolio, T.A., Collins, F.S., Cox, N.J., Goldstein, D.B., Hindorff, L.A., Hunter, D.J., et al. (2009). Finding the missing heritability of complex diseases. *Nature*, 461, 747–753.

Mistry, S., Harrison, J.R., Smith, D.J., Escott-Price, V., and Zammit, S. (2018). The use of polygenic risk scores to identify phenotypes associated with genetic risk of schizophrenia: systematic review. *Schizophrenia Research*, 197, 2–8.

Munafò, M.R. (2006). Candidate gene studies in the 21st century: meta-analysis, mediation, moderation. *Genes, Brain and Behavior*, 5, 3–8.

Neale, M.C. (1997). Mx: statistical modelling, 3rd edn. Box 980126 MCV, Richmond VA 23298.

Neale, M.C. and Cardon, L.R. (1992). *Methodology for genetic studies of twins and families*. Dordrecht: Kluwer Academic Publishers.

Network and Pathway Analysis Subgroup of Psychiatric Genomics Consortium (2015). Psychiatric genome-wide association study analyses implicate neuronal, immune and histone pathways. *Nature Neuroscience*, 18, 199–209.

O'Reilly, P.F., Hoggart, C., Pomyen, Y., Calboli, F.C.F., Elliot, P., Jarvelin, M.R., and Coin, L.J. (2012). MultiPhen: joint model of multiple phenotypes can increase discovery in GWAS. *PLoS One*, 7, e34861.

Price, A.L., Zaitlen, N.A., Reich, D., and Patterson, N. (2010). New approaches to population stratification in genome-wide association studies. *Nature Reviews Genetics*, 11, 459–463.

Plomin, R., DeFries, J.C., McClearn, G.E., and McGuffin, P. (2001). *Behavioral genetics*, 4th edn. New York: Worth Publishers.

Plomin, R., Haworth, C.M.A., Meaburn, E.L., Price, T.S., Wellcome Trust Case Control Consortium, and Davis, O.S.P. (2013). Common DNA markers can account for more than half of the genetic influence on cognitive abilities. *Psychological Science*, 24, 562–568.

Rijsdijk, F.V. and Sham, P.C. (2002). Analytic approaches to twin data using structural equation models. *Briefings in Bioinformatics*, 3, 119–133.

Ripke, S., Neale, B.M., Corvin, A., Walters, J.T.R., Farh, K.-H., Holmans, P.A., et al. (2014). Biological insights from 108 schizophrenia-associated genetic loci. *Nature*, 511, 421–417.

Sham, P.C. (1998). *Statistics in human genetics*. London: Arnold.

Sladek, R., Rocheleau, G., Rung, J., Dina, C., Shen, L., Serre, D., et al. (2007). A genome-wide association study identifies novel risk loci for type 2 diabetes. *Nature*, 445, 881–885.

Stranger, B.E., Stahl, E.A., and Raj, T. (2011). Progress and promise of genome-wide association studies for human complex trait genetics. *Genetics*, 187, 367–383.

Tabor, H.K., Risch, N.J., and Myers, R.M. (2002). Candidate-gene approaches for studying complex genetic traits: practical considerations. *Nature Reviews Genetics*, 3, 391–397.

Trzaskowski, M., Dale, P.S., and Plomin, R. (2013). No genetic influence for childhood behavior problems from DNA analysis. *Journal of the American Academy of Child and Adolescent Psychiatry*, 52, 1048–1056.

Visscher, P.M., Brown, M.A., McCarthy, M.I., and Yang, J. (2012). Five years of GWAS discovery. *American Journal of Human Genetics*, 90, 7–24.

Walter, S., Marden, J.R., Kubzansky, L.D., Mayeda, E.R., Crane, P.K., Chang, S.C., et al. (2016). Diabetic phenotypes and late-life dementia risk: a mechanism-specific Mendelian randomization study. *Alzheimer's Disease and Associated Disorders*, 30, 15–20.

Wellcome Trust Case Control Consortium (2007). Genome-wide association study of 14,000 cases of seven common diseases and 3,000 shared controls. *Nature*, 447, 661–678.

Wray, N.R., Ripke, S., Matthiesen, M., Trzaskowski, M., Byrne, E.M., Abdellaoui, A., et al. (2018). Genome- wide association analyses identify 44 risk variants and refine the genetic architecture of major depressive disorder. *Nature Genetics*, 50, 668–681.

Yang, J., Benyamin, B., McEvoy, B.P., Gordon, S., Henders, A.K., Nyholt, D.R., et al. (2010). Common SNPs explain a large proportion of the heritability for human height. *Nature Genetics*, 42, 565–569.

Yang, J., Lee, S.H., Goddard, M.E., and Visscher, P.M. (2011). GCTA: a tool for genome-wide complex trait analysis. *American Journal of Human Genetics*, 88, 76–82.

Zhou, X. and Stephens, M. (2014). Efficient algorithms for multivariate linear mixed models in genome-wide association studies. *Nature Methods*, 11, 407–409.

Chapter 20

Gene–environment interaction

Craig Morgan, Marta Di Forti, and Helen L. Fisher

Introduction

For all major mental disorders there are many factors that, in combination and through multiple pathways, increase or decrease the risk of onset. These include, to varying degrees, genetic and environmental factors. These are no longer seen as competing explanations and, in recent years, interest has shifted decidedly to how genes and environments combine (interact) in the aetiology of mental disorders, with a consequent upsurge of related research (Belsky et al., 2014; Iyegbe et al., 2014; Uher, 2014). However, investigating how genes and environments combine is not straightforward and throws up a number of conceptual puzzles and methodological challenges (Moffitt et al., 2005; Schwartz, 2006; Kendler and Gardner, 2010; Zammit et al., 2010a, 2010b). This chapter provides an introduction, from an epidemiological perspective, to the study of gene–environment interaction. It begins by providing a working definition of gene–environment interaction, rooted in a sufficient causes framework, and then considers, in turn, the prominent puzzles and challenges, including statistical modelling of interaction, the main study designs (including strengths and weaknesses), measurement of environmental exposures, and required sample sizes. The chapter finishes with consideration of the implications of recent advances in genetics for studies of gene–environment interaction. One final introductory note: in this chapter, by environment we mean all factors external to individuals, which can include both social factors (e.g. trauma, discrimination, and life events) and non-social factors (e.g. obstetric complications, viral infection, pollution, and drug use).

Gene–environment interaction

It used to be that almost everyone had some distant relative who had smoked every day and lived to a ripe old age. This was—and maybe still is—used by individuals to justify continued smoking in the face of overwhelming evidence of an increased risk of lung cancer, many other illnesses, and premature death. However, it stems from a common feature of causal factors for many non-infectious diseases, including all major mental disorders: that these factors are neither necessary nor sufficient; they increase risk, but do not determine onset. What this further means is that, for a disorder to occur, other factors or causal partners must be present. The effect of one risk factor, then, commonly depends on the presence of other factors. This, in essence, is what we mean by interaction.

To round this out further, it must then be that it is combinations of causal factors, via effects on the same biological mechanism, that together constitute a sufficient cause of disorder (Rothman et al., 2013). Moreover, there can be multiple sufficient causes (i.e. clusters of component causal factors) for the same outcome. This can be represented visually using causal pies, in which each segment represents a component cause and each pie constitutes a sufficient cause (i.e. if all component causes are present, the disorder will occur) (Figure 20.1) (Rothman et al., 2013). Note that this framework uses a counterfactual definition of cause, in which a cause is any factor without which the disorder would not have occurred (Schwartz, 2006). In this model, all component factors are causes (i.e. in the absence of any one of the factors within each sufficient cause the disorder would not have occurred).

From this perspective, gene–environment interaction is present when the effect of a genotype on an outcome depends on the presence of some environmental factor(s) or vice versa (Uher, 2014).

An example can be used to illustrate this. It is well established that childhood maltreatment increases the risk of antisocial behaviour. However, not all those who experience

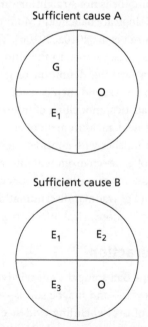

Figure 20.1 Hypothetical causal pies, each representing a sufficient cause of mental disorder.
Note: each pie constitutes a sufficient cause of disorder. Each segment is a component cause or risk factor. For a disorder to occur, each component cause within a sufficient cause must be present. If a component cause is not present, a disorder will not occur because of this sufficient cause. A component cause may be part of more than one sufficient cause. In 'Sufficient cause A', genotype and some environmental risk factor (plus other unmeasured risk factors) are causal partners. In 'Sufficient cause B', a number of environmental risk factors (plus other unmeasured risk factors) are causal partners.

E, environmental risk factor; G, genotype; O, other unmeasured risk factors.

abuse and neglect in childhood go on to be inconsiderate, disruptive, and violent. Using data from the Dunedin Multidisciplinary Health and Development Study, Caspi and colleagues (2002) sought to examine whether, in men ($n = 442$), variations in responses to maltreatment were dependent on variations in the monoamine oxidase A gene (*MAOA*). This gene was chosen because previous studies, in both animals and humans, had found associations between functional variants of *MAOA* and aggression. The analyses were restricted to men because *MAOA* is on the X chromosome and antisocial behaviours are more common in men (Uher, 2011). What Caspi and colleagues found was that the association between maltreatment and antisocial behaviour was stronger in those with the low-activity variant of *MAOA*, compared with those with the high-activity variant. For people with the high-activity variant, maltreatment had only a modest impact on antisocial behaviour (Caspi et al., 2002). This finding has since been replicated in a number of studies (Uher, 2011). The key point for our purposes is that the effect of maltreatment on antisocial behaviour is dependent on the presence of a certain functional variant of the *MAOA* gene: they are causal partners.

This example is instructive for at least two further reasons. First, the implication is that both maltreatment and *MAOA* are acting on the same biological mechanism to cause antisocial behaviour. Second, it illustrates the value of research on gene–environment interaction (and more broadly on the interaction of two or more risk factors). Such research can help to elucidate causal mechanisms and, from this, inform strategies for prevention and intervention.

Types of gene–environment interaction

There are at least three plausible ways in which genes and environments might interact (Figure 20.2) (Ottman, 1990, 1996; Hernandez and Blazer, 2006). First, genotype might amplify the effect of an environmental factor on disorder, while itself having only a modest or no direct effect, as in the earlier example of maltreatment and *MAOA* (model A). This may be the most common form of interaction (Kendler, 2011). Second, an environmental factor might amplify the effect of genotype on disorder, while itself having no direct effect (e.g. a small amount of cannabis may disproportionately increase the risk of psychosis in the presence of genes that increase levels of dopamine in the brain) (model B). Third, both genotype and environment may only have an effect when both are present (e.g. genes that are associated with increased stress response may have an effect only when an individual is exposed to stress and vice versa) (model C). While these specify different processes, all share the characteristic that, at an observational level, the effects of one factor (whether genes or environment) depend on the presence of the other.

There are other ways in which genes and environments may be involved in the aetiology of mental disorder (e.g. independent effects, on a causal path, correlated). These are beyond the scope of this chapter. However, it is important to note that gene–environment correlation (rGE), that is, where genes influence exposure to environments, is common and can confound gene–environment interactions (Kendler, 2011). It is difficult, statistically,

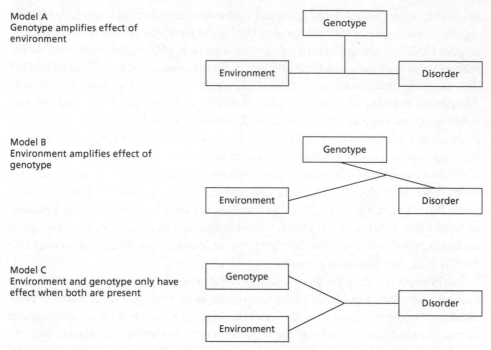

Figure 20.2 Models of how genes and environments may interact in the onset of mental disorder.

Source data from: Ottman, R., An epidemiologic approach to gene-environment interaction. *Genet Epidemiol*, 1990. 7(3): p. 177–85.; Ottman, R., Gene-environment interaction: definitions and study designs. *Prev Med*, 1996. 25(6): p. 764–70; Hernandez, L.M. and D.G. Blazer, *Genes, Behaviour and the Social Environment: Moving Beyond the Nature/Nurture Debate*. 2006, Washington DC, USA: National Academies Press.

to discount confounding by rGE in models of gene–environment interaction. However, it is at least possible to test separately whether genotype and environment are associated, which provides some indication of possible rGE (van Os et al., 2008) and some study designs (e.g. extended children of twins (Narusyte et al., 2008)) can be used to disentangle rGE from true environmental effects.

Further, environmental factors can influence the regulation of genes via epigenetic processes, that is, heritable changes in gene expression that do not involve changes in DNA sequence. Epigenetic processes may confound gene–environment interactions and constitute one pathway through which genes and environments combine to increase the risk of mental disorders (Klengel and Binder, 2015). This is an area of increasing interest and is important in providing a plausible mechanism for the co-participation of genes and environments in the onset of disorders.

Statistical modelling of gene–environment interaction

A fundamental issue in the study of gene–environment interaction concerns how, statistically, evidence for the presence or absence of substantive (or biological) interaction should be evaluated. The problem is that statistical tests for interaction are scale dependent; that is, using the same data, researchers can reach entirely different conclusions about the presence or absence of interaction solely based on the scale used, that is, whether additive or multiplicative (Schwartz, 2006; Schwartz and Susser, 2006; Zammit et al., 2010b).

For example, if it is assumed that the effects of two independent exposures on an outcome are additive, then in the presence of both exposures, interaction is indicated by a combined effect which is *greater than the sum* of the two independent effects. To make this concrete, consider Table 20.1. If, in this example, the risk of schizophrenia is 10% in those with a family history of disorder (i.e. a proxy for genetic risk), 3% in those who use cannabis (an environmental risk factor), and 1% in those with neither, then it would be expected that the effect (i.e. risk difference) in those exposed to both would be the sum of the effects of each alone (i.e. 9% + 2% = 11%; see Table 20.1). A combined effect greater than this would be evidence, on an additive scale, of interaction. In Table 20.1, the combined effect (i.e. risk difference between those exposed to both and those exposed to neither) is 29%. On an additive scale, then, there is evidence of interaction.

Alternatively, if it is assumed that the effects of two independent exposures on an outcome are multiplicative, then in the presence of both factors interaction is indicated by a combined effect which is *greater than the product* of the two independent effects. Note, moving from an additive scale to a multiplicative scale involves moving from risk differences to risk (or odds, rate, etc.) ratios. Continuing the previous example (Table 20.1), if the risk ratio for family history is 10 (i.e. 10%/1%) and for cannabis use is 3 (i.e. 3%/1%), then it would be expected that the effect in those exposed to both would be the product of the effects of each alone (i.e. 10 × 3 = 30). A combined effect greater than this would be evidence, on a multiplicative scale, of interaction. In Table 20.1, the combined effect (i.e. risk ratio in those exposed to both vs those exposed to neither) is indeed 30. On a multiplicative scale, then, there is no evidence of interaction: the same data but a different conclusion. As Schwartz puts it: 'This state of affairs is disconcerting, to say the least' (2006, p. 314).

Table 20.1 Hypothetical example to illustrate scale dependence of statistical interaction

	Schizophrenia		Total	Risk	Risk difference	Risk ratio
	Yes	No				
Both	30	70	100	0.30 (30%)	0.30 − 0.01 = 0.29 (29%)	0.30/0.01 = 30
Family history	10	90	100	0.10 (10%)	0.10 − 0.01 = 0.09 (9%)	0.10/0.01 = 10
Cannabis	3	97	100	0.03 (3%)	0.03 − 0.01 = 0.02 (2%)	0.03/0.01 = 3
Neither	1	99	100	0.01 (1%)	ref	ref
Total	44	356	400	–	–	–

Interaction contrast ratio = 18 (i.e. $RR_{A\ and\ B}$ − $RR_{A\ only}$ − $RR_{B\ only}$ + 1 = 30 − 10 − 3 + 1 = 18); ref, reference category.

To make matters worse, if both exposures have an effect on the outcome, there will always be a statistical interaction on at least one of the scales (Schwartz, 2006).

This has led to considerable confusion about the appropriate scale for assessing interaction in studies of the combined effects of genes and environments and it has been questioned whether there is value in modelling interaction at all (Kendler and Gardner, 2010; Zammit et al., 2010a, 2010b). The confusion in part stems from the fact that choice of scale is usually determined by statistical considerations (Kendler, 2011; Uher, 2011). For example, linear regression tests for interaction on an additive scale; however, in gene–environment research (and indeed much epidemiology) the outcome is often binary (e.g. presence vs absence of disorder) rather than continuous. For binary outcomes, logistic regression is the appropriate statistical model. However, logistic regression ultimately tests interaction on a multiplicative scale. This is because logistic regression, for statistical reasons, models the log odds of disorder or exposure and tests for additive interaction of log odds ratios. As readers may recall, addition on the log scale is equivalent to multiplication on the arithmetic scale. Therefore, when transformed back to the arithmetic scale, logistic regression tests for interaction on a multiplicative scale. Statistical—rather than theoretical—considerations, then, usually dictate the scale used to assess evidence for interaction.

Interaction within a sufficient causes framework

In light of the previous discussion, epidemiologists have sought to develop a basis for deciding on which scale to model interaction that is not based on statistical considerations. This has been most carefully articulated by Sharon Schwartz, who has shown that, within what is termed a 'sufficient causes framework', evidence that two exposures combine or interact (i.e. are causal partners) is indicated if the combined effect of two exposures is greater than the sum of the individual effects (Schwartz, 2006; Schwartz and Susser, 2006).[1] This suggests that substantive (i.e. biological, psychological, etc.) interaction is best approximated, statistically, by departure from the additive effects of two variables (i.e. interaction on an additive scale). There is not space to rehearse fully the detailed logic used in reaching this conclusion and interested readers are referred to the relevant papers and texts by Schwartz (Schwartz, 2006; Schwartz and Susser, 2006) and others (e.g. Rothman et al., 2013). The key point for our purposes is that there is now a conceptual framework for investigating interaction that does not rely on statistical considerations to determine the scale used.

Further, within this framework, departure from additivity can be estimated using a formula that calculates an interaction contrast ratio (ICR) (or relative excess risk due to interaction), which contrasts the effects in those exposed to various combinations of genotype and environment (i.e. $ICR = Risk_{A \text{ and } B} - Risk_{A \text{ only}} - Risk_{B \text{ only}} + 1$, where A is

---

1 Note, however, that lack of departure from additivity does not necessarily indicate absence of interaction (see Schwartz and Susser, 2006).

genotype and B is environment) (Schwartz, 2006; Rothman et al., 2013). In this model, deviation from additivity is indicated by an ICR greater than 0. This approach, moreover, allows use of ratios, including odds ratios derived from logistic models (including from case–control data), to estimate the relative excess risk due to interaction for combinations of dichotomous, ordinal, and continuous exposures (e.g. for odds ratios, $ICR = OR_{A\ and\ B} - OR_{A\ only} - OR_{B\ only} + 1$, where A is genotype, B is environment, and OR is odds ratio) (Schwartz and Susser, 2006). To illustrate this, we can apply the formula to the data in Table 20.1. This produces an ICR of 18 (i.e. $RR_{A\ and\ B} - RR_{A\ only} - RR_{B\ only} + 1 = 30 - 10 - 3 + 1 = 18$, where RR is relative risk), which, being substantially above 0, provides strong evidence of interaction on an additive scale (i.e. the combined effect of a family history and cannabis use is substantially higher than the sum of the individual effects of each alone). This, moreover, can be illustrated visually, as in Figure 20.3 (Morgan et al., 2014).

Study designs

Studies to investigate gene–environment interaction utilize a range of designs (Hernandez and Blazer, 2006; Plomin et al., 2008). These include adoption and twin studies and standard observational studies (i.e. cohort studies and case–control studies). A key distinction among them is the way in which the genetic component is measured.

Family, adoption, and twin studies

All of these study designs make use of the simple fact that biological relatives, to varying degrees, share genetic variations. Family relatedness, then, is used as a proxy marker of genetic risk.

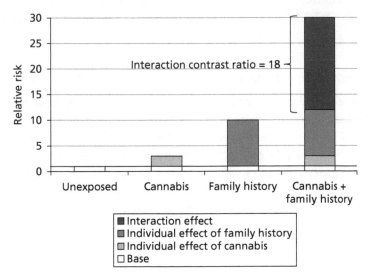

Figure 20.3 Graphical presentation of combined effects of two variables.

Family studies

The most straightforward of these studies, using standard cohort or case–control designs, simply include a variable for a family history of disorder as a marker of genetic risk or liability and use this to examine putative gene–environment interactions. Two brief examples illustrate this approach. First, van Os and colleagues (2004) used a family history of schizophrenia in a first-degree relative to examine putative interaction between genetic risk and urbanicity (an established environmental risk factor for schizophrenia) in a large cohort derived from Danish population registers. They found some evidence, on an additive scale, for interaction, such that the effect of a family history was greater at higher levels of population density (their measure of urbanicity). Second, Fisher and colleagues (2014) used history of psychotic disorder in a parent to examine putative interaction between genetic risk and physical abuse in childhood in a sample of 172 cases with a first-episode psychosis and 246 controls. They found no evidence, on an additive scale, of interaction; that is, there was no evidence that the combined effect of abuse and family history was greater than the effect of each alone. It is likely, however, that this study was under-powered to detect an interaction effect (see later).

There are notable limitations to such studies. Perhaps the most pertinent is that family history is, at best, an imperfect proxy for genetic risk. Indeed, it may be that disorders affect multiple members of a family for reasons other than genetic, such as shared exposure to environmental factors. It is also possible that parents pass on a genetic vulnerability for disorder to their children without overtly manifesting the disorder themselves (i.e. the phenotype is not expressed in the parent perhaps due to lack of environmental exposure) (Gottesman and Bertelsen, 1989). Further, the presence of a family history is usually established retrospectively and based on participant or informant reports, with the consequent risk of recall bias (e.g. cases or informants of cases more often remembering a relative with a disorder than controls). Nevertheless, studies of reported family history can at least provide initial evidence of interaction that can be pursued using more robust designs.

Adoption and twin studies

Adoption studies make use of the fact that adoptees do not grow up with their biological parents. The basic premise is that, if adopted early in life, resemblances of adoptees to their biological parents are more likely to be due to shared genes than to shared environments. In other words, the presence of a disorder in a biological parent of an adoptee indicates a high genetic risk and absence indicates a low genetic risk. This assumption accepted, the standard design for investigating putative gene–environment interaction is to compare outcomes in a sample of high and low genetic risk adoptees by exposure to some environmental risk factor (Plomin et al., 2008).

Tienari and colleagues (2004), for example, used this type of design to examine whether the effect of family environment on the risk of schizophrenia was dependent on genetic risk. First, they assessed family communication patterns (dichotomized into low dysfunction and high dysfunction) in a sample of adoptees of mothers with a diagnosis of a schizophrenia spectrum disorder (high genetic risk; $n = 145$) and a sample of adoptees of mothers without a diagnosis of a schizophrenia spectrum disorder (low genetic risk; $n = 158$). Next, they followed the adoptees, up to 21 years later, to determine who developed a schizophrenia spectrum disorder. What they found was that the effect of dysfunctional family communication patterns on the odds of disorder at follow-up was indeed dependent on level of genetic risk. In the high genetic risk group, the odds of disorder were around ten times greater in the high-dysfunction than in the low-dysfunction group (odds ratio 10.00; 95% confidence interval 3.26–30.69); in the low genetic risk group, the odds of disorder for each level of family dysfunction were roughly the same (odds ratio 1.11; 95% confidence interval 0.37–3.39). Note, Tienari and colleagues (2004) assessed the interaction effect by fitting an interaction term to a logistic regression model and found evidence indicating interaction on a multiplicative scale (i.e. greater than multiplicative and therefore also greater than additive).

Twin studies make use of the fact that there are two types of twin pairs: monozygotic (MZ) sharing 100% of genetic variants, and dizygotic (DZ) sharing 50% of genetic variants. The basic premise is that, if genetic factors are important for a trait or outcome, identical (MZ) twins will be more similar on the trait or have higher rates of the outcome than non-identical or fraternal (DZ) twins. This means the occurrence of a trait or outcome in one twin can be used as an index of genetic risk in the co-twin. This has been used as a basis for investigating gene–environment interaction within twin studies (Plomin et al., 2008).

Kendler and colleagues (1995), for example, used this type of design to examine whether the impact of stressful life events on risk of major depression was dependent on genetic risk. Using longitudinal data on female–female twin pairs from the Virginia Twin Registry (n in analyses = 2164 individuals), they sought to test the hypothesis that the association between stressful life events and major depression would be greater in those at higher genetic risk compared with those at lower genetic risk. Participants were assigned to one of four categories signifying increasing genetic risk for major depression: (1) MZ twin, co-twin unaffected; (2) DZ twin, co-twin unaffected; (3) DZ twin, co-twin affected; (4) MZ twin, co-twin affected. What the authors found was that, over an average of around 18 months of follow-up, the risk of major depression was indeed greatest among those at highest genetic risk who were exposed to a severe life event (14.6% vs, for example, 6.2% in those at lowest genetic risk who were exposed to a severe life event). There was evidence of interaction on the additive scale, but not on the multiplicative scale, a finding that further emphasizes the scale dependence of statistical interactions (Kendler et al., 1995).

Adoption and twin studies are more effective than family studies in separating genetic and environmental effects and, as such, allow for more robust estimates of gene–environment interaction. There are, nonetheless, limitations. It remains possible, for example, that assumed genetic effects may partly reflect shared environmental effects (e.g. MZ twins being treated more similarly than DZ twins). There are, moreover, limitations to the representativeness of samples and, therefore, the generalizability of findings. Adoptees and twins are not typical of the general population. Further, adoption and twin studies still only provide proxy measures of total genetic effects. They consequently provide no information about the specific genes nor the biological pathways and mechanisms involved.

Candidate gene studies

The breath-taking advances in molecular genetics over the past decade or so have enabled the investigation of gene–environment interaction, in cohort and case–control studies, using direct measures of specific candidate genes, that is, genes either associated with a disorder or involved in a relevant biological pathway. Further advances that enable genome-wide scans for risk genes now allow direct measures or estimates of combined genetic risk (polygenic risk scores; e.g. International Schizophrenia Consortium (2009)) that can be used in gene–environment interaction research (see 'Advances in genetics of mental disorder').

There have been a large number of studies testing candidate gene–environment interactions in relation to a range of mental health outcomes. These have been summarized in a number of recent reviews (e.g. Iyegbe et al., 2014; Uher, 2014). The seminal work on this was conducted by Caspi, Moffitt, and colleagues using data from the Dunedin Multidisciplinary Health and Development Study (New Zealand). Their findings concerning the interaction between variants of the *MAOA* gene and childhood maltreatment in the development of antisocial behaviour have already been described (Caspi et al., 2002). Perhaps more informative for understanding the challenges and issues in studying gene–environment interactions (see later sections), is their work on interactions between functional polymorphisms in the promoter region of the serotonin transporter (5-HTT) gene (*SLC6A4*) and life events in the onset of depression and suicidality (Caspi et al., 2003). The decision to focus on 5-HTT was based on findings from animal and human functional neuroimaging studies that suggest the 5-HTT gene is associated with physiological responses to stress (Uher, 2011). In brief, they found that people with one or two copies of the short allele of the 5-HTT gene were more sensitive to the effects of life events; that is, associations between number of life events and depressive symptoms, depressive disorder, and suicidality were all strongest in those with a short allele of the 5-HTT gene (e.g. see Figure 20.4). There was also evidence of a similar interaction effect for childhood maltreatment and depression. Notably, there was no evidence of a main effect of 5-HTT genotype on risk of depression (Caspi et al., 2003).

An important strength of candidate gene studies is that they provide information about the biological mechanisms that may be involved in the aetiology of disorder and on which both genes and environments may act (e.g. findings discussed earlier in this chapter suggest genes and stress may increase risk of depression via combined effects on the serotonin system). This noted, there remain limitations and challenges. Two related issues, in

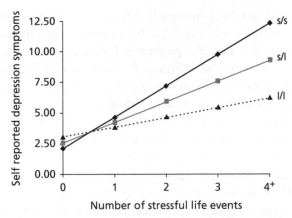

Figure 20.4 Interaction between 5-HTT serotonin transporter gene and depression. Note: the effect of life events on depression symptoms was strongest among those with a short allele (s) on the 5-HTT serotonin transporter gene compared to long (l) (p for interaction term = 0.02).

Reproduced with permission from Caspi, A. et al. Influence of life stress on depression: moderation by a polymorphism in the 5-HTT gene. *Science*, 301(5631), 386–9. Copyright © 2003, American Association for the Advancement of Science. DOI: 10.1126/science.1083968.

particular, come to the fore and merit further discussion: measurement of environmental exposures and required sample sizes.

Measurement of environmental exposures

Advances in molecular genetics now allow for cheap, automated, and precise generation and analyses of genotype data for large samples of individuals. The latest genome-wide association study (GWAS) for schizophrenia, for example, included data on 36,989 cases and 113,075 controls and it is likely that these numbers will expand further in the coming years (Schizophrenia Working Group of the Psychiatric Genomics Consortium, 2014). By contrast, measurement of environmental exposures (and of phenotypes, i.e. symptoms and diagnoses) is expensive, less standardized, and prone to error (Shanahan and Bauldry, 2011). As a consequence, many gene–environment studies rely on crude and simplified proxy measures of environmental exposures (e.g. urbanicity (van Os et al., 2004)). This has important implications.

The effects of environmental factors, especially socioenvironmental, on mental health outcomes often depend on the timing, duration, and severity of exposure (Shanahan and Bauldry, 2011). For example, the effects of stressful life events unsurprisingly are stronger in the months following exposure and the effects of childhood adversities are stronger the more severe and persistent they are. Further, there is substantial evidence that it is cumulative exposure to multiple stressors and adversities over time that is particularly important in the onset of many mental disorders (Shanahan and Bauldry, 2011). Consequently, the use of broad markers of single (socio-) environmental exposures that do not consider these other dimensions will almost certainly underestimate effects and make them harder to detect and to replicate. Compounding this, there is often considerable inconsistency in how the same exposures are measured. The findings on the interaction between 5-HTT and life events in the onset of depression and subsequent attempts to replicate them are particularly instructive here and illustrate the problems of imprecise and inconsistent measurement of environmental exposures. One reason why this finding has proved contentious is that some studies have succeeded and others have failed to replicate it. In their reviews, Uher and colleagues (Uher and McGuffin, 2008, 2010; Uher, 2011) compared findings from attempted replications by method used to measure life events. Of the 35 studies reviewed, 25 replicated or partly replicated and 10 failed to replicate the initial findings of Caspi and colleagues (Uher and McGuffin, 2008, 2010; Uher, 2011). All of the studies that failed to replicate used self-report questionnaires to measure life events, rather than interviews or some objective source (e.g. social service records) (Uher, 2011). This is a striking finding and inevitably raises the question of whether failure to replicate is a function of weaker measurement, perhaps in part due to the loss of power that results from measurement error.

Sample size, statistical power, and accuracy of measurement

A major challenge for studies of gene–environment interaction is sample size. In general, it has been estimated that, to detect multiplicative interactions, samples are required that are four times larger than to detect main effects (Smith and Day, 1984). The required samples to detect additive interactions may be larger still (Garcia-Closas and Lubin, 1999; Hernandez and Blazer, 2006). This is a daunting prospect. Direct estimates, for example, suggest that, to detect a moderate candidate gene–environment interaction that explains around 5% of the variance in outcome, samples with around 10,000 individuals are required (Uher, 2011).

The sample size required to detect candidate gene–environment interaction is determined by a number of parameters, including the expected magnitude of the interaction, allele frequency, and measurement error in the environmental exposure (Hernandez and Blazer, 2006). The relevance of measurement error to statistical power, however, is often overlooked. As discussed previously, it may be that this partly lies behind inconsistencies in findings on 5-HTT, stress, and depression. What follows from this is that there are two ways to increase power in studies of gene–environment interaction: (1) increase sample size and (2) improve measurement of environmental exposures. The first strategy is probably only achievable with increasingly crude proxy measures of distal environmental exposures, which, paradoxically, will probably introduce more measurement error. It has been suggested, then, that a more efficient approach may be to focus on increasing the validity and precision of measures of environmental exposures, particularly proximal exposures (Wong et al., 2003; Hernandez and Blazer, 2006). Such studies are underway (e.g. European Network of National Networks studying Gene-Environment Interactions in Schizophrenia (EU-GEI), 2014). Further, more precise measurement of proximal environmental exposures may provide more valuable information about the types and nature of exposures that increase risk and the putative mechanisms through which they might work.

Strategies for investigating gene–environment interaction

A useful framework to guide studies of gene–environment interaction, that addresses many of the methodological issues discussed here, has been set out by Moffitt and colleagues (2005). This comprises seven steps that emphasize the importance of formulating, at the outset, clear hypotheses that centre on testing interactions, on a specified scale, of plausible candidate genes, and carefully measured proximal environmental factors. The steps are: (1) consult quantitative behavioural genetic studies; (2) identify environmental risk factors; (3) optimize measurement of environmental risk factors; (4) identify candidate genes (or polygenic risk score for disorder or for candidate biological pathway); (5) test for interaction, with scale specified a priori; (6) examine whether interaction extends beyond the initial triad of gene(s), environmental risk factor, and disorder; and (7) replication and meta-analysis.

Advances in genetics of mental disorder

Any template for conducting gene–environment interaction studies, such as that proposed by Moffitt and colleagues (2005), will of course require modifications to accommodate new discoveries, particularly in the rapidly advancing field of the genetics of mental disorders. The advent of GWASs, for example, has important implications for research on gene–environment interaction.

First, GWASs allow polygenic risk scores to be derived, which provide an estimate of cumulative genetic risk (International Schizophrenia Consortium, 2009). This, crudely, involves summing the effects of all genes found to be associated, in GWAS analyses, with a disorder at a specified threshold of probability. Such scores, moreover, can be derived for clusters of genes known to be involved in specific biological pathways (e.g. dopamine) that may be linked to a disorder (e.g. schizophrenia). This opens up the possibility of investigating interactions between phenotypic or pathway-specific polygenic risk scores and environmental exposures. In so far as most mental disorders are likely polygenic and involve multiple genes of small effect (Sullivan et al., 2012), this approach may be more fruitful than the painstaking examination of one candidate gene at a time. Polygenic risk scores also afford greater statistical power and once a score is established in a large discovery sample it can subsequently be used in much smaller independent samples to examine gene–environment interactions. This noted, Jaffee and Price (2012) have cautioned that this approach may not necessarily be any more helpful than using family history to understand the mechanisms underlying gene–environment interaction because polygenic risk scores aggregate information across thousands of single nucleotide polymorphisms and in essence provide a more expensive 'black box' genetic risk estimate than a family history of mental disorder.

Second, it is possible to extend genome-wide scans for risk genes to genome-wide searches for gene–environment interactions (Uher, 2014). There have been some attempts to do this for some disorders (e.g. Cornelis et al., 2012); however, there are currently considerable challenges confronting such efforts, not least the limited availability of suffi- ciently large samples that have both genetic and environmental data. The required sample sizes may prove prohibitive, at least for now. This noted, it is likely that efforts in this direction will be a feature of future research on gene–environment interactions. Possible approaches to maximize samples, for example, include pooling data from studies with both genetic and environmental data and using linked population register data, such as that available in Denmark (Borglum et al., 2014; Uher, 2014). One important difference between this approach and the strategy set out by Moffitt and colleagues (2005) is that genome-wide interaction studies, like GWASs, are hypothesis free. Analyses will, conse- quently, have to account for a greater probability of type I error and be more cautious in interpreting findings, a requirement that further underscores the challenge of generating sufficiently large samples.

Conclusion

All major mental disorders are influenced by combinations of risk factors that, alone, are neither necessary nor sufficient to cause onset. This poses the question of which factors combine to increase risk and how. Considerable interest and research has focused on gene–environment interaction, that is, the extent to which the effect of genes depends on the presence of environmental factors and vice versa. Further, while not the focus of this chapter, it is pertinent to note that there are plausible mechanisms with some emerging supportive evidence (e.g. environmental effects on gene expression via epigenetic mech- anisms) that may account for how, at a biological level, genes and environments interact (Plomin et al., 2008; Pishva et al., 2014). The focus in this chapter has been on providing an introduction, from an epidemiological perspective, to approaches to, and challenges inherent in, investigating gene–environment interaction. As a still-emerging and fast- developing field, methods and strategies will continue to evolve.

References

Belsky, D.W., Suppli, N.P., and Israel, S. (2014). Gene-environment interaction research in psychiatric epidemiology: a framework and implications for study design. *Social Psychiatry and Psychiatric Epidemiology*, **49**, 1525–1529.

Borglum, A.D., Demontis, D., Grove, J., Pallesen, J., Hollegaard, M.V., Pedersen, C.B., et al. (2014). Genome-wide study of association and interaction with maternal cytomegalovirus infection suggests new schizophrenia loci. *Molecular Psychiatry*, **19**, 325–333.

Caspi, A., McClay, J., Moffitt, T.E., Mill, J., Martin, J., Craig, I.W., et al. (2002). Role of genotype in the cycle of violence in maltreated children. *Science*, **297**, 851–854.

Caspi, A., Sugden, K., Moffitt, T.E., Taylor, A., Craig, I.W., Harrington, H., McClay, J., et al. (2003). Influence of life stress on depression: moderation by a polymorphism in the 5-HTT gene. *Science*, **301**, 386–389.

Cornelis, M.C., Tchetgen, E.J., Liang, L., Qi, L., Chatterjee, N., Hu, F.B., and Kraft, P. (2012). Gene-environment interactions in genome-wide association studies: a comparative study of tests applied to empirical studies of type 2 diabetes. *American Journal of Epidemiology*, **175**, 191–202.

European Network of National Networks studying Gene-Environment Interactions in, Schizophrenia (2014). Identifying gene-environment interactions in schizophrenia: contemporary challenges for integrated, large-scale investigations. *Schizophrenia Bulletin*, **40**, 729–736.

Fisher, H.L., McGuffin, P., Boydell, J., Fearon, P., Craig, T.K., Dazzan, P., et al. (2014). Interplay between childhood physical abuse and familial risk in the onset of psychotic disorders. *Schizophrenia Bulletin*, **40**, 1443–1451.

Garcia-Closas, M. and Lubin, J.H. (1999). Power and sample size calculations in case-control studies of gene-environment interactions: comments on different approaches. *American Journal of Epidemiology*, **149**, 689–692.

Gottesman, I.I. and Bertelsen, A. (1989). Confirming unexpressed genotypes for schizophrenia. Risks in the offspring of Fischer's Danish identical and fraternal discordant twins. *Archives of General Psychiatry*, **46**, 867–872.

Hernandez, L.M. and Blazer, D.G. (eds.) (2006). *Genes, behaviour and the social environment: moving beyond the nature/nurture debate*. Washington, DC: National Academies Press.

International Schizophrenia Consortium (2009). Common polygenic variation contributes to risk of schizophrenia and bipolar disorder. *Nature*, **460**, 748–752.

Iyegbe, C., Campbell, D., Butler, A., Ajnakina, O., and Sham, P. (2014). The emerging molecular architecture of schizophrenia, polygenic risk scores and the clinical implications for GxE research. *Social Psychiatry and Psychiatric Epidemiology*, **49**, 169–182.

Jaffee, S.R. and Price, T.S. (2012). The implications of genotype-environment correlation for establishing causal processes in psychopathology. *Development and Psychopathology*, **24**, 1253–1264.

Kendler, K.S. (2011). *A conceptual overview of gene-environment interaction and correlation in a developmental context*. In: Kendler, K.S., Jaffee, S., and Romer, D. (eds). *The dynamic genome: the role of genes and environments in youth development*, pp. 5–28. Oxford: Oxford University Press.

Kendler, K.S. and Gardner, C.O. (2010). Interpretation of interactions: guide for the perplexed. *British Journal of Psychiatry*, **197**, 170–171.

Kendler, K.S., Kessler, R.C., Walters, E.E., MacLean, C., Neale, M.C., Heath, A.C., and Eaves, L.J. (1995). Stressful life events, genetic liability, and onset of an episode of major depression in women. *American Journal of Psychiatry*, **152**, 833–842.

Klengel, T. and Binder, E.B. (2015). Epigenetics of stress-related psychiatric disorders and gene x environment interactions. *Neuron*, **86**, 1343–1357.

Moffitt, T.E., Caspi, A., and Rutter, M. (2005). Strategy for investigating interactions between measured genes and measured environments. *Archives of General Psychiatry*, **62**, 473–481.

Morgan, C., Reininghaus, U., Reichenberg, A., Frissa, S.; SELCoH study team, Hotopf, M., and Hatch, S.L. (2014). Adversity, cannabis use and psychotic experiences: evidence of cumulative and synergistic effects. *British Journal of Psychiatry*, **204**, 346–353.

Narusyte, J., Neiderhiser, J.M., D'Onofrio, B.M., Reiss, D., Spotts, E.L., Ganiban, J., and Lichtenstein, P. (2008). Testing different types of genotype-environment correlation: an extended children-of-twins model. *Development and Psychology*, **44**, 1591–1603.

Ottman, R. (1990). An epidemiologic approach to gene-environment interaction. *Genetic Epidemiology*, **7**, 177–185.

Ottman, R. (1996). Gene-environment interaction: definitions and study designs. *Preventative Medicine*, **25**, 764–770.

Pishva, E., Kenis, G., van den Hove, D., Lesch, K.P., Boks, M.P., van Os, J., and Rutten, B.P. (2014). The epigenome and postnatal environmental influences in psychotic disorders. *Social Psychiatry and Psychiatric Epidemiology*, **49**, 337–348.

Plomin, R., DeFries, J.C., McClearn, G.E., and McGuffin, P. (2008). *Behavioural genetics*, 5th edn. New York: Worth Publishers.

Rothman, K.J., Greenland, S., and Lash, T.L. (2013). *Modern epidemiology*, 3rd edn. Philadelphia, PA: Lippincott Williams & Wilkins.

Schizophrenia Working Group of the Psychiatric Genomics Consortium (2014). Biological insights from 108 schizophrenia-associated genetic loci. *Nature*, **511**, 421–427.

Schwartz, S. (2006). *Modern epidemiologic approaches to interaction: applications to studies of genetic interactions*. In: Hernandez, L.M. and Blazer, D.G. (eds). *Genes, behaviour and the social environment: moving beyond the nature/nurture debate*, pp. 310–337. Washington, DC: National Academies Press.

Schwartz, S. and Susser, E. (2006). *Relationships among causes*. In: Susser, E., Schwartz, S., Morabia, A., and Bromet, E. (eds). *Psychiatric epidemiology: searching for the causes of mental disorders*, pp. 62–74. Oxford: Oxford University Press.

Shanahan, M.J. and Bauldry, S. (2011). *Improving environmental markers in gene-environment research: insights from life-course sociology*. In: Kendler, K.S., Jaffee, S., and Romer, D. (eds). *The dynamic genome and mental health: the role of genes and environments in youth development*, pp. 59–78. Oxford: Oxford University Press.

Smith, P.G. and Day, N.E. (1984). The design of case-control studies: the influence of confounding and interaction effects. *International Journal of Epidemiology*, **13**, 356–365.

Sullivan, P.F., Daly, M.J., and O'Donovan, M. (2012). Genetic architectures of psychiatric disorders: the emerging picture and its implications. *Nature Reviews Genetic*, **13**, 537–551.

Tienari, P., Wynne, L.C., Sorri, A., Lahti, I., Läksy, K., Moring, J., et al. (2004). Genotype-environment interaction in schizophrenia-spectrum disorder. *British Journal of Psychiatry*, **184**, 216–222.

Uher, R. (2011). Gene-environment interactions. In: Kendler, K.S., Jaffee, S., and Romer, D. (eds). *The dynamic genome and mental health: the role of genes and environments in youth development*, pp. 29–58. Oxford: Oxford University Press.

Uher, R. (2014). Gene-environment interactions in common mental disorders: an update and strategy for a genome-wide search. *Social Psychiatry and Psychiatric Epidemiology*, **49**, 3–14.

Uher, R. and McGuffin, P. (2008). The moderation by the serotonin transporter gene of environmental adversity in the aetiology of mental illness: review and methodological analysis. *Molecular Psychiatry*, **13**, 131–146.

Uher, R. and McGuffin, P. (2010). The moderation by the serotonin transporter gene of environmental adversity in the etiology of depression: 2009 update. *Molecular Psychiatry*, **15**, 18–22.

van Os, J., Pedersen, C.B., and Mortensen, P.B. (2004). Confirmation of synergy between urbanicity and familial liability in the causation of psychosis. *American Journal of Psychiatry*, **161**, 2312–2314.

van Os, J., Rutten, B.P., and Poulton, R. (2008). Gene-environment interactions in schizophrenia: review of epidemiological findings and future directions. *Schizophrenia Bulletin*, **34**, 1066–1082.

Wong, M.Y., Day, N.E., Luan, J.A., Chan, K.P., and Wareham, N.J. (2003). The detection of gene-environment interaction for continuous traits: should we deal with measurement error by bigger studies or better measurement? *International Journal of Epidemiology*, **32**, 51–57.

Zammit, S., Lewis, G., Dalman, C., and Allebeck, P. (2010a). Examining interactions between risk factors for psychosis. *British Journal of Psychiatry*, **197**, 207–211.

Zammit, S., Owen, M.J., and Lewis, G. (2010b). Misconceptions about gene-environment interactions in psychiatry. *Evidence-Based Mental Health*, **13**, 65–68.

Chapter 21

Bio-informatics and psychiatric epidemiology

Nicola Voyle, Maximilian Kerz, Steven Kiddle, and Richard Dobson

Introduction

Chapter 18 provides an overview of the statistical methods needed to explore, analyse, and interpret data collected in epidemiological studies. In this chapter we highlight the methodologies which are increasingly being applied to large datasets or 'big data', with an emphasis on bio-informatics.

Data collection

The first stage of any analysis is to collect data from a well-designed study. We begin by looking at the raw data that arises from epidemiological studies and highlighting the first stages in creating clean data that can be used to draw informative conclusions through analysis. We move on to describe big data and associated challenges before emphasizing the importance of reproducibility in research.

Data formats

Raw data can come in many different types and formats, ranging from hand-written laboratory sheets and unformatted Excel files, to images. In order to analyse and explore data it is vital to fully understand the structure and content of your raw data set. Depending on its nature, and the type of analyses you would like to run, an initial pre-processing step is recommended or even unavoidable. Examples of pre-processing steps include transforming qualitative data into machine-readable categories or using an image analysis pipeline to extract important features of an image and cast them into a structured, tabular format.

Data exploration

The aim of data exploration is to use descriptive methods to get a statistical and visual impression of the data (Sayad, 2011). Exploratory statistics allow quantification and visualization of qualitative variables, such as categorical data, as well as continuous variables. Perhaps most importantly, data exploration is the first step in identifying new patterns and/or associations. Data exploration is of particular importance in large data samples where a preliminary impression of the data helps to identify potential confounding factors, anomalies, and missing data (Podsakoff et al., 2003).

Data cleaning

Data collection and aggregation into a master data set can result in irregularities and missingness. Human error during data collection and participant drop outs during a longitudinal study are examples that can result in the former. The process of removing or accounting for these impurities within the data set is known as *data cleaning*.

The extent of data cleaning depends on the specific method that you are aiming to apply and ranges from basic methods to advanced pre-processing. Among the most common mistakes that lead to impure data sets is failure to look at the data at all, or in tabular form only. Basic data exploration and plots can easily identify missing values, label switching, and unit mismatches. A further advantage of exploratory plots is an indication of skewness that can reveal biases within the data (Kuhn and Johnson, 2013). These can then be accounted for before applying additional analyses.

Missing data

Missingness in statistics is defined as the lack of data for a variable in an observation. It is a common phenomenon in the realm of data analysis and is grouped into three categories: missing completely at random (MCAR), missing at random (MAR), and missing not at random (MNAR), also known as informative missingness (van Buuren, 2012).

♦ MCAR: the probability of being missing is equal for all observations. In other words, the cause for missingness is unrelated to the data.

♦ MAR: the probability of being missing is equal for a particular observation only.

♦ MNAR: the probability of being missing varies depending on another observation.

An example of MNAR would be an increasing drop-out rate in a clinical trial based on the administered concentration of an experimental drug. Even though the data exhibits increasingly more missingness, it is highly informative on drug adherence in patients (Kuhn and Johnson, 2013).

Treating missingness is a challenging topic that can range from simple data removal to application of prediction models for imputation. Depending on the nature of the data, as well as the type and extent of missingness, different methods should be applied (Schafer and Graham, 2002). The exact intricacies of treating missingness in data are beyond the scope of this chapter; an overview of methods to deal with missing data are discussed in chapter 18.

Big data

Big data is vaguely defined. However, the most commonly cited definition of big data is by Laney (2001) as 'high volume, velocity and variety information that demand cost-effective, innovative forms of information processing for enhanced insight and decision making'. Additionally, variability within a data type is an important characteristic of big data and should be added to the definition. There is no clear boundary to when conventional data turn into big data; however, any combination of complexity, size, and advanced analytics technology satisfies the definition by Laney (2001). In fact, data sets do not even need to be particularly big, just complex, to be considered big data.

Reproducibility

Reproducibility allows re-running an analysis and always obtaining the same result when applied to the same data set. This is particularly important for the validity and generalizability of your analysis should you want to publish your results. Unfortunately, reproducing complex analyses is associated with challenges, such as software updates that change the outcome of an analysis, incomplete or non-existent documentation, and failing to record intermediary results.

Detailed documentation and scripted analyses are a great way to ensure that your research is reproducible. This will not only benefit you but also the community of psychiatric epidemiology.

Classification versus regression

It is likely that the data collection and cleaning covered in previous sections has been to answer a specific research question. Before moving forward it is important to identify whether the question you are answering is a *classification* or *regression* question:

◆ Classification: allocation of an observation to one of several groups. For example, classifying a brain scan as positive or negative for a defined pathology.

◆ Regression: predicting a continuous outcome for an observation. For example, predicting hippocampal volume from a magnetic resonance imaging scan.

Throughout this chapter we will refer to classification, however, most methods can also be applied in a regression setting.

Feature identification and selection

Once a data set has been processed (if not before), an analysis plan needs to be created. Conventional statistical methods (not covered in this chapter) require the number of variables in the data set to be less than the number of samples. However, *machine learning* algorithms do not have such a limitation. Machine learning algorithms use induction to learn; they aim to improve prediction based on the data provided. Although they can handle many thousands of predictors, it is often computationally expensive to do so. Additionally, models with many predictors are very hard to interpret. Therefore, we aim to reduce the number of variables we use in modelling via *feature selection*. Feature selection removes redundancy and noise from data leaving only the most discriminatory features while reducing problems of dimensionality. Guyon and Elisseeff (2003) provide a good introduction to feature selection techniques.

Method selection

After selecting features to include in the analysis, or planning the feature selection techniques to use alongside modelling, the modelling algorithm must be selected. The choice of algorithm is important and should be tailored to the question you are looking to answer and the data you have. Do you have more predictor variables than samples? Some methods (e.g. support vector machines (SVMs)) are good at coping with high-dimensionality datasets with a small number of samples; however, this may require large amounts of computer memory. Do you have balanced training data? Some methods, such as SVMs and decision trees, are sensitive to imbalance in the training dataset and should therefore be avoided if you have unbalanced data. Where possible, it is preferable to test a number of classifiers to identify the most appropriate choice for the specific problem.

Supervised versus unsupervised machine learning

The most common types of machine learning algorithms are *supervised learning* and *unsupervised learning*. Supervised learning takes a set of examples that are labelled and creates a set of rules to classify samples where the status is unknown (see Box 21.1 for an example). In contrast, unsupervised learning models a set of inputs where labelled examples are not available. The algorithm finds a way of clustering the data based upon the known features and then provides descriptions for these clusters.

In the following sections, we will introduce some vital concepts before discussing some supervised and unsupervised algorithms that are among the most commonly used within the field of bioinformatics.

Important concepts

Training, testing, and validation

A common problem of supervised learning methods is over-fitting. An algorithm can be trained for too long on one particular data set so that it fails to generalize the information learned to similar data sets. A number of methods are available for evaluating machine learning results and showing the results are general enough to be applied to other data (Hand et al., 2001). To successfully train a supervised learning algorithm, one should aim to generate three data sets from the original data set:

Box 21.1 Supervised learning example

Predicting whether a non-synonymous single nucleotide polymorphism (nsSNP) is disease related is a question that can be addressed via machine learning methods. Supervised learning is appropriate because the aim is to assign an nsSNP to one of a number of classes. It is possible to use a set of nsSNPs where the disease status is known as a training set to form a set of rules. These rules can then be used to make a prediction for nsSNPs where the function is unknown.

- A *training set*: used to train the algorithm.
- A *validation set*: to track how well the algorithm is generalizing and to perform parameter tuning.
- A *test set*: an unseen data set on which the finalized algorithm's performance is tested.

As machine learning algorithms require substantial training data, the usual distribution of the training, validation, and testing sets is 2:1:1. However, in the case of limited data availability, different *cross-validation* methods can be used.

Cross-validation

In cross-validation, the data is divided into a number (*n*) of 'folds'. Each fold is treated as the validation dataset in turn, with the remaining $n - 1$ folds being used as training data. Cross-validation is especially useful for smaller datasets (Kohavi, 1995). The performance of the classifier on each fold is measured and then a final accuracy is calculated based upon the average of all *n* folds.

Bootstrap

Sampling from a whole dataset, with replacement, creates a bootstrap sample. The bootstrap sample is the same size as the original dataset and contains, on average, one-third of all observations in the whole dataset. The observations not included in the bootstrap sample are called the out-of-bag data. As sampling with replacement creates the bootstrap sample, it can contain repeated instances (Efron and Tibshirani, 1994).

Bootstrapping is a useful tool to maintain the size of your training dataset while also creating validation data. The performance of the classifier is calculated by averaging the accuracy from the out-of-bag data of each bootstrap sample.

Hyper-plane

A hyper-plane is a subspace with one less dimension than the whole space under consideration. This is easiest to imagine in small dimensions. For example, if we consider a problem in two dimensions (e.g. plotting age against height), a hyper-plane is any one-dimensional line running through the space. Similarly, if we consider a problem in three dimensions (e.g. plotting age against height and weight), a hyper-plane is any two-dimensional plane.

Unsupervised methods

Unsupervised learning has a long and distinguished history within modern epidemiology. For example, John Snow, a physician in the mid-nineteenth century, is famous for discovering the source of cholera outbreaks, which were at the time believed to be due to 'bad air'. To achieve this he used an unsupervised data analysis method. During the 1854 cholera outburst in Soho, London, John Snow recorded the location of deaths onto a map of Soho, showing that deaths were clustered around an intersection of Broad Street. He later identified the source as an infected water pump (Johnson, 2006).

Unsupervised machine learning extends the concept of looking for patterns to complex multidimensional datasets. Like John Snow's map, it seeks to identify patterns within datasets. Patterns extracted from data using unsupervised machine learning can also be used later in supervised approaches to identify the underlying causes of various patterns, analogous to John Snow adding information on water pumps onto his maps.

Principal components analysis

A commonly used unsupervised approach to data analysis is principal components analysis (PCA). For example, PCA is often used in genetic epidemiology to take into account population stratification and systematic differences in allele frequencies that are often due to ancestry (Price et al., 2006). It can also be invaluable for visualizing outliers (Price et al., 2006) and batch effects (Alter et al., 2000) in high-dimensional datasets, for example, whole-genome gene expression data. As such, it is often used as part of the important 'quality control' process.

PCA takes a set of possibly correlated variables and returns a set of principal components (PCs), which are orthogonal hyper-planes that explain maximal variance in the predictors. A useful feature of the PCs is that they are given in rank order for the proportion of total variation they explain; PC 1 explains more of the variation in a dataset than PC 2 does. A useful consequence of this is that it is often possible to summarize a large proportion of the total variance using only two or three principal components allowing high-dimensional datasets to be summarized in two- or three-dimensional plots. For example, Figure 21.1 shows the effect of ancestry on PCA applied to genetic data. The proportion of variance that each PC explains can be visualized in a 'scree plot', helping you to choose the number of PCs to use for plotting or further analysis. More details on PCA are reviewed in Jolliffe (2014).

Clustering

Methods such as PCA can be used to summarize variability in a dataset, often showing that data points can be divided into 'groups' or 'clusters'. The general definition of a cluster is that objects within a cluster are more similar to each other than they are to objects outside of that cluster. But how do you automate the assignment of data points to clusters? And how many clusters exist?

The problem of assigning data points to clusters is an unsupervised machine learning problem, for which many different approaches exist. One of the most commonly used approaches is *hierarchical clustering*, which generates a hierarchy tree with a data point lying at the end of every branch (Ward, 1963). The branches for the most similar data points are connected first, and this is repeated until eventually all data points are connected. Data points are separated into clusters by applying a threshold to the tree. The problem with this approach is that as branches are combined one at a time, the final grouping may not always be optimal.

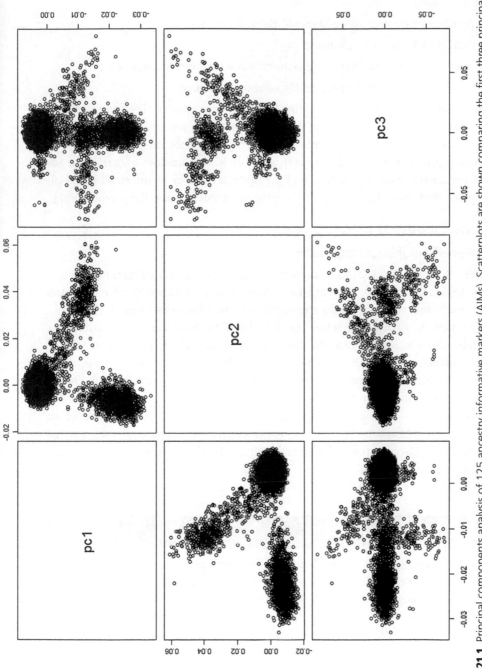

Figure 21.1 Principal components analysis of 125 ancestry informative markers (AIMs). Scatterplots are shown comparing the first three principal components (pc1–pc3). Individuals are represented by one circle in each scatterplot. The first three principal components summarize the majority of the variability in ancestry, and help to distinguish individuals of European, African American, Hispanic, and Asian descent.

Figure generated by Dr William S. Bush, Assistant Professor at Case Western Reserve University, Cleveland Ohio. http://www.gettinggeneticsdone.com/2011/10/new-dimension-to-principal-components_27.html.

A common alternative to hierarchical clustering is called *K-means* (Jain, 2010). This involves looking for K clusters in the data, where K is a number. The K-means procedure proceeds as follows:

- Data points are randomly assigned into K different clusters.
- The mean of each cluster is calculated.
- Each data point is assigned to belong to the cluster whose mean it is closest to.
- Steps 2–3 are repeated until an acceptable solution is reached.

K-means solutions are often more optimal than a hierarchical clustering solution. However, to perform K-means, a 'mean' must be definable for your dataset. Where this is not possible, alternatives such as K-centres or affinity propagation can be used.

For both approaches, you need to specify a threshold or a number of clusters in advance. A commonly used approach to find the optimal number or threshold is the silhouette plot, which provides a visualization of the quality of clusters (Rousseeuw, 1987).

Supervised methods

The *k*-nearest neighbours algorithm

The *k*-nearest neighbours (KNN) is arguably the simplest supervised learning method (Altman, 1992). The basic idea is that a new observation is classified to the modal class of the *k* closest observations from the training data (where *k* is some integer). There are a number of methods to define what we mean by 'closest' but these are not discussed here. The example given in Box 21.2 should clarify this idea. In order to perform an analysis using this method we must choose a suitable value for *k*. This is known as parameter tuning and is usually performed by using several rounds of cross-validation to choose the value that gives the best results. If *k* is too low the model can over-fit to the training data and conversely, if *k* is too high, the model may under-fit. Although KNN provides a method with very simple intuition the model fit can be hard to interpret; it is solely based on training data so there is no description of the model. Furthermore, it can become computationally expensive on large datasets.

Box 21.2 KNN example

We have a group of patients presenting with memory impairment; they have been classified as having either dementia or short-term memory loss. Suppose that for each of them we have only two pieces of clinical information: age and hippocampal volume from a magnetic resonance imaging scan. We could plot this information and colour code by the subject's classification. When a new patient enters the clinic presenting with memory impairment and with these two measures available we can add them to the plot. We can consider the five patients who are closest to the new patient on the graph and output the most common class from these five subjects as the classification.

Decision trees

Decision trees are supervised classifiers composed of a graph (tree structure) of decisions (Quinlan, 1993). Each point in the tree where a decision is made is called a node and the result of each decision determines which branch to follow. The decisions are usually simple single attribute tests to divide the data. A leaf represents the predicted class based on values at the nodes on the path from the root (the first decision point). Decision trees have an advantage over many classifiers in that they produce interpretable rules. Once a tree has been built, new instances can be classified by starting at the root and following a path down to a leaf. An example of a decision tree can be seen in Figure 21.2 where a patient is classified as being at high or low risk of psychosis based on a number of attributes.

When the attribute at a node is categorical, there will be one branch for each attribute value. If the attribute is continuous, a decision will be made based on whether the instance

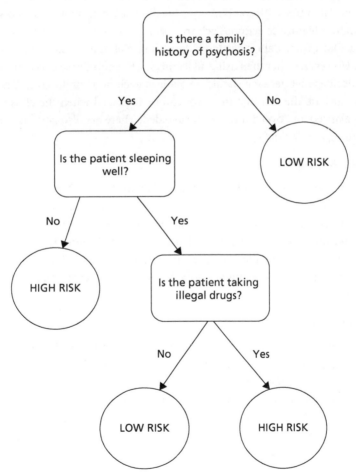

Figure 21.2 An example of a decision tree used to classify a patient as being at high or low risk of psychosis. The diagram shows decisions at the nodes and final classification at the leaves.

is above or below a specific cut-off value. There are a number of methods for deciding which attribute should be used at each node but they are not discussed here.

A decision tree is complete when some criterion about the terminal nodes has been met, for example, when all the terminal nodes contain samples from only one class. At this point the tree is often 'pruned' to prevent it being too specific to the training dataset. The aim is to produce a tree that is general enough to be applied to any new instances that require classification, avoiding over-fitting. The algorithms are efficient and therefore able to handle large volumes of data. However, one drawback to this approach is that the partitioning can cause interesting relationships between attributes to be lost.

Random forests

Random forest (RF) is a supervised classifier consisting of multiple decision trees (Breiman, 2001). The final class assigned to an observation is the modal class selected by the multiple decision trees. RF combines two machine learning methods: bootstrap sampling and random feature selection. Each tree is created from a bootstrap sample of the training data. Out-of-bag data is used to obtain an unbiased estimate of the error during the training. However, rather than using all features, RF randomly selects a subset of input variables to decide what decision should be made at each node of the tree. Advantages of RF classifiers include the fact that the error can be balanced when the class population sizes are imbalanced and over-fitting can be avoided. There are also good methods available for handling missing data.

Partial least squares

Partial least squares (PLS) modelling is very similar to PCA. Where PCA looks for orthogonal hyper-planes that explain maximal variance in the predictors, PLS looks to explain maximal covariance between the predictors and the outcome (Wold, 2004). It is this reliance on the outcome measure that means PLS modelling is supervised and is particularly suited for prediction problems. PLS modelling is useful when the number of predictors is greater than the number of samples as it reduces the size of the predictor space by creating components.

Support vector machines

SVMs are a supervised learning classifier developed by Corte and Vapnik (1995). They have been shown to be very accurate in many disciplines including bioinformatics, benefitting from the ability to handle high-dimensional data with a small number of instances, finding a good balance between training set accuracy and test data error. For a given set of training vectors labelled with two classes, a SVM can find the optimal linear hyper-plane that maximizes the margin between the two classes. An example of SVM classification in two dimensions is given in Figure 21.3.

SVMs can be extended to provide non-linear classification through the application of a kernel function and to multiclass classification but that is not discussed here.

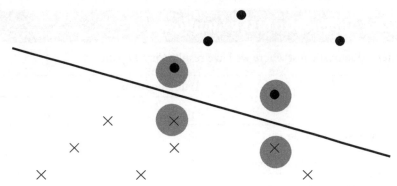

Figure 21.3 An example of a SVM classifying between two classes (circles and crosses). The points acting as support vectors are highlighted.

Training a classifier

The process of building a model with initial data is called training.

An important point to consider when training a classifier is the presence (or lack thereof) of balanced data. The number of instances belonging to each class in the training set may be imbalanced resulting in a danger that the classifier will have a preference for selecting the most populated class because the classifier assumes that there is a greater chance of an instance belonging to this class (Barandela et al., 2003). The result is that performance is reduced for the minority dataset. However, it may be the case, such as when detecting fraudulent telephone calls, for example, that detecting the minority case is of greater importance (Fawcett and Provost, 1997).

Drawing conclusions from modelling

It is necessary to summarize the results of model testing using informative metrics. These metrics should quantify how well a model fits the test data. Some of the material here has already been covered in Chapter 2, but is reproduced here, as an important consideration in the application of modelling techniques.

Accuracy, sensitivity, and specificity

There are four possible scenarios that could arise when classifying a new observation using a trained classifier. In this case we consider the example of a diagnostic test:

◆ A person with the disease is correctly classified as having the disease.

◆ A person without the disease is correctly classified as not having the disease.

◆ A person with the disease is misclassified as not having the disease.

◆ A person without the disease is misclassified as having the disease.

These are the four key features that determine how well a classification test has performed and they can be summarized using three metrics. The accuracy is defined as the

Box 21.3 Diagnostic test example

Consider a diagnostic test where we have results for 100 patients.

		True diagnosis	
		Disease	No disease
Diagnostic test	Disease	30	5
	No disease	20	45

Accuracy = (30 + 45)/100 = 75%.
Sensitivity = 30/50 = 60%.
Specificity = 45/50 = 90%.
Positive predictive value = 30/35 = 85.7%.
Negative predictive value = 45/65 = 69.2%.

percentage of all patients who are correctly classified and is perhaps the most intuitive and general of these metrics. It can be split into the percentage of patients with the disease who are correctly classified as having the disease (sensitivity) and the percentage of patients without the disease who are correctly classified as not having the disease (specificity), see Box 21.3 for an example.

It is important to look at all three of these metrics, as often a high sensitivity will coincide with a low specificity and vice versa. However, the nature of your question will determine which of these metrics is most important. When interpreting accuracy, sensitivity and specificity remember that these metrics are not affected by the prevalence of a disease.

Negative predictive value and positive predictive value

Two further metrics are often used to describe the performance of a classifier: negative predictive value (NPV) and positive predictive value (PPV).

- NPV: the percentage of negative predictions that are true negatives.
- PPV: the percentage of positive predictions that are true positives.

Unlike accuracy, sensitivity, and specificity, NPV and PPV will change if the prevalence of a disease changes. PPV will fall as the prevalence of a disease decreases while NPV will rise. This should make sense as a lower prevalence means, over the whole population, a positive result is less likely (Loong, 2003).

Receiver operating characteristic analysis

In most cases, when a classifier is built, the underlying method works by creating a probability of assigning a sample to a certain class. If this probability is above a predefined threshold then the sample is allocated to the class in question. It is therefore interesting to

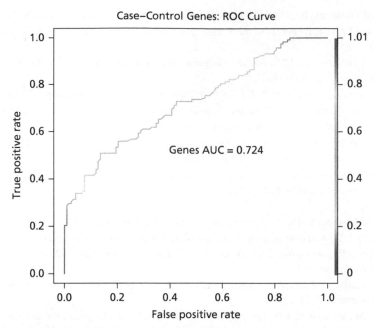

Figure 21.4 An example of an ROC curve generated from a random forest model. The model uses gene expression data to classify subjects as having Alzheimer's disease or being control subjects.

vary the threshold to see if we can create a test that best answers the question we are studying. A good way to visualize the effect of changing this threshold is through a receiver operating characteristic (ROC) plot. These plots usually have the false-positive rate (1 – specificity) on the x-axis and the true positive rate (sensitivity) on the y-axis. They are often summarized by measuring the area under the curve (AUC) (Figure 21.4). A perfect test would have sensitivity and specificity of 1 meaning the AUC would also be 1, as we create a unit square. We therefore look to maximize the AUC to get as close to this perfect test as possible. It is useful to remember that a test that is randomly guessing between two classes should, by chance, achieve an AUC of around 0.5 so any classifier should aim to out-perform this.

References

Alter, O., Brown, P.O., and Botstein, D. (2000). Singular value decomposition for genome-wide expression data processing and modeling. *Proceedings of the National Academy of Sciences of the United States of America*, **97**, 10101–10106.

Altman, N.S. (1992). An introduction to kernel and nearest-neighbor nonparametric regression. *The American Statistician*, **46**, 175–185.

Barandela, R., Sánchez, J.S., García, V., and Rangel, E. (2003). Strategies for learning in class imbalance problems. *Pattern Recognition*, **36**, 849–851.

Breiman, L. (2001). Random forests. *Machine Learning*, **45**, 5–32.

Cortes, C. and Vapnik, V. (1995). Support-vector networks. *Machine Learning*, **20**, 273–297.

Efron, B. and Tibshirani, R. (1994). *An introduction to the bootstrap*. Boca Raton, FL: CRC Press.

Fawcett, T. and Provost, F. (1997). Adaptive fraud detection. *Data Mining and Knowledge Discovery*, 1, 291–316.

Guyon, I. and Elisseeff, A. (2003). An introduction to variable and feature selection. *Journal of Machine Learning Research*, 3, 1157–1182.

Hand, D.J., Mannila, H., and Smyth, P. (2001). *Principles of data mining*. Cambridge, MA: MIT Press.

Jain, A.K. (2010). Data clustering: 50 years beyond K-means. *Pattern Recognition Letters*, 31, 651–666.

Johnson, S. (2006). *The ghost map*. New York: Riverhead Books.

Jolliffe, I. (2014). Principal component analysis [Wiley StatsRef: Statistics Reference Online]. https://onlinelibrary.wiley.com/doi/abs/10.1002/9781118445112.stat06472

Kohavi, R. (1995). A study of cross-validation and bootstrap for accuracy estimation and model selection. *Proceedings of the 14th International Joint Conference on Artificial Intelligence*, 2, 1137–1143.

Kuhn, M. and Johnson, K. (2013). *Applied predictive modeling*. New York: Springer.

Laney, D. (2001). 3D data management: controlling data volume, velocity, and variety. https://blogs.gartner.com/doug-laney/files/2012/01/ad949-3D-Data-Management-Controlling-Data-Volume-Velocity-and-Variety.pdf

Loong, T.W. (2003). Understanding sensitivity and specificity with the right side of the brain. *British Medical Journal*, 327, 716–719.

Podsakoff, P.M., MacKenzie, S.B., Lee, J.Y., and Podsakoff, N.P. (2003). Common method biases in behavioral research: a critical review of the literature and recommended remedies. *Journal of Applied Psychology*, 88, 879–903.

Price, A.L., Patterson, N.J., Plenge, R.M., Weinblatt, M.E., Shadick, N.A., and Reich, D. (2006). Principal components analysis corrects for stratification in genome-wide association studies. *Nature Genetics*, 38, 904–909.

Quinlan, J.R. (1993). *C4.5: Programs for machine learning*. San Mateo, CA: Morgan Kaufmann Publishers.

Rousseeuw, P.J. (1987). Silhouettes: a graphical aid to the interpretation and validation of cluster analysis. *Journal of Computational and Applied Mathematics*, 20, 53–65.

Sayad, S. (2011). *Real time data mining*. Cambridge, ON: Self-Help Publishers.

Schafer, J.L. and Graham, J.W. (2002). Missing data: our view of the state of the art. *Psychological Methods*, 7, 147–177.

van Buuren, S. (2012). *Flexible imputation of missing data*. New York: Chapman and Hall/CRC Press.

Ward, J.H. (1963). Hierarchical grouping to optimize an objective function. *Journal of the American Statistical Association*, 58, 236–244.

Wold, H. (2004). *Partial least squares*. Chichester: John Wiley & Sons, Inc.

Chapter 22

Health economics
for psychiatric epidemiology

Margaret Heslin, Paul McCrone,
and Daniel Chisholm

The relationship of health economics and psychiatric epidemiology

This chapter examines the interface between psychiatric epidemiology and health economics, particularly in relation to mental health service planning and evaluation. We discuss the issues inherent in conducting an economic evaluation and conclude with a summary of the applications of economic analyses.

The use of health economics in mental health research is a relatively recent phenomenon. The most common form is in experimental designs in which economic evaluations are conducted alongside randomized controlled trials (RCTs) to examine the cost-effectiveness of new interventions. However, health economics can do far more than this, from estimating the burden of a disorder to exploring fairer ways of allocating resources.

While the ultimate objectives of the two disciplines of health economics and epidemiology may differ, both are essentially pitched at understanding the consequences of disorder and its treatment at the level of the population at risk. As such, the two disciplines can be viewed as offering complementary perspectives to mental health policy, planning, and evaluation.

Estimating the burden of psychiatric disorders

Epidemiological perspective: burden of disease studies

The link between health economics and epidemiology is well illustrated by efforts to measure the burden of disease at national and global levels. The Global Burden of Disease study, initially conducted by the World Health Organization (WHO) and the World Bank, set out to provide estimates of incidence, prevalence, duration, and case fatality for all major contributors to mortality and morbidity, which could be used to generate summary measures of population health to inform resource allocation decisions (Murray and Lopez, 1996). The main summary measure used was the disability-adjusted life year (DALY), consisting of years of life lost (YLLs) by premature death and years of life lived with disability (YLDs). The disability component of this summary health measure (YLDs) was weighted according to the severity of the disorder's sequelae, using methods drawn from the field of health economics (health state preference or utility measurement). On a scale of 0–1 (where 0 represents no disability or full health and 1 represents complete disability or death), disability caused by major depression was found to be equivalent to blindness or paraplegia, whereas active psychosis was estimated as somewhere between paraplegia and quadriplegia in severity of disability. Following this incorporation of disability into disease burden estimates, mental disorders ranked as high as cardiovascular and respiratory diseases, and exceeded all malignancies combined or HIV (Murray and Lopez, 1996). The most recent WHO estimates of the Global Burden of Disease study show that mental, neurological, and substance use disorders contribute more than 10% of all DALYs lost, and close to 25% of all YLDs (WHO, 2018). Table 22.1 provides the proportion of DALYs lost due to a range of disorders and across a range of geographically and epidemiologically determined world regions. Although there remain important gaps in the availability of epidemiological data in certain regions of the world, as well as ongoing methodological debate about the derivation of disability weights, this study posed new challenges to mental health policy by highlighting unmet and growing needs in both developed and developing countries (Patel, 2000).

Economic perspective: cost-of-illness studies

Disease burden has also been gauged from an economic perspective for many years by 'cost of illness' and other economic impact studies, which attempt to attach monetary values to a variety of societal costs associated with a particular disorder, often expressed as an annual estimate aggregated across all involved agencies. In so doing, such studies extend beyond the purely health consequences of disease by also showing the economic and social impacts of disease. Since no measures of outcome enter into these analyses, cost-of-illness studies are not true economic evaluations as the latter involves the *comparison of costs to outcomes attained*. However, cost-of-illness studies can serve as a benchmark against which to compare the costs of future interventions.

Psychiatric disorders impose a range of costs on individuals, households, employers, and society as a whole. A proportion of these costs are self-evident, including the varied contributions made by service users, employers, and taxpayers/insurers towards the costs of treatment and care, and the productivity losses resulting from impaired work performance or inability to work. However, there are other significant costs that are not so readily quantifiable, including informal care inputs by family members and friends, treatment side effects, and excess premature mortality. Most recent cost-of-illness studies attempt to account for these costs, with lost productivity being the biggest item in most studies as others are more problematic to estimate. Where a comprehensive estimate of overall economic burden for depression has been attempted, for example, total estimated costs (prices in the year 2000) amounted to £9 billion in the UK, and $83 billion in the US (Greenberg et al. 2003; Thomas and Morris, 2003). A common feature of these studies has

Table 22.1 Proportion of DALYs attributable to mental, neurological, and substance use disorders, by WHO region for the year 2016

Region[a]	World	Africa	The Americas	Eastern Mediterranean	Europe	South-East Asia	Western Pacific
Population (millions)	7462	1020	992	664	916	1948	1890
DALYs lost all causes (millions)	2668	599	287	251	300	713	510
Proportion of DALYs lost to all mental, behavioural and neurological disorders	10.1%	4.9%	15.7%	9.2%	14.5%	8.8%	12.8%
1. Common mental disorders (depression, anxiety, eating disorders)	2.7%	1.4%	4.1%	2.8%	3.5%	2.4%	3.4%
2. Severe mental disorders (bipolar, psychotic disorders)	0.8%	0.3%	1.2%	0.7%	1.0%	0.7%	1.4%
3. Substance use disorders (alcohol and drug use disorders)	1.5%	0.6%	3.3%	1.2%	2.9%	1.0%	1.6%
4. Neurodevelopmental disorders (Autism, Asperger syndrome and childhood behavioural disorders)	0.6%	0.4%	0.8%	0.6%	0.6%	0.6%	0.7%
5. Idiopathic intellectual disorders	0.4%	0.3%	0.2%	0.4%	0.2%	0.5%	0.4%
6. Other mental and behavioural disorders	0.4%	0.2%	0.5%	0.3%	0.5%	0.4%	0.6%
7. Alzheimer's and other forms of dementia	1.3%	0.3%	1.9%	0.7%	2.5%	0.7%	2.4%
8. Epilepsy	0.6%	0.6%	0.6%	0.6%	0.5%	0.6%	0.5%
9. Headache disorders (migraine and non-migraine headache disorders)	1.4%	0.6%	1.9%	1.5%	1.9%	1.5%	1.4%
10. Other neurological conditions (including Parkinson's disease and multiple sclerosis)	0.5%	0.1%	0.8%	0.2%	0.5%	0.3%	0.2%

[a] For a list of countries by region, go to https://www.who.int/healthinfo/global_burden_disease/estimates/en/index1.html

Source data from *Global Health Estimates 2016: Disease burden by Cause, Age, Sex, by Country and by Region*, 2000–2016. World Health Organization.

been that the lost productivity costs exceed the direct costs of care and treatment, sometimes by as much as six or seven times.

A key document in the UK attempted to estimate the current and projected cost of eight key areas/disorders: depression, anxiety disorders, schizophrenic disorders, bipolar disorder, eating disorders, personality disorders, child/adolescent disorders, and dementias (McCrone et al., 2008). It estimated the total cost of these disorders to be £49 billion in 2007 accounting for service costs and lost earnings, with this being predicted to rise to £61 billion in 2026 (£88 billion with real pay and price effects).

Cost-of-illness studies in mental health have focused mainly on schizophrenia, depression, and dementia in a handful of countries and thus have limited relevance to the economic burden associated with a broader range of psychiatric disorders in the global population. Some researchers are concerned that the *human capital approach* to costing lost productivity, based on the assumption that when an individual is absent from work there is a corresponding reduction in national productivity, leads to overestimation since lost work may be 'made-up' when the individual returns, or replacement workers can be employed temporarily (see, e.g. Drummond 1992). An alternative approach, the *friction-cost* method, takes these counterbalancing influences into account. For example, Goeree and colleagues (1999), in Canada, estimated that the cost of lost productivity resulting from schizophrenia-related mortality was $1.53 million, as opposed to $105 million if the human-capital approach had been used.

Due to these methodological complexities with cost-of-illness studies, DALYs currently constitute the more internally consistent and globally applicable metric for assessment of the burden of disease. However, it is important to emphasize that cost-of-illness and burden of disease estimates alone provide insufficient information for allocating resources or setting priorities.

Applying health economics to mental health

Much of the need for a health economics perspective arises out of the *scarcity of resources* relative to needs, which translates into a requirement to make choices about how to allocate resources. At the level of mental health purchasers, resource scarcity prompts the need to gather evidence with which to evaluate the clinical and cost-effectiveness of new and current therapies. At a more aggregated level, the challenge of resource scarcity leads governments to consider the overall (allocative) efficiency of mental health spending, including revisions to funding arrangements for healthcare providers.

Macro-analyses: assessment of mental health system financing

Core functions of a health system include the generation and allocation of resources, the provision of services, and overall stewardship of these various components (WHO, 2000, 2007). Concerning the health financing function, all health financing systems, however organized, share three key features (WHO, 2010): revenue collection (i.e. how financial contributions are collected from different sources, and via what mechanism (tax, insurance, etc.); pooling (i.e. how financial contributions are pooled together so that the risk of having to pay for healthcare is not borne by each contributor individually); and purchasing/provision (i.e. how contributions are used to purchase or provide health services). Since the economic evaluation of (mental) healthcare services and interventions essentially concerns itself with the last of these key health financing issues, it is addressed in the following section under 'micro-level' analysis.

In terms of generating and pooling resources for mental health, recent results of a global Atlas survey show that that government is by far the most commonly cited main source of funds (first ranked in 79% of the 120 countries responding to this item (WHO 2015)). In 18% of countries, however, households are ranked as the main source of funds (mainly through direct out-of-pocket payments, but could also be via private health insurance cover). It is widely acknowledged that out-of-pocket payments are a regressive form of health financing (they penalize those least able to afford care) and represent an obvious channel through which impoverishment may occur. Specifically, they lead in many cases to health spending levels that have been labelled 'catastrophic' because they cause households to reallocate their budgets away from other essential needs such as education, food, and housing. Accordingly, health economic analysis can complement epidemiological research on the rates and impacts of mental illness across socioeconomic groups by assessing out-of-pocket expenditures and economic impacts of illness at the household level (Lund et al., 2011; Chisholm et al., 2015).

A health economics perspective can also inform the question of how many human, financial, and other resources need to be generated in order to scale-up services and meet programme goals. Again, epidemiological estimates of the number of cases in the population in need of services form the foundation of such resource planning and costing exercises (Box 22.1).

Micro-analyses: economic evaluation of mental healthcare interventions

Economic evaluation provides a set of principles and analytical techniques used to assess the relative costs and consequences of different interventions or treatment strategies. Despite the need for cost-effectiveness evidence, there remains a paucity of mental health economic evaluations from both developed and developing countries (Levin and Chisholm, 2016), although this is changing. The majority have been concerned with specific treatment modalities for psychoses and affective disorders, in particular the cost-effectiveness of different psychotropic drugs and, more recently, various psychotherapeutic approaches (see Box 22.2 for some examples).

Pharmacotherapy

Most economic studies have focused on the cost-effectiveness of newer classes of antidepressant and antipsychotic medications over their older counterparts. Synthesis of the available evidence indicates that these newer psychotropic drugs may have fewer adverse side effects but are not significantly more efficacious, and that the higher acquisition costs of the newer drugs are offset by a reduced need for other care and treatment (Knapp

Box 22.1 Scaling up mental health services

Many low- and middle-income countries do not assign adequate financial resources for care of mental, neurological, and substance use disorders and as a result, many people with mental health disorders who need treatment, do not receive it. This has led to increased interest in 'scaling-up' services to increase the coverage level (the percentage of people who need treatment and are actually receiving it). Estimation of the necessary financial resources needed for scaling up is therefore an important task. To aid in this, WHO and other partners have developed a strategic planning and costing tool called OneHealth, which enables epidemiologically based assessment of resource needs associated with the scale-up of a defined set of evidence-based mental health-care interventions for priority disorders (Chisholm et al., 2017).

The OneHealth tool is an excellent example of how epidemiology and health economics can work in tandem. Epidemiological data on the incidence and remission rates of a disorder, the efficacy and adherence rates of treatments, and the health impacts of disorders and treatments (mortality, healthy years lived) can be combined with demographic data and economic data on the costs of treatments (price of drugs, cost of inpatient stays, staff costs) to produce a comprehensive picture of the economic and health impacts.

et al., 1999; Rosenbaum and Hylan, 1999). However, some evidence suggests that some of the newer antipsychotics may be more effective and have less side effects with the cost-effectiveness remaining unclear (Bagnall et al., 2003). The inconclusive evidence arising out of experimental and simulated studies to date suggests that the choice of drug, particularly in localities where evidence has not been accrued, remains a question of preference and affordability.

Psychological interventions

Encouraging evidence is emerging in relation to the cost-effectiveness of psychotherapeutic approaches to the management of psychosis and a range of mood and stress-related disorders, with or without pharmacotherapy (Miller and Magruder, 1999; Bird et al., 2010; Koeser et al., 2015). A consistent research finding is that psychological interventions lead to improved satisfaction and treatment concordance compared to usual care alone, which contributes significantly to reduced rates of relapse, hospitalization, and unemployment. For example, controlled cost–outcome trials of family therapy for schizophrenia carried out in the UK, US, and China each identified appreciably greater reductions in relapse rates, hospital readmission, and family burden for study subjects in receipt of the family intervention (Knapp et al., 1999). As with the newer psychotropic medications, the prevailing, if not fully substantiated view is that the additional costs of psychological treatments are countered by decreased levels of other health service contact.

Box 22.2 Illustrative cost-effectiveness trials of mental healthcare interventions

Although the volume of completed studies remains modest, particularly in middle- and low-income countries, there is increasing economic evidence to support the argument that interventions for schizophrenia, depression, and other mental disorders are not only available and effective but also affordable and cost-effective.

Schizophrenia care

Controlled cost–outcome trials of family therapy for schizophrenia carried out in the UK, US, and China have each identified greater reductions in relapse rates, hospital readmission, and family burden for study subjects in receipt of the family intervention as compared to standard care. In the China study, for example, researchers developed a family-based intervention appropriate to the Chinese context and showed that, in comparison to patients receiving standard care, such an approach reduced the need for inpatient hospital care, improved employment, and saved an estimated US $149 per family (Xiong et al., 1994). In Thailand, Phanthunane and colleagues (2011) showed that despite the higher costs of including family psychoeducation, the inclusion of this psychosocial support element increases adherence to and outcomes from medication and is the most cost-effective option. Analysis of these factors helped Thailand to prioritize a strategy to use generic newer drugs as the first-line treatment, ideally in combination with family interventions, to increase health gains and lower hospitalization costs.

Depression and anxiety

A series of prospective trials undertaken in Seattle and elsewhere in the US have shown that important gains in clinical outcomes and functioning can be achieved for a modest investment via the pursuit of disease management and quality improvement programmes for depression in primary care settings (Rosenbaum and Hylan, 1999; Simon et al., 2001; Gilbody et al., 2006). In India, a study of a task-shifting approach to the treatment of depression and/or anxiety (MANAS trial) involved trained lay health workers to provide psychosocial interventions as part of primary care. The intervention was found to be cost-effective and cost saving, and it overcame barriers posed by a shortage of mental health professionals (Buttorff et al., 2012).

Alcohol misuse

A controlled trial of brief physician advice to problem drinkers in primary care carried out in the US produced a cost–benefit ratio of 1:5.6, with savings made up of reduced use of hospital services and avoided crime and motor accidents in broadly equal measure (Fleming et al., 2000).

Box 22.3 The LEGs study

The LEGs study (Perez et al., 2015) aimed to determine the clinical and cost-effectiveness of a high-intensity and low-intensity intervention that aided general practitioners in detecting either those individuals at risk of developing psychosis or those who already were experiencing a first episode of psychosis in primary care. This allowed patients to be referred on to appropriate secondary care. The study found that the high-intensity intervention referred more 'true-positive' cases to secondary services than either the low-intensity treatment or the practice as usual, but also referred more 'false-positive' cases. The economic evaluation reported that the high-intensity intervention was more cost-effective than both the other groups as it was more effective at identifying patients at high risk of developing psychosis or with a first episode of psychosis and was also associated with lower total costs per practice. The high-intensity intervention actually cost more to provide but 'paid' for itself as it reduced the number of late presenters (individuals whose psychosis is not identified early and are more costly to treat) and it reduced the costs of treating individuals at high risk who are treated early.

Pathways to care and implementation

An economic evaluation is very useful for telling us which treatment might be more cost-effective compared to alternatives, but that is generally within the narrow scope of an RCT. These type of evaluations rarely take into account other important factors such as the cost associated with actually implementing a new treatment (e.g. the cost of training staff in the new treatment) or facilitating access to the intervention (e.g. the pathway to care). The Liaison and Education in General Practices (LEGs) study (Perez et al., 2015) is an example of how economic evaluations can go beyond the comparison of two treatments and inform decision-making on screening processes (Box 22.3).

Conducting an economic evaluation

The merit of an economic study in terms of its coverage and generalizability is determined to a significant extent by three parameters: study design, type of economic evaluation, and perspective (Table 22.2).

Study design

RCTs are regarded as the 'gold standard' of clinical and economic evaluation, since changes in outcome measures are attributable to the intervention, as opposed to other possible explanatory factors or 'confounding' variables. Where it is not practical to carry out an experimental study, observational studies may have better external validity by preserving the context in which care is provided, but shift the focus of the analysis towards identifying associations between the intervention and changes in costs or outcomes (Black, 1996).

Table 22.2 Study design parameters

Parameter 1: type of clinical data (what ratings are based on)	Parameter 2: costing scope/ perspective (what costs are included)	Parameter 3: type of economic evaluation (how costs and outcomes are combined)
Non-empirical (e.g. claims database)	Single care agency (e.g. health service only)	Cost-minimization analysis (CMA) (outcomes are the same)
Observational (e.g. cross-sectional study)	All formal care agencies (e.g. voluntary sector included)	Cost-effectiveness analysis (CEA) and cost-consequences analysis (e.g. cost per change in depression score)
Quasi-experimental (e.g. retrospective study)	Formal and informal care agencies (e.g. lost employment included)	Cost–utility analysis (CUA) (e.g. quality-adjusted life year)
Experimental (e.g. RCT)	All societal costs (e.g. user/carer distress included)	Cost–benefit analysis (CBA) (all costs and outcomes monetized)

Mode of economic evaluation

Cost-minimization analysis is the simplest economic evaluation and establishes the least costly method of achieving given outcomes. However, it is only appropriate if all outcomes are known or found to be identical, which is unlikely given the multidimensional nature of mental health outcome studies.

A much more common type of economic evaluation in the field of mental healthcare is *cost-effectiveness analysis*, which assesses the outcome of an intervention combined with costs, expressed in terms of cost per reduction in symptom level, or cost per life saved. Where there is more than a single measure of outcome being investigated, as is often the case in psychiatry, it is more correctly called a *cost-consequences analysis*. This kind of economic evaluation has the advantage of presenting an array of outcome findings to decision-makers (Box 22.4).

Box 22.4 Types of economic analyses

- Cost-minimization analysis—the least costly method of achieving the same known outcome.
- Cost-effectiveness analysis—cost per unit of (principal) outcome.
- Cost-consequences analysis—cost per unit of (several) outcomes.
- Cost–utility analysis—cost per unit of 'utility' (summary measure allowing comparison across different fields of healthcare).
- Cost–benefit analysis—converts outcomes into monetary units to establish if monetarized benefits exceed costs.

Cost–utility analysis has considerable appeal for decision-makers since it generates a combined index of the mortality and quality of life effects of an intervention, upon which priorities can then be based. This would allow, for example, cost–utility findings for an intervention for schizophrenia to be compared to an intervention for asthma or cancer.

Cost–benefit analysis includes all costs and outcomes valued in monetary units, thereby allowing assessment of whether a particular course of action is worthwhile, based on a simple decision rule that benefits must exceed costs. The difficulty of this approach is quantifying all outcomes in monetary terms, and consequently is rarely found in mental healthcare evaluation. Nevertheless, methodologies have now been developed which aim to obtain direct valuations of health outcomes by patients or the general public, such as 'willingness-to-pay' techniques, where an individual states the amount they would be prepared to pay to achieve a given health state (Healey and Chisholm, 1999).

These modes of economic evaluation enable the relative efficiency of different interventions to be determined. However, comparing the efficiency of different services can produce problematic results. The Oregon prioritization exercise in the United States, for example, resulted in tooth-capping receiving a higher ranking than appendectomies (Hadorn, 1991). The general public will often want to prioritize interventions that preserve life, although they could be relatively inefficient. This 'rule of rescue' needs to be considered alongside evidence from economic evaluations.

Costing perspective

A key decision to make at the design stage of an economic study relates to the perspective of the evaluation. The perspective dictates which resources should be included in the estimation of the costs. Not only are costs associated with the health and social care support of users (direct costs) included, but also knock-on effects (indirect costs) such as the impact on someone's ability to work. The chosen perspective depends on the disorder area, who the stakeholders are, and who the target audience is and can vary from narrow to wide. For example, a new treatment for hay fever, which is not likely to influence ability to work and mainly involves National Health Service (NHS) prescribing is likely to have a narrow perspective of the NHS. However, a new treatment for schizophrenia, which has the potential to influence the ability to work by promoting recovery, and is treated by a whole range of healthcare and social service, is likely to take a wider societal perspective that assesses the impact of the intervention on all involved agencies. Since comprehensive mental healthcare requires multidisciplinary inputs, the adoption of a single-agency perspective is not appropriate for most evaluations and the most suitable perspective will seek to identify the costs falling to the multiplicity of care agencies involved, plus any costs incurred by users or carers.

Measurement of resource utilization

Measurement of individuals' resource use can be undertaken in three main ways: use of a retrospective service use questionnaire/interview, use of a prospectively kept diary, or examination of patient records. Sole reliance on patient records is difficult as health services often use multiple and non-connected databases or paper records, and non-health resource use can be dispersed across a number of agencies. However, they can act as useful validation of data obtained through self-report.

The service use needs of people with mental health disorders are variable. For people with common mental disorders this may be quite modest, focusing on primary healthcare-based counselling or psychological therapy. In contrast, the needs of users with more severe mental disorders, such as schizophrenia, are likely to encompass a wide range of services, such as psychiatric inpatient and outpatient hospital services, social care, housing or residential care, structured day care support, and activities and sheltered employment. The extensive range of services that people with mental health problems may use means that most evaluations should adopt a wide coverage, emphasizing the usefulness of an instrument that is similarly broad based.

Calculation of unit costs

For each item of resource utilization, a unit cost estimate is required, such as a cost per inpatient day, day care attendance, or professional contact. Theoretically, the appropriate level of cost analysis is 'over the long run' and 'at the margin', since it is the *incremental change* in resources implied by an intervention that is of interest. The difficulty associated with deriving costs in this way often results in a reliance on average revenue costs, adjusted to include capital and overhead elements. Economic theory suggests that in the long run these average costs may be approximately equal to long-run marginal costs (Knapp 1993). In some countries and for certain services, unit cost data of this kind have been calculated, otherwise they need to be computed from sources such as national/local government statistics, health authority figures, and specific facility accounts. In practical terms, the main categories of cost that need to be quantified are:

- wages of professional staff
- facility operating costs where the service is provided such as cleaning and catering
- overhead costs such as personnel and finance
- capital costs of the buildings and equipment where the service is provide.

The aggregation of these components amounts to the total cost of a service and this total is divided by the appropriate unit of service provision, such as number of patient contacts, to give the unit costs.

Measurement of outcomes

Intermediate outcomes, also known as process indicators, should not normally be the focus of the analysis, since positive changes in attendance or detection rates, for example, may not necessarily result in improved patient welfare or mental health. Final outcomes are concerned with detecting changes in the physical, psychological, or social well-being of individuals, and commonly revolve around the measurement of symptoms, functioning and disability, quality of life, and service satisfaction. Further population-level assessments of outcome are the composite indices of health such as the quality adjusted life-year (QALY) or DALY, which weight time spent in a certain state of health by the severity of the health state. With the further development and refinement of cost–utility methods, such measures of outcome are being more routinely included as a corollary to more condition- or domain-specific measures.

Comparative analysis of costs and outcomes

Economic evaluation compares the costs and outcomes of a mental healthcare intervention in an explicit framework, enabling decision-makers to assess whether the intervention offers a good use of resources. An analysis of costs or outcomes alone does not provide such information. In analytical terms, there are a number of possible scenarios:

- If one intervention is both less costly and more beneficial than a comparison intervention, one can immediately conclude that this intervention is preferable.

- If the costs and outcomes are equivalent, then either is acceptable.

- If costs alone are equivalent, then the more effective intervention is preferable, and if clinical outcomes are equivalent, then the cheaper intervention is preferable.

When the evidence shows that one intervention is more costly and more effective, we need to assess whether the additional costs are worth the greater effectiveness. This can be established by calculating an incremental cost-effectiveness ratio (Box 22.5). A negative cost-effectiveness ratio has little meaning since it implies that one intervention is dominant over, or dominated by the other in terms of cost or outcome.

The usefulness of economic analysis depends on the validity of the evidence about the study population, which is never perfect. A key stage of an economic evaluation is a *sensitivity analysis*, which involves the introduction of alternative values to key study parameters to assess the robustness of the conclusions.

The uptake of services is highly variable, so that pooled individual service use and cost data tend to be highly positively skewed, reflecting the heavy use of services by a small number of individuals. As parametric statistical approaches may not be appropriate, non-parametric approaches or data transformation may be required. The median is commonly used as the key measure of central tendency, or data is transformed onto a logarithmic or other scale. While use of the median may be useful for showing the 'typical' cost of a study subject, it is based on ranked data rather than actual values, ignores the influence

---

Box 22.5 The incremental cost-effectiveness ratio

$$\text{Incremental cost-effectiveness ratio} = \frac{\text{Difference in costs between treatments}}{\text{Difference in outcomes between treatments}}$$

This is used to assess whether additional costs are a good investment when one treatment is both more effective and more costly.

of outliers, and does not capture the total or (arithmetic) mean cost of treatment and care (Barber and Thompson, 1998). Likewise, while logarithmic transformation of costs data may resolve the problem of skewness, tests of differences between groups are on the geometric rather than the arithmetic mean. An alternative approach is the non-parametric 'bootstrap', which makes no distributional assumptions, yet is able to generate standard errors and confidence intervals for the parameter of interest (Mooney and Duval, 1993).

Conclusion: the uses and limitations of economic analyses

The results of well-conducted economic evaluations can inform decision-making processes at many levels, from users and caregivers to government and society. However, it is important to mention some limitations of the approach. Conclusions based on a small-sample randomized trial can often only be tentative, while the failure to measure the wider non-health, non-service costs associated with two or more alternative treatments may produce misleading results. There are also a number of ongoing methodological debates such as the alternative techniques available for measuring health state preferences which are essential for both cost–utility and cost–benefit analyses. Given the low priority and stigma that is commonly associated with mental healthcare, a further desirable feature is that more cost-effectiveness data should be available for comparison to interventions for physical conditions, in order to provide a firmer basis for new investment of resources. Even without these limitations, economic evaluation should not be viewed as a panacea for making difficult allocative and policy decisions. It is one additional tool that can facilitate explicit, evidence-based decision-making.

Practical exercises

You are requested by local commissioners to prepare a protocol for the economic evaluation of a group therapy programme for adolescents with repeated self-harm as an alternative to routine care. Construct a two-page summary protocol answering the following questions:

1. What are the specific aims and hypotheses of your planned economic evaluation? What is your chosen study design?

2. What is your chosen scope, duration, and perspective for the evaluation? How might your choice of timescale and viewpoint affect the end results?

3. What are the main categories of cost that you would include in the evaluation? Are there any economic costs that you are not including, and if so, why?

4. What are the key measures of outcome that need to be considered, and by which mode of evaluation will you link these outcomes to cost data?

5. How would you propose to deal with the potential uncertainty surrounding key findings?

Once the exercise has been completed, the following study provides an illustration of how the questions raised were dealt with by a team of researchers in actual clinical practice:

Green JM, Wood AJ, Kerfoot MJ, Trainor G, Roberts C, Rothwell J, Woodham A, Ayodeji E, Barrett B, Byford S, Harrington R. Group therapy for adolescents with repeated self harm: randomised controlled trial with economic evaluation. *BMJ*, 2011 Apr 1;342:d682.

Further reading

Fenwick, E. and Byford, S. (2005). A guide to cost-effectiveness acceptability curves. *British Journal of Psychiatry*, **187**, 106–108.

Green, J.M., Wood, A.J., Kerfoot, M.J., Trainor, G., Roberts, C., Rothwell, J., et al. (2011). Group therapy for adolescents with repeated self harm: randomised controlled trial with economic evaluation. *BMJ*, **342**, d682.

Petrou, A. and Gray, A. (2011). Economic evaluation alongside randomised controlled trials: design, conduct, analysis and reporting. *BMJ*, **342**, d556.

Robinson, R. (1993). Economic evaluation and health care: what does it mean? *BMJ*, **307**, 670–673.

References

Bagnall, A.-M., Jones, L., Ginnelly, L., Lewis, R., Glanville, J., Gilbody, S., et al. (2003). A systematic review of atypical antipsychotic drugs in schizophrenia. *Health Technology Assessment*, **7**, 1–93.

Barber, J. and Thompson, S. (1998). Analysis and interpretation of cost data in randomised controlled trials: review of published studies. *British Medical Journal*, **317**, 1195–200.

Bird, V., Premkumar, P., Kendall, T., Whittington, C., Mitchell, J., and Kuipers, E. (2010). Early intervention services, cognitive-behavioural therapy and family intervention in early psychosis: systematic review. *British Journal of Psychiatry*, **197**, 350–356.

Black, N. (1996). Why we need observational studies to evaluate the effectiveness of health care. *British Medical Journal*, **312**, 1215–1218.

Buttorff, C., Hock, R., Weiss, H., Naik, S., Araya, R., Kirkwood, B.R., et al. (2012). Economic evaluation of a task-shifting intervention for common mental disorders in India. *Bulletin of the World Health Organization*, **90**, 813–821.

Chisholm, D., Heslin, M., Docrat, S., Nanda, S., Shidhaye, R., Upadhaya, N., et al. (2017). Scaling-up services for psychosis, depression and epilepsy in sub-Saharan Africa and South Asia: development and application of a mental health systems planning tool (OneHealth). *Epidemiology and Psychiatric Sciences*, **26**, 234–244.

Chisholm, D., Johansson, K.A., Raykar, N., Megiddo, I., Nigam, A., Strand, K.B., et al. (2015). Moving toward universal health coverage for mental, neurological, and substance use disorders: an extended cost-effectiveness analysis. In: Patel, V., Chisholm, D., Dua, T., Laxminarayan, R., and Medina-Mora, M.E. (eds.). *Disease control priorities (third edition): Volume 4, Mental, neurological, and substance use disorders*, pp. 237–252. Washington, DC: World Bank.

Drummond, M. (1992). Cost-of-illness studies: a major headache? *Pharmacoeconomics*, **2**, 1–4.

Fleming, M.F., Mundt, M.P., French, M.T., Manwell, L.B., Stauffacher, E.A., and Barry, K.L. (2000). Benefit-cost analysis of brief physician advice with problem drinkers in primary care settings. *Medical Care*, **38**, 7–18.

Gilbody, S., Bower, P., Fletcher, J., Richards, D., and Sutton, A.J. (2006). Collaborative care for depression. *Archives of Internal Medicine*, **166**, 2314–2321.

Goeree, R., O'Brien, B., Blackhouse, G., Agro, K., and Goering, P. (1999). The valuation of productivity costs due to premature mortality: a comparison of the human-capital and friction-cost method for schizophrenia. *Canadian Journal of Psychiatry*, **44**, 464–472.

Greenberg, P.E., Kessler, R.C., Birnbaum, H.G., Leong, S.A., Lowe, S.W., Berglund, P.A., and Corey-Lisle, P.K. (2003). The economic burden of depression in the United States: How did it change between 1990 and 2000? *Journal of Clinical Psychiatry*, **64**, 1465–1475.

Hadorn, D.C. (1991). Setting health care priorities in Oregon: cost-effectiveness meets the rule of rescue. *Journal of the American Medical Association*, **265**, 2218–2225.

Healey, A. and Chisholm, D. (1999). Willingness to pay as a measure of the benefits of mental health care. *Journal of Mental Health Policy and Economics*, **2**, 55–58.

Koeser, L., Donisi, V., Goldberg, D.P., and McCrone, P. (2015). Modelling the cost-effectiveness of pharmacotherapy compared with cognitive–behavioural therapy and combination therapy for the treatment of moderate to severe depression in the UK. *Psychological Medicine*, **45**, 3019–3031.

Knapp, M.R.J. (1993). Background theory. In: Netten A. and Beecham, J. (eds.) *Costing community care: theory and practice*, pp. 9–24. Aldershot: Ashgate.

Knapp, M.R.J., Almond, S., and Percudani, M. (1999). Costs of schizophrenia. In: Maj, M. and Sartorius, N. (eds.). *Evidence and experience in psychiatry (Volume 1)*, pp. 407–454. London: John Wiley and Sons.

Levin, C. and Chisholm, D. (2016). Cost and cost-effectiveness of interventions, policies, and platforms for the prevention and treatment of mental, neurological, and substance use disorders. In: Patel, V., Chisholm., D., Dua, T., Laxminarayan, R., and Medina-Mora, M.E. (eds.). *Disease control priorities (third edition): Volume 4, Mental, neurological, and substance use disorders*, pp. 219–236. Washington, DC: World Bank.

Lund, C., De Silva, M., Plagerson, S., Cooper, S., Chisholm, D., Das, J., et al. (2011). Poverty and mental disorders: breaking the cycle in low-income and middle-income countries. *Lancet*, **378**, 1502–1514.

McCrone, P, Dhanasiri, S., Patel, A., Knapp, M., and Lawton-Smith, S. (2008). *Paying the price: the cost of mental health care in England to 2026*. London: The King's Fund.

Miller, N. and Magruder, K. (eds.) (1999). *Cost-effectiveness of psychotherapy*. New York: Oxford University Press.

Mooney, C. and Duval, R. (1993). *Bootstrapping: a nonparametric approach to statistical inference*. London: Sage Publications.

Murray, C.J.L. and Lopez, A.D. (1996). *The global burden of diseases: a comprehensive assessment of mortality and disability from diseases, injuries and risk factors in 1990 and projected to 2020*. Boston, MA: Harvard School of Public Health, WHO, and World Bank.

Patel, V. (2000). The need for treatment evidence for common mental disorders in developing countries. *Psychological Medicine*, **30**, 743–746.

Perez, J., Jin, H., Russo, D.A., Stochl, J., Painter, M., Shelley, G., et al. (2015). Clinical effectiveness and cost-effectiveness of tailored intensive liaison between primary and secondary care to identify individuals at risk of a first psychotic illness (the LEGs study): a cluster-randomised controlled trial. *Lancet Psychiatry*, **2**, 984–993.

Phanthunane, P., Vos, T., Whiteford, H., and Bertram, M. (2011). Cost-effectiveness of pharmacological and psychosocial interventions for schizophrenia. *Cost Effectiveness and Resource Allocation*, **9**, 1–9.

Rosenbaum, J.F. and Hylan, T. (1999). Costs of depressive disorders: a review. In: Maj, M. and Sartorius, N. (eds.). *Evidence and experience in psychiatry (Volume 2)*, pp. 401–480. London: John Wiley and Sons.

Simon, G.E., Katon, W., VonKorff, M., Unützer, J., Lin, E.H., Walker, E.A., et al. (2001). Cost-effectiveness of a collaborative care program for primary care patients with persistent depression. *American Journal of Psychiatry*, **158**, 1638–1644.

Thomas, C.M. and Morris, S. (2003). Cost of depression among adults in England in 2000. *British Journal of Psychiatry*, **183**, 514–519.

World Health Organization (2000). *The world health report 2000; health systems: making a difference.* Geneva: World Health Organization.

World Health Organization (2007). Everybody business: strengthening health systems to improve health outcomes: WHO's framework for action. https://www.who.int/healthsystems/strategy/everybodys_business.pdf

World Health Organization (2010). *World health report 2010: world health report: health systems financing; the path to universal coverage.* Geneva: World Health Organization.

World Health Organization (2015). *Mental health atlas 2014.* Geneva: World Health Organization.

World Health Organization (2018). Global health estimates 2016 summary tables: DALY by cause, age and sex, by WHO region, 2000–2012. http://www.who.int/healthinfo/global_burden_disease/estimates/en/index1.html

Xiong, W., Phillips, M., Xiong, H., Wang, R., Dai, Q., Kleinman, J., and Kleinman, A. (1994). Family-based intervention for schizophrenic patients in China: a randomised controlled trial. *British Journal of Psychiatry*, **165**, 239–247.

Chapter 23

Life course epidemiology

Marcus Richards and Rebecca Hardy

Introduction

Life course epidemiology investigates the long-term effects on health-related outcomes of exposures during gestation, childhood, adolescence, young adulthood, and later adult life, and across generations (Kuh and Ben Shlomo, 2004). For several reasons, a life course approach is particularly well suited to psychiatric epidemiology. First, effects of exposures on mental health outcomes indeed appear to operate across most of these stages of life, although it is important to recognize that the onset of psychiatric outcomes is far from random with respect to age. For example, almost all impulse control disorders develop in childhood, whereas mood disorders are rare before adolescence, after which they show a steady increase until late middle age (Kessler et al., 2007). Second, several common psychiatric problems themselves show recognizable patterns of continuity and discontinuity (Rutter et al., 2006). For example, adolescent-onset depression shows a high degree of continuity (Rutter et al., 2006), with risk transmissible across generations (Weissman et al., 2006), as does positive well-being (Richards and Huppert, 2011) and cognitive impairment (Richards, 2014). On the other hand, mild adolescent-onset conduct problems often diminish over adulthood after benefitting from turning points such as stable partnership formation and labour market attachment (Moffitt, 1993). A life course approach provides optimum ways to describe these trajectories, and to map them onto studies of relevant influences. Third, many psychiatric disorders have an impact on a wider range of health, economic, and social outcomes, sometimes continuing for decades (Richards and Abbott, 2009). Thus a life course approach is useful for conceptualizing and studying how mental health is embedded in a more holistic context.

This chapter contains four main sections. First we briefly review key concepts in life course epidemiology, with emphasis on their implications for mental disorders. Then we summarize relevant study designs and their advantages and disadvantages, with examples of available resources. Next we review some of the principal analytic tools applied to these resources. Finally, we provide illustrations of three of these tools, applied to the British 1946 birth cohort.

Key concepts in life course epidemiology

Kuh and Ben Shlomo (2004) broadly distinguish critical and sensitive period models from risk accumulation models. The former refer to an exposure (or in the case of hypoxia, for example, interruption of an essential exposure) during a specific period having a lasting effect on an outcome where exposure to the same outcome outside of this window has no such effect. A 'sensitive' period, which should not be used interchangeably, more broadly implies an optimum widow for exposure, although exposure outside of this window may still have an effect on the outcome. Both models may be with or without later effect modification. This is the foundation of the developmental origins (programming) model of chronic disease historically identified with David Barker (1992). For some, this is virtually synonymous with 'life course epidemiology', although this is a misleadingly narrow interpretation in any context. Certainly there is evidence for the role of pre- and peri-natal factors in the aetiology of psychotic, bipolar, autism spectrum, and attention deficit hyperactivity disorders, especially in interaction with genetic and epigenetic modification. However, these are not the strongest predictors of more common psychiatric outcomes within the normal population range. For example, a systematic review and meta-analysis concluded that the association between birth weight and adult depression is modest at best (Wojcik et al., 2013). There is a consensus that higher birth weight is associated with better cognitive development (Shenkin et al., 2004). However, effect sizes are again modest; there is no evidence that they have a long-term impact on cognitive ageing—and by implication, risk of dementia; and effects may be substantially confounded by maternal cognitive ability (Richards, 2014). Birth cohort studies further suggest that adult psychological health is a stronger predictor of midlife affective disorders than childhood psychological health (Clark et al., 2007), and that proximal exposures are more important predictors of adult affective symptoms than distal exposures (von Stumm et al., 2013; Colman et al., 2014), at least within the range typically encountered in the general population. In both cases, however, childhood and adult risk factors are unlikely to be mutually independent, which leads to risk accumulation models in life course epidemiology. Kuh and Ben Shlomo (2004) distinguish four variants, according to whether multiple exposures are indeed mutually independent (Figure 23.1a); or clustered by one or more common factors (such as socioeconomic position; Figure 23.1b); or operate in sequence, with either the final link only having impact (Figure 23.1d), or with additional independent effects of each sequential factor (Fig 23.1c). The two best known examples for understanding mental health that are relevant to the latter possibilities are the stress process (Pearlin et al., 1981) and the chain reaction (Rutter, 1989). Examples include the effects of economic hardship following involuntary job loss (Pearlin, 2010); effects on occupational role of becoming a caregiver (Pearlin, 2010); and the diverse long-term effects of early conduct problems on socioeconomic, social, and health outcomes (Richards and Abbott, 2009). Such a sequence can be a positive one too; for example, Quinton and Rutter (1988) described how institution-reared children with positive school experiences were more likely to develop planning skills in relation to key life decisions, perhaps because success in one arena can enhance self-esteem and self-efficacy leading to resilience (Rutter, 1999).

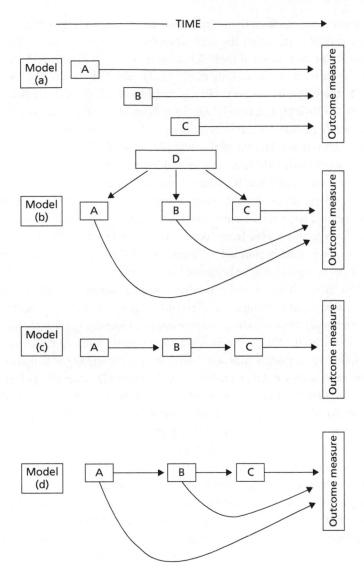

Figure 23.1 Life course causal models.

Reproduced with permission from Kuh, D. and Ben-Shlomo, Y. (eds). *A Life Course Approach to Chronic Disease Epidemiology*. 2nd ed. Oxford University Press (2004). Reproduced with permission of the Licensor through PLSclear.

Study design for psychiatric life course epidemiology

A life course study refers to 'a cohort study that has information from at least one stage of development (gestation, childhood or adolescence) and in adult life' to distinguish it from a general cohort or longitudinal study followed up over a shorter period (Hardy and Kuh, 2009). Given the definition of 'life course' that opens this chapter, we might naturally anticipate that the birth cohort study is the preeminent design for this approach. A birth cohort consists of a sample born in close temporal proximity and a birth cohort study follows the study members from their birth onwards. For example, the three adult British birth cohorts were all born within the same week of their respective years. These cohorts are the Medical Research Council (MRC) National Survey of Health and Development (NSHD, the 1946 birth cohort) (Kuh et al. 2011); the National Child Development Study (NCDS, the 1958 birth cohort) (Power and Elliott, 2006); and the British Cohort Study (BCS70, the 1970 birth cohort) (Elliott and Shepherd, 2006). Two British birth cohorts subsequently recruited are the Avon Longitudinal Study of Parents and Children (ALSPAC, also known as Children of the 90s) (Fraser et al., 2012); and the eponymous Millennium Cohort Study (MCS) (Connelly and Platt 2014). From New Zealand, and of particular interest for mental health research, members of the Dunedin Multidisciplinary Health and Development Study were born between 1972 and 1973 (e.g. Moffitt et al., 2011). These cohorts have been continuously followed since birth; however, some birth cohorts have been reconstructed from records, or revived from earlier studies that were interrupted or not originally planned for long-term follow-up. Examples of studies reconstructed from records that have been used for mental health research are the Lothian 1921 and 1936 birth cohorts, and the Swedish 1969 Conscription Cohort. The Lothian cohorts were constructed by using archival records of the Scottish Mental Surveys of 1932 and 1947, then tracing those who had sat these tests and recruiting a sample for follow-up in later life (Deary et al., 2012). The Swedish 1969 Conscription Cohort was randomly selected for follow-up in midlife from a national database originally obtained during conscription into compulsory military service between 18 and 20 years of age (e.g. Allebeck and Allgulander, 1990). Another example of a revived study (also referred to as a historical cohort study) relevant to mental health research include the New England Family Studies, which are following up in adulthood part of the Collaborative Perinatal Project that originally ran to age 7 years (e.g. Seidman et al., 2013).

As we will see, there are disadvantages with the birth cohort design, although there is little question of its power in the context of mental health research. Some advantages, such as prospective follow-up and representative sampling from the source population, are common to other epidemiological designs. A special advantage of the birth cohort, arising from the narrow age range, is the ability to study within-person age-related change which, unlike in age-heterogeneous cross-sectional studies, is not confounded with secular or birth cohort effects. So, for example, when studies recruit across a wide age range (e.g. the Adult Psychiatric Morbidity Survey), a comparison of age-specific prevalence rates of specific disorders are mixed with cohort and/or period effects. Period effects refer to factors that vary according to calendar time and affect all ages simultaneously. For example, a severe natural disaster (such as the 2004 Indian Ocean earthquake and tsunami, and the 2005 hurricane Katrina in the US) or a major human-engineered traumatic event (such as the 9/11 terrorist attack in the US) is likely to have an impact across ages. On the other hand, a policy change leading to increased unemployment will of course primarily affect people of labour market age, although there may be indirect mental health effects on children via quality of parenting, and on elderly people via availability for caring. In epidemiology, such an interaction due to a period effect that is differentially experienced across age groups has been conceptualized as a cohort effect. Methodological changes in outcome definitions, classifications, or method of data collection can also lead to period effects (Keyes and Li, 2012). Comparison of different birth cohorts with the same or similar assessments made at comparable ages can be informative about changes in prevalence of disorders. A meta-analysis of 26 studies of children born between 1965 and 1996 showed that the prevalence of depression based on a structured psychiatric interview up to age 18 was stable over these years (Costello et al., 2006). This is a complex issue however; more granular work suggests a rise in adolescent emotional problems in the UK from the mid 1970s to the turn of the twenty-first century (Collishaw et al. 2004), although the opposite trend for the first decade of the twenty-first century (Collishaw et al. 2015). Incidentally, the meta-analysis of Costello and colleagues (2006) also demonstrates the importance of concurrent assessment of depression, since previous indications of a secular increase in this disorder were likely to be artefactual; evidence for this apparent increase was mostly based on recall of depressive episodes in cross-sectional studies, where older participants were more vulnerable to 'recall failure' from a longer recollection interval than younger participants (Collishaw et al., 2015). The authors concluded that previous perceptions of an 'epidemic' of child or adolescent depression may be due to increased awareness of a disorder that had been underdiagnosed by clinicians. On the other hand, the MRC Cognitive Function and Ageing Study which recruited two samples of participants aged 65 and older, between 1989 and 1994, and between 2008 and 2011 showed that those later born had a lower risk of prevalent dementia than those born earlier in the past century (Matthews et al., 2013).

Along with the advantages, it is equally important to highlight methodological disadvantages of life course designs. First, birth cohorts are highly costly of financial and human resources to establish and maintain. Typically, scientific justification and scientific returns are maximized through a multidisciplinary structure. This allows mental health to be set in its social and biomedical context, but can be at the expense of domain-specific measurement time, particularly for time-consuming psychiatric diagnostic schedules, when demands have to be balanced against those of measuring other health domains. However, this challenge has in turn been met by the development of more streamlined instruments for community-based research such as the revised Clinical Interview Schedule (CIS-R) (Lewis et al., 1992), from which clinical psychiatric diagnoses can be derived. The financial expense of a large cohort can also limit the frequency of assessment waves, to the extent that opportunities to capture adverse psychiatric events can be missed. A lengthy interval between waves not only increases the burden of recall of these events themselves, but will almost certainly exceed the reporting window of the symptom assessment instrument. Second, while not a problem that is specific to birth cohorts, care needs to be taken as a cohort is followed over a long time that measures are always age-appropriate. Clearly the kind of measure used to capture behaviour in relation to childhood mental state is very different to the kind of measure used to elicit symptoms in adulthood; which in turn may not capture emotional problems common in old age such as loneliness. This, however, limits the extent to which true repeated measures can be obtained, although there are techniques that allow for this in analysis, which will be addressed in the final section. Third, although these cohorts are exquisitely suited for research into common mental disorders, they are less well equipped for investigation of rare psychiatric outcomes. Nevertheless, even the smallest of the British birth cohorts, NSHD, was able to study determinants of the relatively rare disorders of depersonalization (33 cases) (Lee et al., 2012) and schizophrenia (30 cases) (Jones et al., 1994), and the association between affective symptoms in early midlife and premature mortality (Henderson et al., 2011). Finally, and in common with most types of longitudinal study, birth cohorts are vulnerable to bias from selective attrition over time, with losses of study members who are relatively less socially advantaged and less healthy. This problem has received increasing attention in recent years, with corresponding emphasis on participant engagement and retention strategies to prevent attrition as well as on compensatory statistical methods. This leads to our final section, on analytic strategies in life course epidemiology.

Analytic strategies in life course epidemiology

The statistical analysis of life course data is complex and challenging as it aims to study how risk factors from across the whole of life jointly influence later health. It should be stated from the outset that there are no longitudinal statistical techniques unique to life course epidemiology; that is, these techniques are generally applicable to most kinds of longitudinal data. Life course analyses will often need to deal with repeated outcome variables or repeated exposure variables or both. Models for the analysis of repeated outcome measures are well developed; for example, random effects models are in widespread use. Methodology is less standard when attempting to relate one time-varying measure to another and the most appropriate method will depend on the specific research question of interest. Regardless of the statistical approach taken, analyses require understanding of the underlying pathways, and careful consideration of confounding, intermediate variables, and potential biases. Directed acyclic graphs can be used to express assumptions made about potential confounding and mediating variables, and to help identify variables to be controlled for in analyses (e.g. Greenland et al., 1999).

The workhorse for testing a simple association between an earlier life exposure and subsequent mental health outcome, or between mental health and other outcomes, is the generalized linear model. Such models are straightforward to implement, but have several limitations in addressing more complex life course hypotheses. They are unable to estimate multiple associations relating to pathways simultaneously, and cannot easily deal with repeated, and thus correlated, measures of the same exposure over time. Path analysis is a popular approach which is able to estimate direct associations between an exposure and an outcome simultaneously as well as the indirect effect through a mediator. Where latent variables are incorporated, to reduce the number of variables or to help correct measurement error in the observed variables, this is called structural equation modelling. When considering how a continuous repeated exposure, such as body size, influences a distal health outcome, a multitude of different statistical approaches have been proposed. The approaches range from simpler methods based on multivariable regression (Cole, 2007), through two-stage processes where firstly either characteristics of the growth curves (Tilling et al., 2011), or latent classes (Gaysina et al., 2011; Silverwood et al., 2013), are extracted and then related to the outcome, to full multivariate models in, for example, a structural equation model (De Stavola et al., 2006). Examples using some of these more complex models are illustrated in the following section.

Missing data are unavoidable in longitudinal and life course studies and can lead to biased estimates if not accounted for correctly. Statistical methods for dealing with missing data are well developed, although implementation can be complex in a life course setting. Multilevel models (estimated using maximum likelihood) allow for missing data in the outcome, provided that the data are missing at random and full information maximum likelihood is often implemented within structural equation models. Multiple imputation is one of the most popular methods of dealing with missing data (e.g. Sterne et al., 2009) and can be implemented in many statistical packages, and is particularly recommended when missing observations occur in the covariates. As cohorts age, the potential bias as a result of the high mortality rates and the increased likelihood of missing data being non-ignorable, alternative approaches need to be considered. In the context of longitudinal studies, joint models (e.g. Muniz-Terrera et al., 2011) which assess both survival and the evolution of the longitudinal ageing process simultaneously, while informing us about the association between both processes, may be useful.

Three examples of life course modelling of mental health from the British 1946 birth cohort

1. Longitudinal profiles of emotional symptoms: latent class analysis

This example illustrates how profiles of emotional symptoms over the life course can be identified when changing measures of mental health are used using latent class analysis (Colman et al., 2007). The data consisted of four types of age-appropriate measure representing emotional problems: teacher behavioural ratings at ages 13 and 15 years, subjected to classical linear factor analysis with one factor identified as internalizing emotions and behaviours; the Present State Examination at age 36 (a structured clinical interview schedule); the Psychiatric Symptom Frequency Scale at age 43 (an interview-based symptom scale); and the 28-item General Health Questionnaire at age 53 (a self-report symptom scale). From these measures, six life course profiles were defined. In order of frequency these were life course absence of symptoms (44.8%), repeated moderate symptoms (33.6%), adult-onset moderate symptoms (11.3%), adolescent symptoms with good adult outcome (5.8%), adult-onset severe symptoms (2.9%), and repeated severe symptoms (1.7%). These trajectories are illustrated in Figure 23.2.

To arrive at these final trajectories, the constituent measures were first modelled by confirmatory factor analysis. Factors were scored using a regression method, and regression

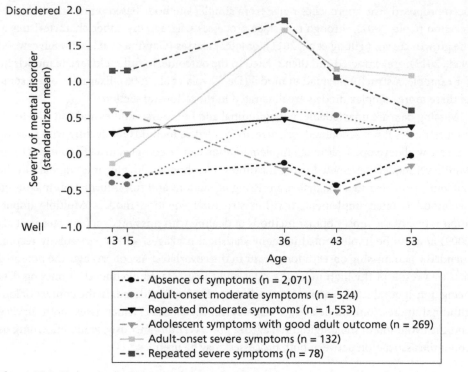

Figure 23.2 Six longitudinal classes of depressive and anxious symptomatology from age 11 to 53 years; the British 1946 birth cohort.

Reproduced with permission from Colman, I. et al. A longitudinal typology of symptoms of depression and anxiety over the life course. *Biological Psychology*, 62(11), 1265–1271. Copyright © 2007 Society of Biological Psychiatry. Published by Elsevier Inc. All rights reserved. DOI: https://doi.org/10.1016/j.biopsych.2007.05.012.

estimates were treated as continuous measures of depressive and anxious symptomatology at the five ages. Since all these measures exhibited floor effects, they were then converted into four-category ordinal variables, with the first group representing lack of symptoms (1st to 50th percentile); the second group representing occasional symptoms (51st to 75th percentile); the third group representing moderate symptoms (76th to 90th percentile); and the fourth group representing severe symptoms (91st to 100th percentile). Finally, latent class analysis was applied based on the hypothesis that these ordinal measures are indicators of unobserved latent classes underpinning a more valid typology of observed longitudinal symptom courses than a classification based on manifest characteristics alone. Latent class analysis estimates class membership probabilities for each individual using Bayes' theorem. Because the appropriate number of (unobserved) latent classes was initially unknown, seven classes were explored to derive the most parsimonious model, tested by multiple goodness-of-fit indices. The analysis included all individuals who had at least one of the five assessments of symptoms of depression and anxiety (n = 4627). Individuals who did not have all five assessments (1801 had five assessments, 952 had four, 650 had three, 952 had two, and 272 had one) were assigned to their most likely class on the basis of the available information and parameter estimates obtained under a missing at random assumption. These derived classes can then be used to investigate earlier life antecedents of longitudinal profiles of emotional symptoms. For example, those in the no-symptom and persistent severe symptom classes had, respectively, the highest and lowest birth weights; the next lowest mean birth weights were in those with repeated moderate symptoms and with adolescent-onset symptoms with good adult outcome, perhaps illustrating an early sequela of slow fetal growth. Class membership (or probabilities of membership) can also be used to relate life course symptoms with another health outcome (e.g. change in body mass index (Gaysina et al. 2011)). In this way, the latent class analysis can be seen as a way of summarizing the repeated exposure measures.

2. Life course pathways to depression: structural equation modelling (SEM)

As noted earlier, proximal influences on risk of depression are generally stronger than distal influences, unless the latter are extreme, such as severe abuse. This is demonstrated in a SEM that links pathways between early life factors and affective symptoms across adulthood via affective symptoms in adolescence and adult social position (Colman et al., 2014). The latent variables in the model illustrated here are neurodevelopment, consisting of four developmental milestones of age at sitting, standing, walking, and speaking words other than derivations of 'mother' or 'father'; acute stress in adulthood, consisting of adverse life events at ages 36, 43, and 53 years; emotional problems in adolescence; and the outcome of affective symptoms in adulthood. The components of the latter two latent variables are as described in example 1 previously. Observed variables also in the model were birth weight, crowding in the home at age 4 years (representing early deprivation), separation from the mother for more than 28 days before the age of 4 years, parental divorce during childhood, and adult occupational social class. The analytic sample consisted of 4627 study members with at least one assessment of affective symptoms. Models were estimated separately for males and females using robust weighted least squares estimation under a missing completely at random assumption. Figure 23.3 summarizes results for females. Note that the coefficients are standardized regression weights, and that all paths are mutually statistically independent. By standard convention, latent variables are represented as ellipses, and observed variables as rectangles.

It can be seen that easily the strongest influence on adult affective symptoms was from proximal stressful events. Independently, there were two separate paths of lesser magnitude to the outcome: one leading from early deprivation through parental divorce and low adult social position; and the other leading from birth weight through neurodevelopment and adolescent emotional problems, with neurodevelopment additionally influenced by early deprivation. The only variable with neither a direct nor indirect path to the outcome was separation from the mother. This pattern is broadly similar in males, except that separation from the mother rather than parental divorce or adult social class mediated the path from early deprivation (not shown).

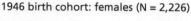

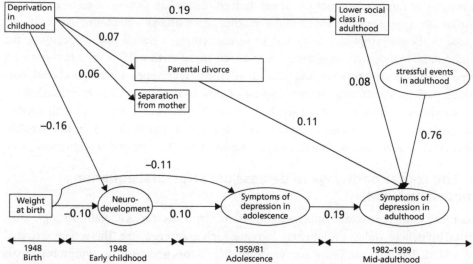

Figure 23.3 Significant pathways to symptoms of depression and anxiety among 2226 females in the British 1946 birth cohort. Values are standardized path coefficients.

Reproduced with permission from Colman, I. et al. Early development, stress and depression across the life course: pathways to depression in a national British birth cohort. *Psychological Medicine*, 44(13), 2845–2854. © Cambridge University Press 2014. DOI: https://doi.org/10.1017/S0033291714000385.

3. Consequences of adolescent mental health: latent growth modelling

Our third example is distinct from the first two examples in two ways. First, by focusing on associations between adolescent mental health and midlife memory it investigates long-term consequences of mental health. Second, this example involves repeated measures of the memory outcome. Latent growth modelling was used to estimate paths from adolescent mental health and verbal memory intercept at age 43 years, and memory slope over two further measurement points, at ages 53 and 60–64 years (Xu et al., 2013). Exploratory factor analysis was used to partition teacher ratings of adolescent mental health into emotional problems, conduct problems, and self-organization. SEM incorporating latent growth analyses then estimated simultaneous paths between these adolescent factors and memory intercept and slope, with educational attainment as a potential mediator. Also incorporated in the model were paths from cognition at age 8 years to the adolescent mental health factors, educational attainment, and memory intercept and slope, to control for possible selection effects by cognitive ability. All variables except educational attainment were modelled as latent variables. Goodness of fit was found to be adequate by a range of indices, as was measurement invariance of the latent memory variables using maximum likelihood. The model indicated negligible associations between adolescent emotional and conduct problems and memory intercept and slope, but a strong association between adolescent self-organization and memory intercept (but not slope). This was largely mediated by educational attainment although a modest residual association remained. This path was independent of childhood cognition, although the latter strongly predicted self-organization. This model is shown in Figure 23.4.

Conclusion

Life course epidemiology provides a powerful framework for studying determinants, trajectories and consequences of mental health across multiple stages of the life course in the general population. Life course epidemiology helps to clarify distinctions between sensitive period and accumulation models, with potential implications for intervention. Arguably the principal resource for life course epidemiology is the birth cohort, since these have the advantages of general population representation; prospective follow-up; narrow age bands that allow for the study of age-related change which is not confounded by cohort effects; and, typically, measures across multiple biomedical and social domains, thus enabling mental health to be studies in a holistic context. As these birth cohorts age, they will be in a strong position to shed light into a corner that still remains dimly lit in psychiatric epidemiology: how risk of mental disorders and their consequences for physical health, daily function, and survival are patterned over the third age.

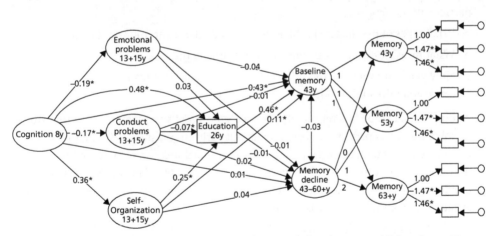

Figure 23.4 Longitudinal path diagram representing associations between childhood cognition, adolescent mental health, educational attainment, and memory at 43 years (baseline) and from 43 to 60–64 years (rate of decline). * p <0.01. For ease of reading paths from gender are omitted from this figure. The rectangular boxes on the right in grey represent three memory task trials at each age.

Practical exercises

Please answer the following questions:

1. The Adult Psychiatric Morbidity Surveys of 2000 and 2007 provide comprehensive descriptions of psychiatric disorders for private household-dwelling residents in England aged between 16 and 74 years.

   a. What kinds of information would be added to these descriptions from the methods typically used in life course studies?

   b. What information is likely to be lost with a complete switch to these life course approaches?

2. A 2016 report from the UK Office for National Statistics using the Annual Population Survey (the 'census') shows that psychological well-being tends to decrease from early adulthood to midlife and is at its lowest around ages 45–60 years.

   a. What are the limitations on interpreting these as valid age effects?

   b. How might a life course study overcome these limitations?

   c. What limitations might such a design face in turn?

3. A large national birth cohort has been followed up to age 12 years, and you have now been invited as a specialist to develop its capacity to assess mental health. The birth cohort study is multidisciplinary, the budget is constrained, and there are concerns about participant burden.

   a. What types of psychiatric problem do you consider most important to capture?

   b. What measures would you consider for capturing these?

   c. How viable are these methods likely to be as the cohort transitions through adolescence and into adulthood?

4. A longitudinal study has repeatedly assessed emotional symptoms in the same study members, and has previous information about early circumstances (e.g. father's occupation), educational attainment, labour market attachment, and partnership formation. You are interested not only in testing for the kind of trend in emotional symptoms previously described in question 2, but also in whether change in symptoms is influenced by any of the earlier experiences.

   a. What methods would you use to address these questions?

   b. What are the statistical assumptions of these methods, and are they likely to be met with these kinds of data?

Further reading

Colman, I., Jones, P.B., Kuh, D., Weeks, M., Naiker, K., Richards, M., and Croudace, T.J. (2014). Early development, stress and depression across the life course: pathways to depression in a national British birth cohort. *Psychological Medicine*, 44, 2845–2854.

Koenen, K.C., Rudenstein, S., Susser, E., and Galea, S. (eds.). (2014). *A life course approach to mental disorders*. Oxford: Oxford University Press.

Kuh, D., Richards, M., Cooper, R., Hardy, R., and Ben-Shlomo, Y. (2014). Life course epidemiology, ageing research, and maturing cohort studies: a dynamic combination for understanding healthy ageing. In: Kuh, D., Cooper, R., Hardy, R., Richards, M., and Ben-Shlomo, Y. (eds.). *A life course approach to healthy ageing*, pp. 3–15. Oxford: Oxford University Press.

References

Allebeck, P. and Allgulander, C. (1990). Psychiatric diagnoses as predictors of suicide. A comparison of diagnoses at conscription and in psychiatric care in a cohort of 50,465 young men. *British Journal of Psychiatry*, 157, 339–344.

Barker, D.J.P. (1992). *Fetal and infant origins of adult disease*. London: British Medical Journal.

Clark, C., Rodgers, B., Caldwell, T., Power, C., and Stansfeld, S. (2007). Childhood and adulthood psychological ill health as predictors of midlife affective and anxiety disorders: the 1958 British Birth Cohort. *Archives of General Psychiatry*, 64, 668–678.

Cole, T. (2007). The life course plot in life course analysis. In: Pickles, A., Maughan, B., and Wadsworth, M. (eds.). *Epidemiological methods in life course research*, pp. 137–155. Oxford: Oxford University Press.

Collishaw, S. (2015). Annual research review: secular trends in child and adolescent mental health. *Journal of Child Psychology and Psychiatry*, 56, 370–393.

Collishaw, S., Maughan, B., and Pickles, A. (2004). Recent trends in UK child and adolescent mental health. *British Journal of Psychiatry*, 185, 350–351.

Colman, I., Jones, P.B., Kuh, D., Weeks, M., Naiker, K., Richards, M., and Croudace, T.J. (2014). Early development, stress and depression across the life course: pathways to depression in a national British birth cohort. *Psychological Medicine*, 44, 2845–2854.

Colman, I., Ploubidis, G., Wadsworth, M.E.J., Jones, P.B., and Croudace, T.J. (2007). A longitudinal typology of symptoms of depression and anxiety over the life course. *Biological Psychology*, 62, 1265–1271.

Connelly, R. and Platt, L. (2014). Cohort profile: UK Millennium Cohort Study (MCS). *International Journal of Epidemiology*, 43, 1719–1725.

Costello, E.J., Erkanli, A., and Angold, A. (2006). Is there an epidemic of child or adolescent depression? *Journal of Child Psychology and Psychiatry*, 47, 1263–1271.

Deary, I.J., Gow, A.J., Pattie, A., and Starr, J.M. (2012). Cohort profile: the Lothian Birth Cohorts of 1921 and 1936. *International Journal of Epidemiology*, 41, 1576–1584.

De Stavola, B.L., Nitsch, D., dos Santos S, I, McCormack, V., Hardy, R., Mann, V., et al. (2006). Statistical issues in life course epidemiology. *American Journal of Epidemiology*, 163, 84–96.

Elliott, J. and Shepherd, P. (2006). Cohort profile: 1970 British Birth Cohort (BCS70). *International Journal of Epidemiology*, 35, 836–843.

Fraser, A., Macdonald-Wallis, C., Tilling, K., Boyd, A., Golding, J., Davey Smith, G., et al. (2013). Cohort profile: the Avon Longitudinal Study of Parents and Children: ALSPAC mothers cohort. *International Journal of Epidemiology*, 42, 97–110.

Gaysina, D., Hotopf, M., Richards, M., Colman, I., Kuh, D., and Hardy, R. (2011). Symptoms of depression and anxiety, and change in body mass index from adolescence to adulthood: results from a British birth cohort. *Psychological Medicine*, 41, 175–184.

Greenland, S., Pearl, J., and Robins, J.M. (1999). Causal diagrams for epidemiologic research. *Epidemiology*, 10, 37–48.

Hardy, R. and **Kuh, D.** (2009). Discussant chapter—the practicalities of undertaking family-based studies. In: Lawlor, D.A. and Mishra, G.D. (eds.). *Family matters: designing, analysing and understanding family-based studies in life course epidemiology*, pp. 181–191. Oxford: Oxford University Press.

Henderson, M., Hotopf, M., Shah, I., Hayes, R.D., and **Kuh, D.** (2011). Psychiatric disorder in early adulthood and risk of premature mortality in the 1946 British Birth Cohort. *BMC Psychiatry*, **11**, 37.

Jones, P.J., Rodgers, B., **Murray, R.,** and Marmot, M. (1994). Child development risk factors for adult schizophrenia in the British 1946 birth cohort. *Lancet*, **344**, 1398–1402.

Kessler, R.C., Amminger, G.P., Aguilar-Gaxiola, S., Alonso, J., Lee, S., and Ustun, T.B. (2007). Age of onset of mental disorders: a review of recent literature. *Current Opinion in Psychiatry*, **20**, 359–364.

Keyes, K.M. and Li, G. (2012). Age–period–cohort modeling. In: Li, G. and Baker, S.P. (eds.). *Injury research: theory, methods, and approaches*, pp. 409–426. New York: Springer.

Kuh, D. and Ben Shlomo, Y. (2004). *A life course approach to chronic disease epidemiology*, 2nd edn. Oxford: Oxford University Press.

Kuh, D., Pierce, M., Adams, J., Deanfield, J., Ekelund, U., Friberg, P., et al. (2011). Cohort profile: updating the cohort profile for the MRC National Survey of Health and Development: a new clinic-based data collection for ageing research. *International Journal of Epidemiology*, **40**, e1–e9.

Lee, W., Kwok, C.H.T., Hunter, E., Richards, M., and David, A.S. (2012). Prevalence and childhood antecedents of depersonalization syndrome in a UK Birth Cohort. *Social Psychiatry and Psychiatric Epidemiology*, **47**, 253–261.

Lewis, G., Pelosi, A.J., Araya, R., and Dunn, G. (1992). Measuring psychiatric disorder in the community: a standardized assessment for use by lay interviewers. *Psychological Medicine*, **22**, 465–486.

Matthews, F.E., Arthur, A., Barnes, L.E., Bond, J., Jagger, C., Robinson, L., et al. (2013). A two-decade comparison of prevalence of dementia in individuals aged 65 years and older from three geographical areas of England: results of the Cognitive Function and Ageing Study I and II. *Lancet*, **382**, 1405–1412.

Moffitt, T. (1993). Adolescent-limited and life-course-persistent antisocial behaviour: a developmental taxonomy. *Psychological Review*, **100**, 674–701.

Moffitt, T.E., Arseneault, L., Belsky, D., Dickson, N., Hancox, R.J., Harrington, H., et al. (2011). A gradient of childhood self-control predicts health, wealth, and public safety. *Proceedings of the National Academy of Science of the United States of America*, **108**, 2693–2698.

Muniz Terrera, G., Piccinin, A.M., Matthews, F., and Hofer, S.M. (2011). Joint modeling of longitudinal change and survival: an investigation of the association between change in memory scores and death. *GeroPsych*, **24**, 177.

Pearlin, L. (2010). The life course and the stress process: some conceptual comparisons. *Journal of Gerontology Series B: Psychological Sciences and Social Sciences*, **65B**, 207–215.

Pearlin, L., Menaghan, E.G., Lieberman, M.A., and Mullan, J.T. (1981). The stress process. *Journal of Health and Social Behavior*, **22**, 337–356.

Power, C. and Elliott, J. (2006). Cohort profile: 1958 British birth cohort (National Child Developmental Study). *International Journal of Epidemiology*, **35**, 34–41.

Quinton, D. and **Rutter, M.** (1988). *Parenting breakdown: the making and breaking of inter-generational links*. Aldershot: Avebury.

Richards, M. (2014). Cognitive function over the life course. In: Koenen, K.C., Rudenstine, S., Susser, E., and Galea, S. (eds.). *A life course approach to mental disorders*, pp. 185–193. Oxford: Oxford University Press.

Richards, M. and **Abbott, R.** (2009). Childhood mental health and life chances in post-war Britain: insights from three national birth cohort studies. Centre for Mental Health. http://www.centreformentalhealth.org.uk/pdfs/life_chances_report.pdf

Richards, M. and **Huppert, F.A.** (2011). Do positive children become positive adults? Evidence from a longitudinal birth cohort study. *Journal of Positive Psychology*, **6**, 75–87.

Rutter, M. (1989). Pathways from childhood to adult life. *Journal of Child Psychology and Psychiatry*, **30**, 23–51.

Rutter, M. (1999). Resilience concepts and findings: implications for family therapy. *Journal of Family Therapy*, **21**, 119–144.

Rutter, M., Kim-Cohen, J., and **Maughan, B.** (2006). Continuities and discontinuities in psychopathology between childhood and adult life. *Journal of Child Psychology and Psychiatry*, **47**, 276–295.

Seidman, L.J., Cherkerzian, S., **Goldstein, J.M.**, Agnew-Blais, J., **Tsuang, M.T.**, and **Buka, S.L.** (2013). Neuropsychological performance and family history in children at age 7 who develop adult schizophrenia or bipolar psychosis in the New England Family Studies. *Psychological Medicine*, **43**, 119–131.

Shenkin, S.D., Starr, J.M., and **Deary, I.J.** (2004). Birth weight and cognitive ability in childhood: a systematic review. *Psychological Bulletin*, **130**, 989–1013.

Silverwood, R.J., Pierce, M., **Hardy, R.**, Sattar, N., **Ferro, C.**, Savage, C., et al. (2013). Early-life overweight trajectory and CKD in the 1946 British birth cohort study. *American Journal of Kidney Diseases*, **62**, 276–284.

Sterne, J.A., White, I.R., **Carlin, J.B.**, Spratt, M., **Royston, P.**, Kenward, M.G., et al. (2009). Multiple imputation for missing data in epidemiological and clinical research: potential and pitfalls. *British Medical Journal*, **338**, b2393.

Tilling, K., Davies, N.M., **Nicoli, E.**, Ben-Shlomo, Y., **Kramer, M.S.**, Patel, R., et al. (2011). Associations of growth trajectories in infancy and early childhood with later childhood outcomes. *American Journal of Clinical Nutrition*, **94**, 1808S–1813S.

von Stumm, S., Deary, I.J., and **Hagger-Johnson, G.** (2013). Life-course pathways to psychological distress: a cohort study. *BMJ Open*, **3**, e002772.

Weissman, M., Wickramaratne, P., **Nomura, Y.**, Warner, V., **Pilowsky, D.**, and **Verdeli, H.** (2006). Offspring of depressed parents: 20 years later. *American Journal of Psychiatry*, **163**, 1001–1008.

Wojcik, W., Lee, W., **Colman, I.**, Hardy, R., and **Hotopf, M.** (2013). Foetal origins of depression? A systematic review and meta-analysis of low birth weight and later depression. *Psychological Medicine*, **43**, 1–12.

Xu, M.K., Jones, P.B., **Barnett, J.H.**, Gaysina, D., **Kuh, D.**, Croudace, T.J., and **Richards, M.** (2013). Adolescent self-organization predicts midlife memory in a prospective birth cohort study. *Psychology and Aging*, **28**, 958–968.

Chapter 24

Evidence-based mental health policy

Valentina Iemmi, Nicole Votruba, and
Graham Thornicroft

Introduction

The use of research evidence to inform decisions related to health has been growing since the 1990s. Initially focused on evidence-based medicine, the drive has been expanding to evidence-based healthrelated policymaking. Since 2004, the World Health Organization (WHO) has stressed the importance of putting research into action (WHO, 2004a), supporting evidence-based public health, health services, and health policies (WHO, 2004b). In this view, the WHO has been advocating for the importance of establishing or strengthening knowledge translation of research results to different stakeholders (WHO, 2005a), especially focusing upon the need to pay attention to the diversity of languages and the use of information technologies (WHO, 2009). Evidence-based mental health policy has been fully aligned with this impetus (Cooper, 2003).

This chapter considers evidence-based mental health policymaking with the help of illustrative examples. In the next section of the chapter we shall provide a brief description of evidence-based mental health policy and its rationale. In the third section, we illustrate how mental health research may help to inform mental health policy. In the fourth section we provide examples of the use of research in mental health policy at different organizational levels. Finally, we reflect on the opportunities and challenges of evidence-based mental health policy in the future.

What is evidence-based mental health policy?

Although mental and substance use disorders account for 7.4% of the total global burden of disease (Whiteford et al., 2013), only a small proportion of national health budgets is allocated to the treatment and prevention of mental disorders, ranging from 0.5% in low-income countries to 5.1% in high-income countries (WHO, 2013a). This scarcity raises the question of how to best use the available resources not only *effectively* (what works?), but also *efficiently* (what is the best use of resources?), and *equitably* (are all different groups in the population receiving care according to their needs?).

Research evidence may help inform the very difficult choices that policymakers are confronted with, from the design of new mental health policies to their evaluation (Oxman et al., 2009), such as identifying effective and efficient mental health interventions and deciding which services to offer, how to better deliver them, how to fund them, and how to evaluate their implementation. Thus, evidence may be crucial to allow policymakers to design mental health services and systems that are more effective, efficient, and equitable (Saxena et al., 2007).

Evidence-based healthcare policymaking, and therefore evidence-based mental health policymaking, is 'an approach to policy decisions that aims to ensure that decision-making is well-informed by the best available research evidence' (WHO, 2015a). In evidence-based mental health policymaking, recommendations are produced from a combination of research evidence and expert opinions. Once the research evidence is reviewed, expert opinions are crucial in interpreting the evidence and drawing conclusions. Evidence-based recommendations are then provided to policymakers to help inform their final decisions. The process, in theory, is both *systematic* and *transparent* (Oxman et al., 2009). The research evidence is reviewed systematically in order to allow a comprehensive coverage of relevant studies and their quality. The process is transparent to permit reproducibility and to ensure that bias and conflict of interests do not affect final decisions. Notwithstanding its transparency, other factors may influence the process, such as population characteristics, needs and preferences, availability of human and financial resources, and environmental and organizational contexts (Brownson et al., 2009a).

From mental health research to mental health policy

What is the research cycle?

The 'research cycle' or 'measurement loop' (Tugwell et al., 1985) was initially designed to illustrate the research process applied to health interventions and health services, but may be extended to health policies. The research cycle conceptualizes the research process as an iterative sequence of the following seven stages (Figure 24.1):

1. Identification of the burden of disease, when the burden of disease is quantified (e.g. estimation of the prevalence of depression).

2. Definition of the theories of causation, when possible causes of the burden of disease are identified and assessed (e.g. identification of factors associated with depression).

3. Establishment of the effectiveness, when benefits and harms of potentially feasible interventions are evaluated (e.g. evaluation of the impact of cognitive behavioural therapy for people suffering from depression on clinical outcomes and quality of life).

4. Establishment of the efficiency, when the economic value of potentially feasible (and effective) interventions is evaluated (e.g. evaluation of the cost-effectiveness of cognitive behavioural therapy for people suffering from depression).

5. Implementation, when information from different studies evaluating effectiveness, efficiency, and feasibility are used to draw recommendations to inform decision-makers' choice, and promising interventions are implemented (e.g. implementation

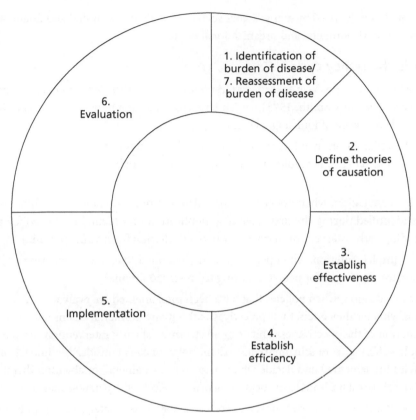

Figure 24.1 The research cycle.

Adapted with permission from Tugwell, P. et al. The measurement iterative loop: a framework for the critical appraisal of need, benefits and costs of health interventions. *Journal of Chronic Diseases,* 38(4), 339–51. Copyright © 1985 Published by Elsevier Inc. DOI: https://doi.org/10.1016/0021-9681(85)90080-3.

of cognitive behavioural therapy along with drug treatment for people suffering from depression).

6. Evaluation, when interventions that have been implemented are monitored and evaluated to appraise whether they have a positive impact on outcomes and costs, without engendering unintended consequences (e.g. evaluation of the effectiveness and cost-effectiveness of cognitive behavioural therapy along with drug treatment for people suffering from depression as implemented).

7. Reassessment of the burden of disease, when the burden of disease after implementation of the interventions is compared with the initial burden of disease (e.g. estimation of the prevalence of depression after the implementation of the intervention). Following this last stage, the cycle will start again with a new sequence of stages.

The seven stages described are a schematic representation of the research process. While they are useful to understand how the research process works, the process is usually more

complicated as influenced by many factors such as availability of human and financial resources, and environmental and organizational contexts.

What is the policy cycle?

The most common approach to understand policy process is the 'stages heuristic' model
(Sabatier and Jenkins-Smith, 1993), which conceptualizes the policy process as a linear
(or cyclical) sequence of four stages (Figure 24.2):

1. Problem identification and issue recognition, when issues to tackle are identified and
   the agenda set (e.g. recognition of the burden of schizophrenia for individuals and
   society).

2. Policy formulation, when policies are formulated in order to address the different issues identified during the first stage (e.g. publication of a mental health policy plan
   including early intervention services for people suffering from schizophrenia).

3. Policy implementation, when policies are implemented (e.g. implementation of early
   intervention services for people suffering from schizophrenia).

4. Policy evaluation, when policies that have been implemented are evaluated in order to
   assess whether they attain their objectives without any unintended consequences (e.g.
   evaluation of the effectiveness and cost-effectiveness of early intervention services for
   people suffering from schizophrenia). Then, policymakers consider the impact of the
   policies implemented and decide whether to continue, amend, or abandon them. The
   end of this last stage leads to the beginning of a new cycle with a new sequence of stages.

As for the research cycle, these four stages are a schematic representation of the policy process which is more complex in reality. While this cycle is useful to understand how the policy
process works, we need to recognize that the process is never as linear (or cyclical) and often
more similar to 'muddling through' (Lindblom, 1959), as influenced by different factors
such as human and financial resources, and environmental and organizational contexts.

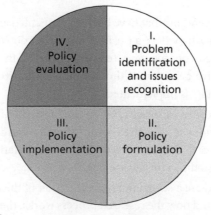

Figure 24.2 The policy cycle.

How are the research cycle and the policy cycle related?

In evidence-based mental health policymaking, each of the four stages constituting the policy cycle are informed by different stages of the research cycle (Figure 24.3). The decisions made during the first stage (problem identification and issue recognition) may be informed by studies identifying the burden of disease and defining the theories of causation (research cycle stages 1–2). The decisions made during the second stage (policy formulation) may be informed by studies evaluating the effectiveness and efficiency of interventions, services, or policies (research cycle stages 3–4). The decisions made during the third stage (policy implementation) may be informed by the synthesis of studies on effectiveness, efficiency, and feasibility of interventions, services, or policies (research cycle stage 5). Finally, the decisions made during the fourth and final stage (policy evaluation) may be informed by studies monitoring and evaluating interventions, services, or policies that have been implemented, and by studies quantifying the burden of disease after implementation (research cycle stage 6). While in evidence-based mental health policymaking research evidence contributes to each stage of the policy cycle, different types of epidemiological and intervention studies may inform different stages.

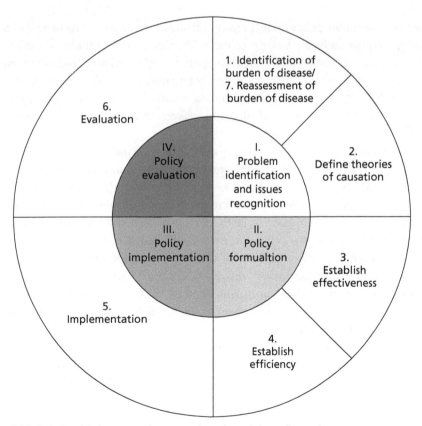

Figure 24.3 Relationship between the research cycle and the policy cycle.

What use are epidemiological studies for policy?

In evidence-based mental health policy, decisions are informed by reviews of the evidence. Systematic literature review and meta-analysis are considered the gold standard to collect and analyse information from original studies, by using an approach that minimizes bias (see Chapter 15). However, sometimes non-systematic literature reviews and rapid evidence assessment may be a better choice when human and financial resources are limited, when information needs to be produced in a short time frame, or when questions asked are better answered by a non-systematic approach (Government Social Research Unit, 2009).

All types of studies described in the chapters of this book may be used to inform different stages of the policy cycle. However, while different study designs may be included in a literature review, a hierarchy of evidence applies according to the robustness of the study design: systematic reviews and meta-analysis, randomized controlled trials, cohort studies, case–control studies, cross-sectional surveys, ecological and cross-level studies, case series and case reports, and expert opinions. While the inclusion of different study designs in the literature review depends on the stage of the policy cycle, their weight depends on the robustness of their study design (and their quality).

The first stage of the policy cycle (problem identification and issue recognition) may be informed by quantitative studies (e.g. cohort studies, case–control studies, cross-sectional surveys, ecological studies, and cross-level studies) and qualitative studies that may inform decision-makers' choices in the absence of quantitative studies. When more robust evidence is lacking, expert opinions—including experts from all stakeholders groups (e.g. service users and carers)—may help decision-makers. In addition, this first stage may be informed by cost-of-illness studies.

The subsequent three stages of the policy cycle (policy formulation, policy implementation, policy evaluation), may be informed preferably by randomized controlled trials, that are considered to be the gold standard for evaluating interventions, services and policies, and by other controlled studies (e.g. non-randomized controlled trials, controlled before–after studies, and controlled interrupted time series studies with multiple points of evaluation after the intervention). In the absence of controlled studies, non-controlled studies (e.g. cross-sectional surveys, ecological studies, and cross-level studies) and qualitative studies may inform decision-makers' choices. When more robust evidence is missing, expert opinions may inform decision-makers' choices. Moreover, those three stages may be informed by economic evaluations, conducted along each of the previous study designs, or economic modelling.

More recently, the increasing number of systematic reviews and meta-analysis of reviews has gained the interest of policymakers. In particular, open-access databases of systematic reviews of interventions have been created (e.g. the Cochrane Library and the Campbell Collaboration Library). Table 24.1 provides examples of different types of studies that may be used to inform the four stages of the policy cycle.

Table 24.1 Example of study types used to inform the policy cycle

Policy cycle	Research cycle	Example of relevant epidemiological studies
I. Problem identification and issue recognition	1. Identification of the burden of disease (and 7. Reassessment of the burden of disease)	◆ Systematic review and meta-analysis of cohort studies to estimate mortality among people with mental disorders, and their differences by type of death and diagnosis (Walker et al., 2015) ◆ Global Burden of Diseases, Injuries, and Risk Factors Study 2010, to estimate the burden of disease attributable to mental and substance use disorders (Whiteford et al., 2013) ◆ National survey to estimate the prevalence of schizophrenia-related disability in the Chinese population, factors associated with differences in prevalence rates between women and men and across geographic regions (Liu et al., 2015) ◆ Cross-sectional surveys to estimate the prevalence of perinatal mental disorders, their determinants, and their association with preventive healthcare use in northern Viet Nam (Fisher et al., 2010) ◆ Cost of illness of dementia globally, including direct and indirect economic costs (Wimo and Prince, 2010) ◆ Cost of illness of schizophrenia in Japan, including direct and indirect economic costs (Sado et al., 2013) ◆ Cost of illness of autism in the UK and US, including direct, indirect, and lifetime societal economic costs (Buescher et al., 2014)
	2. Define theories of causation	◆ Systematic review of epidemiological studies to exam the relationship between poverty and common mental disorders in developing countries (Lund et al., 2010) ◆ Prospective study with 2-year follow-up evaluating the influence of presenteeism on depression and sickness absences due to mental disease in a cohort of Japanese workers (Suzuki et al., 2015) ◆ Longitudinal national survey to study risk factors for poor longitudinal outcomes in individuals with untreated common mental disorders in the US (Henriksen et al., 2015) ◆ Longitudinal surveys to assess unemployment rates among individuals with mental health problems before and during the current economic recession in Europe (Evans-Lacko et al., 2013a) ◆ Longitudinal surveys to study the association between public knowledge, attitudes, and behaviours and the internalization of stigma among people with mental health problems in Europe (Evans-Lacko et al., 2012)

(continued)

Table 24.1 Continued

Policy cycle	Research cycle	Example of relevant epidemiological studies
II. Policy formulation	3. Establish effectiveness	◆ Systematic review and meta-analysis of randomized and non-randomized controlled trials to evaluate the effectiveness of psychosocial interventions for perinatal common mental disorders delivered by providers who are not mental health specialists in developing countries (Clarke et al., 2013) ◆ Randomized controlled trial to evaluate the effectiveness of a community-based care intervention for people with schizophrenia and their caregivers in India (Chatterjee et al., 2014) ◆ Before–after study to evaluate the impact of Time to Change's social marketing interventions on stigma in England (Evans-Lacko et al., 2013b)
	4. Establish efficiency	◆ Economic evaluation alongside a randomized controlled trial to evaluate the effectiveness and cost-effectiveness of cognitive behavioural therapy in adolescents suffering with depression in the Netherlands (Stikkelbroek et al., 2013) ◆ Economic evaluation along a pilot randomized controlled study to evaluate the effectiveness and cost-effectiveness of peer support in addition to usual aftercare for patients during the transition from hospital to home in the UK (Simpson et al., 2014) ◆ Economic modelling to evaluate the cost consequences of early intervention for first-episode psychosis in England in relation to employment, education, homicide, and suicide (Park et al., 2014) ◆ Economic modelling to evaluate the costs and longer-term savings of parenting programmes for the prevention of persistent conduct disorder in England (Bonin et al., 2011)
III. Policy implementation	5. Implementation	◆ See 'Policy formulation (establish effectiveness)' ◆ See 'Policy formulation (establish efficiency)' ◆ Qualitative study exploring reasons for non-adherence to medication in people with schizophrenia in Ethiopia (Teferra et al., 2013) ◆ Qualitative study exploring the health visitors' perceptions on cognitive behavioural therapy to treat postnatal depression (Brown and Reynolds, 2014)

Table 24.1 Continued

Policy cycle	Research cycle	Example of relevant epidemiological studies
IV. Policy evaluation	6. Evaluation	◆ Before–after study to evaluate the impact of the implementation of mental health service recommendations in England and Wales on suicide rates (While et al., 2012) ◆ Retrospective study to evaluate the impact of the Mental Health Act 1983 on the number of voluntary and involuntary admissions for mental disorders in England (Keown et al., 2008) ◆ Longitudinal cohort study to evaluate the effectiveness of early intervention services for people with a first episode of psychosis in England (Birchwood et al., 2014) ◆ Longitudinal study to evaluate the effectiveness of deinstitutionalization of people with long-term mental illness in Australia (Hobbs et al., 2002) ◆ Longitudinal study to evaluate the impact of implementation of deinstitutionalization of psychiatric services on the use of inpatient and outpatient care, and per capita expenditures on psychiatric services in Canada (Sealy and Whitehead, 2004)

Evidence-based mental health policy in context

Evidence-based mental health policy can inform decision-makers at any level, from the clinical level (micro-level), through service provision/healthcare facility level (meso-level) and the whole health system level (macro-level), to the global level (mega-level). While the following sections will provide examples of evidence-based mental health policy at these four levels, we would like to emphasize that all levels are closely interrelated and they help inform each other.

Micro-level

Evidence may help inform decision-makers at the *clinical* level on the best available mental healthcare. An outstanding example is provided by the National Institute for Health and Care Excellence (NICE) in England. NICE, established in 1999, is an independent agency responsible for developing national guidelines to help health and social care professionals 'deliver the best possible care based on the best available evidence' (NICE, 2013a). Clinical guidelines are produced through an iterative process including systematic reviews and meta-analysis of epidemiological and intervention studies, and experts' opinion (NICE, 2014). For example, the NICE guideline on management and support of children and young people on the autism spectrum, developed by a Guideline Development Group of experts on autism using a series of systematic review of the evidence and economic models, summarizes recommendations on the best available psychological, pharmacological, and biomedical interventions aimed to support children and young people on the autism spectrum and their carers (NICE, 2013b).

Similar agencies are developing around the world, such as the National Center for Health Technology Excellence (CENETEC-Salud) in Mexico. The CENETEC-Salud, established in 2004, is an independent agency aiming to produce recommendations on the best care based on the best available evidence to help in informing clinical decisions and guaranteeing the best use of resources. The guidelines are produced with a process similar to the iterative process used by NICE, including review of the evidence and expert opinion. For example, the CENETEC-Salud guideline on diagnosis and treatment of depression in adults provides recommendations on the best diagnostic practices and the best available pharmacological and non-pharmacological interventions for the treatment of depression in adults (Secretaría de Salud, 2009).

Meso-level

Evidence may help inform decision-makers at the *service provision/healthcare facility* level, from commissioners to providers, on the best available mental health services. An ambitious example is the National Service Framework for Mental Health (NSF-MH) in England (Department of Health, 1999). The NSF-MH, published by the Department of Health in 1999, set a 10-year agenda for improving adults' mental healthcare through the description of 'national standards for mental health, what they aim to achieve, how they should be developed and delivered and how to measure performance in every part of the country' (Department of Health, 1999, p. 1). The NSF-MH was based on review of evidence and experts' opinion of an External Reference Group (Thornicroft, 2000). The process helped identify seven standards for mental health (mental health promotion, primary care and access to services (comprising two standards), effective services for people with severe mental illness (comprising two standards), caring about carers, and preventing suicide) that were subsequently implemented across England.

The implementation of the NSF-MH was evaluated through the years using different study designs. For example, a before–after study found a decrease in suicide rates in areas having implemented NSF-MH recommendations (While et al., 2012). Following recommendations of the NSF-MH, crisis resolution and home treatment teams were introduced in England to reduce inpatient admissions and readmissions of people undergoing a severe mental health crisis. An observational study evaluating their implementation found a reduction in hospital admissions across England (Glover et al., 2006). Similarly, following recommendations of the NSF-MH, assertive community treatment (ACT) teams were introduced in England to reduce inpatient admissions of people suffering with severe mental disorders, a high use of inpatient care but difficult engagement with standard mental health services. A randomized controlled trial evaluating the implementation of ACT found no decrease in use of inpatient care 3 years after implementation of ACT, but better engagement with the service (Killapsy et al., 2009).

Macro-level

Evidence may help inform decision-makers at the whole *health system* level, on broader issues from best available models of organization of services and coordination, through workforce organization and training, to funding, quality measurement, and governance. Globally, health systems have overlooked mental disorders for too long. This is reflected in the limited, yet in the last decade, steadily growing number of countries with specific mental health policies. The WHO *Mental Health Atlas* reports in 2011 that only 60% of nations worldwide have a mental health policy, with a large majority of those countries being in high-income settings (WHO, 2011). Mental health policies are specific to each country, and influenced by the specific political, economic, social, and cultural context. For example, in low- and middle-income countries frequently critical factors such as poverty, conflict, or political instability add to the complexity of the process (Sutcliffe and Court, 2005).

An outstanding example of an evidence-based mental health policy at the health system level is presented by Ethiopia. Notwithstanding ranking among the poorest countries in the world (World Bank, 2015) and being so restrained in economic and natural resources, in the last decades Ethiopia has made great efforts and improvements in scaling up the overall health system, as well as mental health system, by leading a challenging evidence-based policy (Wamai, 2009). A first-ever national health policy, and consecutive health sector development plans, were developed from the early 1990s. As part of a mental health policy, in 2012 the Ministry of Health recognized mental health as a major health priority and adopted an ambitious mental health strategy (Federal Democratic Republic of Ethiopia Ministry of Health, 2012). Integrated in the national health policy, the strategy focuses on primary healthcare services and decentralization, in line with global evidence-based mental health recommendations (WHO, 2008, 2013b). The Ethiopian government acknowledges an expected rise in mental illness in the next years, and has defined mental health as a major health priority (Federal Democratic Republic of Ethiopia Ministry of Health, 2012). The gradual implementation of the new evidence-based mental health policy is an important achievement (Fekadu and Thornicroft, 2014). However, the change from a poorly developed mental health system to scaling up mental health services is a large undertaking, particularly considering other competing health system challenges. For Ethiopia to continue following its ambitious goals, research capacity would need to continue to increase and thus the evidence produced by local and regional researchers.

Mega-level

Evidence may help inform decision-makers at the *global* level, on overarching recommendations from the best available care, through models of service provision/healthcare facility, to mental health systems. International organizations as the WHO and the Organization for Economic Cooperation and Development (OECD) have taken a leading role in the field of health and mental health, by providing evidence-based guidelines and policies (Dua et al., 2011; OECD, 2014). While global guidelines and policies can be ground-breaking landmarks, their legislative power depends on the political commitment of each state, as well as the implementability of policies in different political, economic, social, and cultural settings. So far, the majority of the evidence generated and contributing to mental health research and policies came from developed countries, and greatly neglected the evidence on needs and specific conditions in developing countries. While 85% of all people with mental health problems live in low- and middle-income countries, only 10% of the world's medical research addresses these (Lancet Global Mental Health Group, 2007). Thus, evidence-based global mental health policies demand focusing on these neglected parts of the world.

In 2000, the WHO launched the Project Atlas in order to gain and disseminate global evidence on mental health resources (Saraceno and Saxena, 2002). The following year, the WHO *World Health Report 2001* provided a first comprehensive review of the existing evidence on the global burden of mental and substance use disorders, mental health policies, and mental health service provision (WHO 2001a). In the same year, the first global *Mental Health Atlas* was published with information on mental health resources as individual country profiles (WHO, 2001b), and sequentially updated (WHO, 2005b, 2011). In 2005, the WHO Assessment Instrument for Mental Health System (WHO-AIMS) was designed to gather comprehensive information on mental health systems in order to establish mental health country profiles in low- and middle-income countries (WHO 2015b). Similarly, the OECD (2015) produced mental health country profiles for some OECD countries.

With the aim to scale up mental health services especially in low- and middle-income countries, the WHO launched in 2008 the Mental Health Gap Action Programme (mhGAP), designed as a framework for country action, including an integrated package of key interventions for mental, neurological, and substance use disorders to scale up coverage especially in resource-limited settings (WHO 2008, 2010). At present, 'coverage' is conceptualized as simply the proportion of people with mental disorders who receive treatment, and we expect that in the future a more detailed understanding of the levels of coverage will be developed as shown in Figure 24.4 (De Silva et al., 2014).

The mhGAP package provides evidence-based technical guidance, interventions, tools, and training, which must be adapted to national, regional, and local contexts. Priorities in mental, neurological, and substance use disorders have been identified based on the best available scientific and epidemiological evidence, and barriers for scaling up mental healthcare have been considered. A further milestone in evidence-based mental health policymaking is the WHO Mental Health Action Plan 2013–2020, a global strategy setting objectives, targets, and proposed actions for member states and international partners (WHO, 2013b). While the number and extent of evidence-based global mental health policies is growing, epidemiological research needs to continue contributing by keeping both the local and global focus on research.

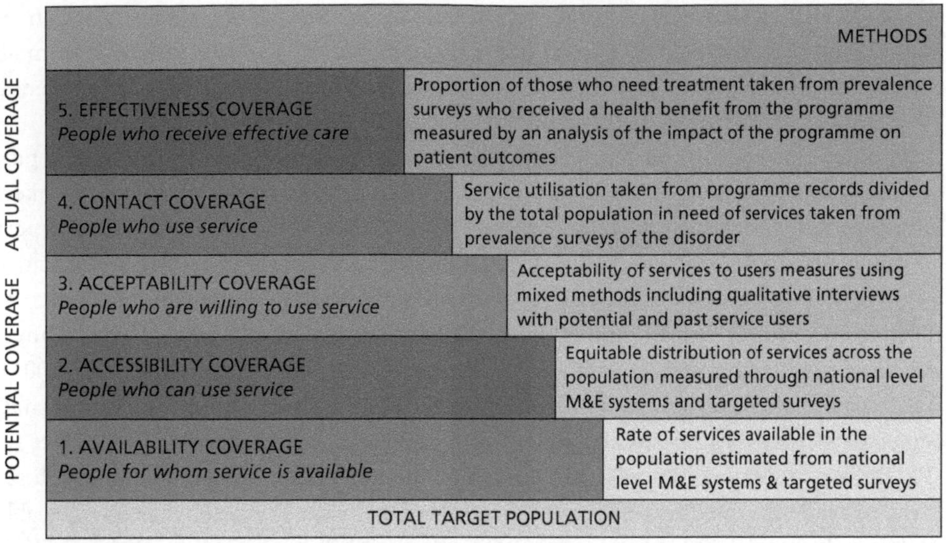

Figure 24.4 Levels of service coverage.

De Silva, M., Cohen, A., and Patel, V. (2014). Evaluation of interventions in the real world. In: Thornicroft, G. and Patel, V. (eds.). Global mental health trials, pp. 282–302. Oxford: Oxford University Press. Adapted from Tanahashi T (1978) Health service coverage and its evaluation. *Bull World Health Organ*, 56(2):295–303. Published by Oxford University Press on behalf of the International Epidemiological Association © The Author 2014. This is an Open Access article distributed under the terms of the Creative Commons Attribution License (http://creativecommons.org/licenses/by/3.0/), which permits unrestricted reuse, distribution, and reproduction in any medium, provided the original work is properly cited. DOI: https://academic.oup.com/ije/article-lookup/doi/10.1093/ije/dyt191.

Opportunities and challenges

Policymaking is a complex, non-linear, and erratic process. Policy decisions are difficult to predict, as details are influenced by a range of stakeholders and circumstances. Evidence-based policymaking attempts and contributes to making the policy process more transparent. Researchers can actively influence evidence-based policymaking, but they need to consider various opportunities and challenges that may favour or hinder the process, such as the quality of the research evidence, the knowledge exchange process, timing and accessibility, stigma, and the heterogeneity of mental health as a policy issue.

The premise for evidence-based policymaking is comprehensive, robust *evidence*, which is mainly provided by systematic reviews, randomized controlled trials, and intervention studies. However, there is still a research gap for some diseases in specific contexts and regions (e.g. suicide (WHO Regional Office for Europe, 2012)) or effectiveness and efficiency, particularly in low- and middle-income settings (Knapp et al., 2006). As the evidence necessarily stems from context-specific observations, it must vice versa be used in a very context-specific way by policymakers (Sutcliffe and Court, 2005). However, underfinancing of the academic and mental health sector in low- and middle-income settings contributes to the lack of context-related evidence from local researchers (Razzouk et al., 2009). More research is needed, providing 'hard' evidence, based on statistical data, as well as 'soft' evidence (Brownson et al., 2009b), such as stakeholder reports or patient monitoring (Mackenzie, 2014). In addition, more public engagement is needed from all stakeholders including service users and carers, as only then can evidence-based mental health policy claim full credibility and authenticity (Collins et al., 2011).

Another challenge lies in the process of *knowledge exchange* from researchers to policymakers. Comprehensive research findings need to be communicated to policymakers in a compact, clear way, understandable for lay audience, for example, in policy papers or policy briefings (Young and Quinn, 2002). Remarkable tools for knowledge exchange in the evidence-based policymaking process are online resources. Social media such as Twitter, Facebook, YouTube, and other social platforms are crucial for research communication, public information campaigns, and targeted dissemination (Stone et al., 2001). Yet, access to the Internet and online tools may constitute an additional technical challenge, particularly for researchers in low- and middle-income countries (Razzouk et al., 2009). In non-democratic political systems, additional challenges can arise through restricted academic freedom and limited freedom of the press. For policymakers to be able to take advantage from the evidence, political continuity and stability of the political system need to be assured, while conflict and volatility have proven to be an obstacle (Sutcliffe and Court, 2005). In addition, over the last decade, multiple evidence-based online tools have been developed to inform the policy process, illustrating how information technology is supporting the drive. Among them, at the micro-level, NICE Pathways (NICE, 2015) is an online tool providing access to NICE clinical guidelines and other NICE tools in England. At the meso-level, PsyMaptic (University of Cambridge, 2015) is an epidemiological prediction tool for first-episode psychosis in England and Wales. At the macro- and mega-levels, GBD Compare (Institute for Health Metrics and Evaluation, 2015) is an online tool for estimating the burden of disease of multiple mental and physical conditions and OneHealth (IHP+, 2015) is an online tool for developing financing scenarios at country level. However, as previously mentioned, access to the Internet may represent a challenge, particularly in low- and middle-income countries (Razzouk et al., 2009).

An important facilitator to the evidence-based policymaking process is *timing* and *accessibility* of the evidence (Oliver et al., 2014). Policymakers often need to decide rapidly on policies they are not experts on, so they need to have access to the specifically required, distinct information quickly and easily (Cable, 2004). Researchers need to use this time window and can facilitate the process by continuous networking and interaction with policymakers (Innvaer et al., 2002). Collaboration with, and continuous involvement of, policymakers during all stages of the research process builds up well-established links and trust, and can facilitate communication (Jenkins et al., 2007).

Networking, together with knowledge sharing and public campaigns, can also facilitate overcoming the additional challenge of *stigma* associated to mental illness which is peculiar to mental health policymaking (Evans-Lacko et al., 2012). An additional global challenge for evidence-based mental health policymaking stands in the complexity and *heterogeneity* of mental health as a policy issue. To date, mental health research has been unable to build a unified voice and framework for public actions, which acts as a major challenge for translating research into policy (WHO, 2013a). The use of a unified voice will facilitate communication.

For more efficient and effective evidence-based policymaking, additional research is needed in mental health policy analysis, particularly on the policy process, and the impact and effectiveness of the use of research to inform the policy process (Oliver et al., 2014). A research gap has also been identified in how to change public and policymakers' attitudes with regard to mental health stigma (Mackenzie, 2014), and more 'action-oriented research' is needed, emanating from mental health workers' priorities, in order to contribute and advise regional health policy and practice (see Chapter 3).

Conclusion

Mental health policy is increasingly supported by research evidence, through a process both systematic and transparent. Research evidence is used to inform decision-makers throughout all stages of the policy process, from problem identification and issue recognition, through policy formulation, to policy implementation, and evaluation. Different types of studies can inform each stage, feeding the multiple aspects of the policy process, including both quantitative and qualitative studies. Evidence can inform decision-makers at every level, from clinical care through service provision/healthcare facility level, to national and global health systems. However, opportunities and challenges need to be considered during the process, such as quality of research evidence, knowledge exchange process, timing and accessibility, stigma, and heterogeneity of mental health as a policy issue. In particular, the use of information technologies is promising in creating a platform for timey and accessible knowledge exchange between researcher and policymakers.

Evidence-based mental health policymaking is crucial to scale up acceptable, effective, efficient, and equitable mental healthcare, services, and systems. However, further evidence to support this process is required not only on mental disorders, mental health interventions, and mental health services, but also on mental health policies and mental health policy process. The call for evidence is paramount in low- and middle-income countries where evidence is particularly scarce. The impact of research on policy has never before been so direct, and the role of researchers in designing and disseminating sound results so crucial.

Practical exercises

1. Policymakers in your country are working on a national plan to improve perinatal maternal mental healthcare. You wish to provide them with the best available evidence in order to facilitate their choices.

   a. Which types of studies would you review to inform them about the *problem*, in terms of burden of perinatal maternal mental health in your country, and in terms of causes of perinatal maternal mental health?

b. Which types of studies would you review to inform them about the *effectiveness* of interventions for perinatal maternal mental health?

c. Which types of studies would you review to inform them about the *efficiency* of interventions for perinatal maternal mental health?

d. Which types of studies would you review to inform them about issues related with the *implementation* of interventions for perinatal maternal mental health?

e. Once the national plan has been published, and recommended services implemented across your country, policymakers are interested in knowing whether the national plan has a positive impact. Which types of studies would you use to inform them about the effectiveness and efficiency of services for perinatal maternal mental health that have been implemented across the country?

2. Imagine that you have received a grant for a project aiming to increase the influence of evidence-based mental health policies in a low-income setting. You need to set up a multidisciplinary team that represents all relevant stakeholders, who would help you in planning and implementing a mental health strategy to scale up mental health services in that country.

a. Who are your relevant stakeholders? How will you involve them?

b. What are the levels of mental health policymaking that you need to consider for your strategy? How will you consider each of the levels in your strategy?

c. What are the essential factors to increase the influence of evidence-based mental health policies? What challenges will you need to consider? Which facilitators can help your work?

References

Birchwood, M., Lester, H., McCarthy, L., Jones, P., Fowler, D., Amos, T., et al. (2014). The UK national evaluation of the development and impact of Early Intervention Services (the National EDEN studies): study rationale, design and baseline characteristics. *Early Intervention in Psychiatry*, 8, 59–67.

Bonin, E.M., Stevens, M., Beecham, J., Byford, S., and Parsonage, M. (2011). Costs and longer-term savings of parenting programmes for the prevention of persistent conduct disorder: a modelling study. *BMC Public Health*, 11, 803.

Brown, M. and Reynolds, P. (2014). Delivery of CBT to treat postnatal depression: health visitors' perceptions. *Community Practitioner*, 87, 26–29.

Brownson, R.C., Fielding, J.E., Maylahn, C.M. (2009a). Evidence-based public health: a fundamental concept for public health practice. *Annual Review of Public Health*, 30, 175–201.

Brownson, R.C., Chriqui, J.F., and Stamatakis, K.A. (2009b). Understanding evidence-based public health policy. *American Journal of Public Health*, 99, 1576–1583.

Buescher, A.V., Cidav, Z., Knapp, M., and Mandell, D.S. (2014). Costs of autism spectrum disorders in the United Kingdom and the United States. *JAMA Pediatrics*, 168, 721–728.

Cable, J. (2004). Evidence and UK politics. In: Young, J. and Court, J. (eds.). *Research and policy in development: does evidence matter?* An ODI Meeting Series, pp. 11–13. London: Overseas Development Institute.

Chatterjee, S., Naik, S., John, S., Dabholkar, H., Balaji, M., Koschorke, M., et al. (2014). Effectiveness of a community-based intervention for people with schizophrenia and their caregivers in India (COPSI): a randomised controlled trial. *Lancet*, **383**, 1385–1394.

Clarke, K., King, M., and Prost, A. (2013). Psychosocial interventions for perinatal common mental disorders delivered by providers who are not mental health specialists in low- and middle-income countries: a systematic review and meta-analysis. *PLoS Medicine*, **10**, e1001541.

Collins, P.Y., Patel, V., Joestl, S.S., March, D., Insel, T.R., and Daar, A.S. (2011). Grand challenges in global mental health: A consortium of researchers, advocates and clinicians announces here research priorities for improving the lives of people with mental illness around the world, and calls for urgent action and investment. *Nature*, **475**, 27–30.

Cooper, B. (2003). Evidence-based mental health policy: a critical appraisal. *British Journal of Psychiatry*, **183**, 105–113.

Department of Health (2009). *The national service framework for mental health: modern standards and service models*. London: Department of Health.

De Silva, M., Cohen, A., and Patel, V. (2014). Evaluation of interventions in the real world. In: Thornicroft, G. and Patel, V. (eds.). *Global mental health trials*, pp. 282–302. Oxford: Oxford University Press.

Dua, T., Barbui, C., Clark, N., Fleischmann, A., Poznyak, V., van Ommeren, M., et al. (2011). Evidence-based guidelines for mental, neurological, and substance use disorders in low- and middle-income countries: summary of WHO recommendations. *PLoS Medicine*, **8**, e1001122.

Evans-Lacko, S., Brohan, E., Mojtabai, R., and Thornicroft, G. (2012). Association between public views of mental illness and self-stigma among individuals with mental illness in 14 European countries. *Psychological Medicine*, **42**, 1741–1752.

Evans-Lacko, S., Knapp, M., McCrone, P., Thornicroft, G., and Mojtabai, R. (2013a). The mental health consequences of the recession: economic hardship and employment of people with mental health problems in 27 European countries. *PLoS One*, **8**, e69792.

Evans-Lacko, S., Malcolm, E., West, K., Rose, D., London, J., Rüsch, N., et al. (2013b). Influence of Time to Change's social marketing interventions on stigma in England 2009-2011. *British Journal of Psychiatry, Supplement*, **55**, s77–s88.

Federal Democratic Republic of Ethiopia Ministry of Health (2012). *National mental health strategy 2012/13–2015/16*. Addis Ababa, Ethiopia: Federal Democratic Republic of Ethiopia Ministry of Health.

Fekadu, A. and Thornicroft, G. (2014). Global mental health: perspectives from Ethiopia. *Global Health Action*, **7**, 25447.

Fisher, J., Tran, T., La, B.T., Kriitmaa, K., Rosenthal, D., and Tran, T. (2010). Common perinatal mental disorders in northern Viet Nam: community prevalence and health care use. *Bulletin of the World Health Organization*, **88**, 737–745.

Glover, G., Arts, G., Babu, K.S. (2006). Crisis resolution/home treatment teams and psychiatric admission rates in England. *British Journal of Psychiatry*, **189**, 441–445.

Government Social Research Unit (2009). *Rapid evidence assessment toolkit*. London: Government Social Research Service.

Henriksen, C.A., Stein, M.B., Afifi, T.O., Enns, M.W., Lix, L.M., and Sareen, J. (2015). Identifying factors that predict longitudinal outcomes of untreated common mental disorders. *Psychiatric Services*, **66**, 163–170.

Hobbs, C., Newton, L., Tennant, C., Rosen, A., and Tribe, K. (2002). Deinstitutionalization for long-term mental illness: a 6-year evaluation. *Australian and New Zealand Journal of Psychiatry*, **36**, 60–66.

Innvaer, S., Vist, G., Trommald, M., and Oxman, A. (2002). Health policy-makers' perceptions of their use of evidence: a systematic review. *Journal of Health Services Research & Policy*, 7, 239–244.

Jenkins, R., McDaid, D., Brugha, T., Cutler, P., and Hayward, R. (2007). The evidence base in mental health policy and practice. In: Knapp, M., McDaid, D., Mossialos, E., and Thornicroft, G. (eds.). *Mental health policy and practice across Europe: the future direction of mental health care*, pp. 100–125. Maidenhead: McGraw Hill Open University Press.

Keown, P., Mercer, G., and Scott, J. (2008). Retrospective analysis of hospital episode statistics, involuntary admissions under the Mental Health Act 1983, and number of psychiatric beds in England 1996-2006. *British Medical Journal*, 337, a1837.

Killaspy, H., Kingett, S., Bebbington, P., Blizard, R., Johnson, S., Nolan, F., et al. (2009). Randomised evaluation of assertive community treatment: 3-year outcomes. *British Journal of Psychiatry*, 195, 81–82.

Knapp, M., Funk, M., Curran, C., Prince, M., Grigg, M., and McDaid, D. (2006). Economic barriers to better mental health practice and policy. *Health Policy and Planning*, 2, 157–170.

IHP+ (2015). OneHealth. International Health Partnership. http://www.internationalhealthpartnership.net/en/tools/one-health-tool

Institute for Health Metrics and Evaluation (2015). GBD Compare. Institute for Health Metrics and Evaluation. http://vizhub.healthdata.org/gbd-compare

Lancet Global Mental Health Group (2007). Scale up services for mental disorders: a call for action. *Lancet*, 370, 1241–1252.

Lindblom, C.E. (1959). The science of "muddling through". *Public Administration Review*, 19, 79–88.

Liu, T., Zhang, L., Pang, L., Li, N., Chen, G., and Zheng, X. (2015). Schizophrenia-related disability in China: prevalence, gender, and geographic location. *Psychiatric Services*, 66, 249–257.

Lund, C., Breen, A., Flisher, A.J., Kakuma, R., Corrigall, J., Joska, J.A., et al. (2010). Poverty and common mental disorders in low and middle income countries: a systematic review. *Social Science & Medicine*, 71, 517–528.

Mackenzie, J. (2014). *Global mental health from a policy perspective: a context analysis characterising mental health and recommending engagement strategies for the Mental Health Innovation Network*. London: Overseas Development Institute.

National Institute for Health and Care Excellence (2013a). NICE charter. NICE. https://www.nice.org.uk/Media/Default/About/Who-we-are/NICE_Charter.pdf

National Institute for Health and Care Excellence (2013b). *Autism: the management and support of children and young people on the autism spectrum (CG 170)*. London: NICE.

National Institute for Health and Care Excellence (2014). *Developing NICE guidelines: the manual*. London: NICE.

National Institute for Health and Care Excellence (2015). NICE pathways. NICE. http://pathways.nice.org.uk

Organisation for Economic Cooperation and Development (2014). *Making mental health count: the social and economic costs of neglecting mental health care*. Paris: OECD.

Organisation for Economic Cooperation and Development (2015). Mental health systems in OECD countries. OECD. http://www.oecd.org/els/health-systems/mental-health-systems.htm

Oliver, K., Innvar, S., Lorenc, T., Woodman, J., and Thomas, J. (2014). A systematic review of barriers to and facilitators of the use of evidence by policymakers. *BMC Health Services Research*, 14, 2.

Oxman, A.D., Lavis, J.N., Lewin, S., and Fretheim, A. (2009). SUPPORT tools for evidence-informed health Policymaking (STP). 1: What is evidence-informed policymaking? *Health Research Policy and Systems*, 7(Suppl 1), S1.

Park, A.L., McCrone, P., and Knapp, M. (2014). Early intervention for first-episode psychosis: broadening the scope of economic estimates. *Early Intervention in Psychiatry*, 10, 144–151.

Razzouk, D., Sharan, P., Gallo, C., Gureje, O., Lamberte, E.E., de Jesus Mari, J., et al. (2009). Scarcity and inequity of mental health research resources in low- and middle-income countries: a global survey. *Health Policy*, 94, 211–20.

Sabatier, P. and Jenkins-Smith, H.C. (eds.) (1993). *Policy change and learning: an advocacy coalition approach*. Boulder, CO: Westview Press.

Sado, M., Inagaki, A., Koreki, A., Knapp, M., Kissane, L.A., Mimura, M., and Yoshimura, K. (2013). The cost of schizophrenia in Japan. *Neuropsychiatric Disease and Treatment*, 9, 787–798.

Saraceno, B. and Saxena, S. (2002). Mental health resources in the world: results from Project Atlas of the WHO. *World Psychiatry*, 1, 40–44.

Saxena, S., Thornicroft, G., Knapp, M., and Whiteford, H. (2007). Resources for mental health: scarcity, inequity, and inefficiency. *Lancet*, 370, 878–89.

Sealy, P. and Whitehead, P.C. (2004). Forty years of deinstitutionalization of psychiatric services in Canada: an empirical assessment. *Canadian Journal of Psychiatry*, 49, 249–257.

Secretaría de Salud (2009). *Diagnóstico y tratamiento del trastorno depresivo de 18 a 59 años de edad*. Mexico: Secretaría de Salud, Mexico City.

http://www.cenetec.salud.gob.mx/descargas/gpc/CatalogoMaestro/161_GPC_TRASTORNO_DEPRESIVO/Imss_161ER.pdf

Simpson, A., Flood, C., Rowe, J., Quigley, J., Henry, S., Hall, C., et al. (2014). Results of a pilot randomised controlled trial to measure the clinical and cost effectiveness of peer support in increasing hope and quality of life in mental health patients discharged from hospital in the UK. *BMC Psychiatry*, 14, 30.

Stikkelbroek, Y., Bodden, D.H., Deković, M., and van Baar, A.L. (2013). Effectiveness and cost effectiveness of cognitive behavioral therapy (CBT) in clinically depressed adolescents: individual CBT versus treatment as usual (TAU). *BMC Psychiatry*, 13, 314.

Stone, D., Maxwell, S., and Keating, M. (2001). *Bridging research and policy: an international workshop*. Warwick: Warwick University.

Sutcliffe, S. and Court, J. (2005). *Evidence-based policymaking: What is it? How does it work? What relevance for developing countries?* London: Overseas Development Institute.

Suzuki, T., Miyaki, K., Song, Y., Tsutsumi, A., Kawakami, N., Shimazu, A., et al. (2015). Relationship between sickness presenteeism (WHO-HPQ) with depression and sickness absence due to mental disease in a cohort of Japanese workers. *Journal of Affective Disorders*, 180, 14–20.

Teferra, S., Hanlon, C., Beyero, T., Jacobsson, L., and Shibre, T. (2013). Perspectives on reasons for non-adherence to medication in persons with schizophrenia in Ethiopia: a qualitative study of patients, caregivers and health workers. *BMC Psychiatry*, 13, 168.

Thornicroft, G. (2000). National service framework for mental health. *The Psychiatrist*, 24, 203–206.

Tugwell, P., Bennett, K.J., Sackett, D.L., and Haynes, R.B. (1985). The measurement iterative loop: a framework for the critical appraisal of need, benefits and costs of health interventions. *Journal of Chronic Diseases*, 38, 339–351.

University of Cambridge (2015). PsyMaptic. http://www.psymaptic.org

Walker, E.R., McGee, R.E., Druss, B.G. (2015). Mortality in mental disorders and global disease burden implications: a systematic review and meta-analysis. *JAMA Psychiatry*, 72, 334–341.

Wamai, R. (2009). Reviewing Ethiopia's health system development. *Japan Medical Association Journal*, 52, 279–286.

While, D., Bickley, H., Roscoe, A., Windfuhr, K., Rahman, S., Shaw, J., et al. (2012). Implementation of mental health service recommendations in England and Wales and suicide rates, 1997–2006: a cross-sectional and before-and-after observational study. *Lancet*, **379**, 1005–1012.

Whiteford, H.A., Degenhardt, L., Rehm, J., Baxter, A.J., Ferrari, A.J., Erskine, H.E., et al. (2013). Global burden of disease attributable to mental and substance use disorders: findings from the Global Burden of Disease Study 2010. *Lancet*, **382**, 1575–1586.

World Health Organization (2001a). *The world health report 2001: mental health: new understanding, new hope*. Geneva: WHO.

World Health Organization (2001b). *Atlas: country profiles on mental health resources 2001*. Geneva: WHO.

World Health Organization (2004a). *World report on knowledge for better health: strengthening health systems*. Geneva: WHO.

World Health Organization (2004b). *The Mexico statement on health research*. Geneva: WHO.

World Health Organization (2005a). *World Health Assembly: resolution on health research*. Geneva: WHO.

World Health Organization (2005b). *Mental health atlas 2005*. Geneva: WHO.

World Health Organization (2008). *mhGAP: Mental Health Gap Action Programme: scaling up care for mental, neurological and substance use disorders*. Geneva: WHO.

World Health Organization (2009). *World Health Organization: the Bamako call to action on research for health*. Geneva: WHO.

World Health Organization (2010). *mhGAP intervention guide for mental, neurological and substance use disorders in non-specialized health settings: Mental Health Gap Action Programme (mhGAP)*. Geneva: WHO.

World Health Organization (2011). *Mental health atlas 2011*. Geneva: WHO.

World Health Organization (2013a). *Investing in mental health: evidence for action*. Geneva: WHO.

World Health Organization (2013b). *Mental health action plan 2013–2020*. Geneva: WHO.

World Health Organization (2015a). Evidence-informed policy-making. http://www.who.int/evidence/about/en

World Health Organization (2015b). WHO-AIMS country reports. http://www.who.int/mental_health/who_aims_country_reports/en/

World Health Organization Regional Office for Europe (2012). *For which strategies of suicide prevention is there evidence of effectiveness?* Copenhagen: WHO Regional Office for Europe.

Wimo, A. and Prince, M. (2010). *World Alzheimer report 2010. The global economic impact of dementia*. London: Alzheimer's Disease International.

World Bank (2015). World development indicators database. http://databank.worldbank.org/data/download/GNIPC.pdf

Young, E. and Quinn, L. (2002). *Writing effective public policy papers: a guide to policy advisers in Central and Eastern Europe*. Budapest: Open Society Institute.

Chapter 25

Psychiatric epidemiology: Looking to the future

Jayati Das-Munshi, Tamsin Ford, Matthew Hotopf, Martin Prince, and Robert Stewart

In the first edition of *Practical Psychiatric Epidemiology*, we devoted some thought in the final chapter to emerging themes and topics that might become increasingly relevant in the future. Looking back on this chapter after 15 years, many of the issues continue to have salience. Indeed, it is reasonable to argue that methods aligned to psychiatric epidemiology have more relevance now than ever before.

Predictions revisited

In the first edition, we highlighted the need for new methodologies alongside generic challenges affecting psychiatric epidemiology, particularly around identifying 'small effect' exposures, such as in genetic epidemiology and in the modelling of multiple aetiological factors for mental health outcomes. We also highlighted challenges in the identification of population-level risk factors: for example, the need to understand the social context, including that of the nation state, social milieu, and constructs such as the 'western' lifestyle. Finally, we highlighted the need to develop newer methods of evaluating interventions, including complex interventions.

As we conclude the second edition, we acknowledge that psychiatric epidemiology continues to draw on generic epidemiological methods. However, the ways in which epidemiological data may be gathered have changed dramatically. For example, the challenge of identifying multiple exposures and relatively small 'effects' and distinguishing real findings from type 1 error are particularly important today in the current era of 'big data'. With relentless and accelerating expansion in data volume and complexity, developments in causal inference, relevant to the modelling of multiple exposures or in identifying population-level risk factors, have enjoyed an ascendency. Methodological advances within the fields of multilevel modelling and a consideration of how the social milieu interacts with individuals have added to our knowledge of social/environmental contexts: in particular, the way in which the social and built environment may play a role in mental health.

The challenges of evaluating complex interventions have as much relevance today as they did 15 years ago. Over the last decade, the definition of 'complex intervention' has rapidly expanded, including, for example, digital interventions, systemic/whole-system-level interventions, advocacy-led interventions, as well as policy interventions which cannot be randomized due to ethical and feasibility concerns (for examples, see Hawton et al., 2013; Erlangsen et al., 2015). Embedding these initiatives within routine clinical settings and using electronic health records to glean long-term real-life outcomes on patients have yet to be fully realized. However, with the expanding influence of evidence-based medicine, the challenges of research, development, and evaluation pathways are more pertinent than ever.

In the first edition, we likened psychiatric epidemiology to a 'toolbox' of methods with research questions generated from outside of the discipline. Arguably interfaces remain with other fields—whether biological sciences, social sciences, or other subjects—and are just as important today. For example, psychiatric epidemiological methods have an important role in informing study design and analysis using large clinical datasets (such as those derived from electronic health records or other administrative sources), even if the research questions still come from outside of the discipline. While epidemiologists may continue to contribute to the research agenda, generating pertinent questions and findings that could have a real impact on clinical care, the interface with other disciplines has become more blurred. Particularly in mental health research, it is increasingly unusual for 'epidemiology' to be carried out in isolation, and epidemiological expertise is increasingly embedded within multidisciplinary academic groupings.

The interface between 'physical' and 'mental' health highlighted in the first edition remains just as relevant today, if not more so. Not only is demographic ageing proceeding ever more rapidly, with all the comorbidity that this entails in later life, but there is also the continuing challenge of improving the general health and substantially reduced life expectancy of people with mental disorders. Epidemiological research has demonstrated this over at least three decades for severe mental illnesses and yet survival-improving interventions remain as elusive as ever in the context of an ever-widening mortality gap. It is well recognized that many chronic physical health conditions share a strong relationship with mental health problems, often with shared determinants acting across the lifespan, and associations between mental and physical health are potentially complex and bidirectional. One could argue that it has been the contribution of psychiatric epidemiology in creating a substantial body of evidence which has irrefutably demonstrated the interlinkages of mental health and physical health over the last 15 years, and which has enabled these issues to be placed at the heart of national and international policy. The challenge now is to develop, deliver, and test interventions at both individual and systems-wide levels to address this need.

Therefore quite a lot can still be reported under the themes laid out in our first edition—the usual mix of continuing activity and the need for further development. The newer horizons that we have chosen to highlight in this second edition reflect the rich diversity of psychiatric epidemiology today. The future of the discipline holds much promise within an increasingly complex world, influenced by rapid developments in technology and strong globalizing forces.

'Big data'

The information revolution presents potentially limitless opportunities for transforming health and healthcare delivery, although the pace of change and lag period between the potential and its realization, can be frustrating. What is undisputed is that psychiatric epidemiology needs to keep apace of developments. Increasing computational capacity and processing speed, and potential access to increasingly large and 'real-world' data sources, present important challenges for study design and the application of epidemiological methods. These include questions around how exploratory we should be, given the scale of the resource, particularly with concerns over type 1 error. In addition, there are ethical considerations relating to privacy and presumed consent for data use which are frequently controversial and yet still rapidly evolving, often faster than is desirable for in-depth consideration. The emergence of 'big data' with all its potential and complexity, is now no longer just of relevance to a limited number of settings but is increasingly an international issue; national electronic health record systems are prevalent across 47% of World Health Organization member states (World Health Organization, 2016). Furthermore, the application of relatively low-cost devices, such as mobile phones, in the collection and recording of patient data means that there is the potential to circumvent some of the traditional problems around cost and feasibility of data collection. Although many commentators have considered the use of these technologies in tracking and containing epidemics, there is a less-realized potential to apply these technologies to mental health and public health interventions—whether recruiting online cohorts *de novo* or using actively and passively collected online data for follow-up and real-time monitoring. Effective interfaces with social sciences continue to be essential for considering and critiquing the use of such data for research, including issues of acceptability and public–academic trust. The systematic consideration of chance, bias, confounding, and causal inference clearly remain as relevant to 'big data' as to any other data source.

'Big data' are often characterized by lists of words beginning with 'V' and which at the time of writing present different degrees of challenge for psychiatric epidemiology. In previous chapters, the 'three Vs' (see Chapter 13) were summarized; over time, additional Vs have been added to characterize these types of data.

Data *volume* is not often a major issue for observational analysis, as most statistical software can handle databases with several million rows (and epidemiologists have historically grown used to the idea of setting a computer running and waiting a few days for the results, from the early days of punch cards onwards); however, challenges start to become more formidable when observational data suggest a need for real-time processing of data on this scale.

Data *velocity* likewise is not currently a major issue for secondary analysis but becomes much more pertinent when interventions become indicated—for example, using or integrating output from health records, social media, or wearables. These in turn exemplify data *variety*, and psychiatric epidemiologists are well placed to advise on challenges around integration of information from widely differing sources, having a long history of collective expertise in, for example, drawing inferences from mixed methods research, multilevel modelling in ecological studies, investigating gene–environment interactions, and other cross-disciplinary endeavours.

Likewise, data *variability* is a well-recognized construct in our field, although the computational challenges remain formidable: for example, characterizing short- and long-term changes in sleep architecture from wearables in order to evaluate these as clinical outcome predictors.

Data *veracity* is perhaps a more novel consideration. It has long been recognized, for example, that suicide recording on death certificates is strongly influenced by the individual and collective behaviour of recording physicians, as well as prevailing social attitudes and stigma. However, it is becoming increasingly important to appreciate, and even investigate, the provenance of different types of information used in new generations of epidemiological research, whether using health records or social media data. In addition, the potential volume of information on data provenance has expanded considerably since the days when diagnoses on a national register had to be taken at face value in the absence of any more in-depth data from actual clinical encounters.

Finally, the more recently suggested sixth and seventh 'big data' Vs, data *visualization* and *value*, are a helpful reminder to epidemiologists that effective research requires effective communication, and there is likely to be a lot to learn about the ways in which this move beyond traditional tables of odds ratios and survival curves, as well as building on already productive collaborations with our health economics colleagues to articulate value impacts beyond relative risks. While some are suggesting that the opportunities of 'big data' have replaced the need for standalone mental health morbidity surveys and cohorts, this is misguided. The benefits of big data analyses and linked data-platforms remain to be fully exploited, while a recent head to head comparison of primary research versus electronic case-note study revealed that each method offers different strengths and weaknesses (Eke et al., 2019), as discussed in Chapter 13. We should be careful not to abandon some tried and tested methodologies too readily in our enthusiasm for the very real opportunities offered by big data techniques.

Importantly, data 'value' also includes the need to justify the existence of 'big data' resources themselves and the role of psychiatric epidemiologists in their use—while we may feel well placed as a specialty to exploit these new opportunities, we may only have a limited period of time to demonstrate this through innovative research output and demonstrable public health and clinical advances as a result.

New technologies, interconnectedness, and science communication

The health application of new technological devices and resources, including the growing but rapidly changing influence of social media, is a development which we did not fully anticipate in the first edition. These innovations are rapidly transforming both the practicalities of study design, particularly measurement, in psychiatric epidemiology, as well as the constructs measured. New technologies—for example, GPS-informed devices to gather health behaviour data—are now increasingly being considered for research in many international settings, as ownership of electronic handheld devices such as mobile phones becomes more prevalent. Furthermore, traditional models of 'social support' and 'social networks' may need to be reframed, now that families and individuals can connect easily over large distances, and as the concept of a 'neighbourhood' takes on an ever more ephemeral guise with national and international interconnectedness.

Methods to communicate research findings are also rapidly evolving to include social media, providing a much more direct link to users of research and the possibility of accelerated translation of findings into policy and action. Conventional peer review is still upheld as the primary means to ensure the scientific veracity of research findings; however, the pace of publishing has been increased through online-only journals and there has been a move to democratize peer review through post-publication review. Post-publication review also allows the possibility of further patient and other stakeholder involvement in research beyond tokenism. What remains unclear is whether the availability of peer reviewers will keep pace with expansions in research output and publication and, if it fails to do so, what alternative solutions are feasible (Stewart, 2015).

Expanding biological data

We anticipated the contribution of whole-genome sequencing to psychiatric epidemiology in the first edition and this is indeed becoming increasingly influential. Fifteen years ago, there was a reasonable distinction to be made between small 'biological' studies with intensively characterized samples and large 'epidemiological' studies with much more limited, and usually questionnaire-derived, information. As biological data acquisition has become much simpler and cheaper, this distinction has become steadily less tenable. At the time of writing, there is no reason to assume that this will not continue and that what is seen as small scale and specialist will in time be routinely applied at low cost across samples of thousands of participants. Over the next 10 years, the application of whole-genome sequencing linked to other data resources has the potential to inform future developments in psychiatric epidemiology, particularly with respect to gene–environment interactions. As discussed by Morgan and colleagues (see Chapter 20), advances in molecular genetics mean that it is now possible to assess directly the role of candidate genes (as opposed to twin or family studies which proxy for genetic risk) and to model potential gene–environment interactions. Epigenetic assays, currently confined to small samples, might translate into measures of exposure routinely collected in the community survey of the future. On the other hand, the susceptibility of these measures to confounding environmental influences might continue to preclude their wider use, just as salivary cortisol assays have never really caught on outside specialist cohorts. Epidemiological issues relating to the precise measurement of the social/environmental exposures and the importance of a priori hypothesis to determine adequate study designs in suitably large samples are still relevant. The opportunity for developing interventions, and particularly the possibility of 'personalizing' medical interventions, has been linked to such developments in genetic epidemiology. However, the extent to which advances in personalized cancer treatments translate to the much more complex phenotypes encountered in mental health remains to be established.

From specific study designs to study platforms and biobanks

While this book has focused on the traditional epidemiological study designs, much of the major investment in biomedical science and general epidemiology has been in developing study platforms of enormous scale which are designed to address many questions. These include UK Biobank ($n = 500,000$) and the US Precision Medicine Initiative (a proposed sample size of 1 million). These platforms do not necessarily sample the population in an epidemiologically pure manner, and for UK Biobank at least, have only recently included much information on psychiatric disorders. However, they have great potential: they collect an enormous scale of information using digitally enabled data collection methods (including web-based questionnaires and cognitive tasks), record linkages to electronic health records, multi-omics analyses, and data from imaging and wearables. Platforms of this nature allow multiple exposures and outcomes to be studied and provide a powerful tool to understand mechanisms of association between exposures and outcomes. We see a future where platforms could be developed, focused at critical points in the development of psychiatric disorders, at considerably lower cost than traditional study designs by linking population resources to provide denominator data (e.g. school data) with health records, enriched with invitations for participants to contribute data via web-based platforms, smartphones, social media, and where possible contributing biosamples. Such platforms will require excellent public involvement and strong relations between participants and researchers.

Globalization, migration, and culture

Globalization may be understood as the increased interconnectedness between individuals across nation states, enhanced through technological advances in communication and transport as well as through finance and international trade (Scholte, 2005). In the first edition of this book, the role of culture in measurement and research within psychiatric epidemiology was highlighted. The updated chapter within this edition by Kohrt and Patel (Chapter 3) underlines the ongoing complexity of assessing 'culture', particularly within a rapidly globalizing world where distance may appear to be shrinking but where 'cultural distance' may remain a challenge. The increasing complexity of global migration, in part a function of globalizing forces such as cheaper transportation and easier communication, but also a feature of broader economic and political change, means that there is an urgency in developing or fine-tuning existing methods to better understand the needs of changing population groups.

More than half of the world's population now live in cities, with further rural–urban migration anticipated in the near future. In countries across the world there are concerns that such movement of people either from rural to urban areas for work, or through labour migration internationally, may have an impact on the mental health and well-being of family members 'left behind' (Gong et al., 2012). Findings from studies which have researched this across international settings have been mixed (Abas et al., 2009, 2013; Siriwardhana et al., 2015; Guoping et al., 2016), which may reflect the diverse contexts of out-migration across studies. How can the toolkit of psychiatric epidemiology be applied to these increasingly complex yet well-recognized situations over the next decade? We anticipate that there will be an increasing (not diminishing) role for psychiatric epidemiologists to better understand and contribute to debates on the mental health consequences of migration, through contributions in study design, measurement, or analytic methods.

Open science

More recently, researchers, funders, and major scientific journals have raised concerns about the lack of reproducibility of scientific findings. This has led many to advocate for open science, in which there is increased transparency in the scientific method. Greater transparency, accessibility, and enhanced collaboration in open science have been further aided through an increasing availability of web-based tools.

Many of the themes underlying the open science movement have a basis in epidemiological principles covered in this book. For example, conducting multiple statistical tests on data until a 'statistically significant' finding emerges not only risks type 1 error (as discussed in Chapter 15) but may underlie at least some of the reasons why certain published findings cannot be readily replicated. As a result, reporting guidelines such as Strengthening the Reporting of Observational Studies in Epidemiology (STROBE) and Consolidated Standards of Reporting Trials (CONSORT) have, for many years, stated a need for investigators to pre-specify analyses and outcomes, in order to protect against selective reporting. Registering study protocols with clearly stated a priori hypotheses and methods prior to conducting a study may protect against so-called p-hacking and are also encouraged by advocates for open science (Bell, 2017). Open science initiatives also include making datasets, statistical code, and other research materials (including peer reviewer reports) readily available, so that researchers may be able to reproduce findings. Free web-based tools, such as the *Open Science Framework*, aid investigators to observe these principles when undertaking research.

While many scientists are committed to making their protocols, data and analytic code available for scrutiny, increasing concerns about information governance and data protection pose a challenge to data access and linkage. Proportionate regulation and timely processing of applications is essential to support appropriate access and use of administrative, survey and cohort data for policy facing research and more importantly for the benefit of those with poor mental health (Editorial. 2019. Smorgasbord or Smaug's hoard? The Lancet Psychiatry, 6, 631).

Conclusions: constancy and evolution

Epidemiology remains the study of the distribution and determinants of health states or events in defined populations and its application to the control of health problems (Porta, 2014). Psychiatric epidemiology has continued to develop and apply these principles in relation to mental health and mental disorders. Maintaining access to methodological training and teaching in psychiatric epidemiology for clinicians, policymakers, and commissioners, as well as other users of research, is as relevant now as it was 15 years ago. There are many old challenges that persist within our specialty, and many exciting new challenges and opportunities on the horizon. We hope that this updated revision provides a useful teaching resource and handbook of methods to support practitioners of the future.

References

Abas, M., Tangchonlatip, K., Punpuing, S., et al. (2013). Migration of children and impact on depression in older parents in rural Thailand, southeast Asia. *JAMA Psychiatry*, 70, 226–233.

Abas, M.A., Punpuing, S., Jirapramukpitak, T., Guest, P., Tangchonlatip, K., Leese, M., et al. (2009). Rural–urban migration and depression in ageing family members left behind. *British Journal of Psychiatry*, 195, 54–60.

Bell, V. (2017). Open science in mental health research. *Lancet Psychiatry*, 4, 525–526.

Eke, H., Janssens, A., Downs, J., Lynn, R. M., Ani, C., & Ford, T. (2019). How to measure the need for transition to adult services among young people with Attention Deficit Hyperactivity Disorder (ADHD): A comparison of surveillance versus case note review methods. *BMC Medical Research Methodology*, 19(1). doi:10.1186/s12874-019-0820-y

Erlangsen, A., Lind, B.D., Stuart, E.A., Qin, P., Stenager, E., Larsen, K.J., et al. (2015). Short-term and long-term effects of psychosocial therapy for people after deliberate self-harm: a register-based, nationwide multicentre study using propensity score matching. *Lancet Psychiatry*, 2, 49–58.

Gong, P., Liang, S., Carlton, E.J., Jiang, Q., Wu, J., Wang, L., et al. (2012). Urbanisation and health in China. *Lancet*, 379, 843–852.

He, G., Xie, J.-F., Zhou, J.-D., Zhong, Z.-Q., Qin, C.-X., and Ding, S.-Q. (2016). Depression in left-behind elderly in rural China: prevalence and associated factors. *Geriatrics & Gerontology International*, 16, 638–643.

Hawton, K., Bergen, H., Simkin, S., Dodd, S., Pocock, P., Bernal, W., et al. (2013). Long term effect of reduced pack sizes of paracetamol on poisoning deaths and liver transplant activity in England and Wales: interrupted time series analyses. *BMJ*, 346, f403.

Porta, M. (ed). (2014). *A dictionary of epidemiology*, 6th edn. New York: Oxford University Press.

Scholte, J.A. (2005). *Globalization: a critical introduction*, 2nd edn. Basingstoke: Palgrave Macmillan.

Siriwardhana, C., Wickramage, K., Siribaddana, S., Vidanapathirana, P., Jayasekara, B., Weerawarna, S., et al. (2015). Common mental disorders among adult members of 'left-behind' international migrant worker families in Sri Lanka. *BMC Public Health*, 15, 299.

Stewart, R. (2015). Scientific theory, the publishing crisis and the wisdom of editors. *Acta Psychiatrica Scandinavica*, 132, 427.

World Health Organization (2016). *Global diffusion of eHealth: making universal health coverage achievable. Report of the third global survey on eHealth*. Geneva: **World Health Organization**. https://www.who.int/goe/publications/global_diffusion/en/

Index

Tables and boxes are indicated by *t* and *b* following the page number

For the benefit of digital users, indexed terms that span two pages (e.g., 52–53) may, on occasion, appear on only one of those pages.

accuracy 226, 354, 369
  diagnostic 13
Acholi Psychosocial Assessment Instrument 42–45
activities 7
adaptive designs 212
adoptees design 329
adoptees' family design 329
adoption studies 329, 350
Adult Psychiatric Morbidity Surveys (APMS) 135
advance directive 62
affected sibling method 333–34
age effects 179
agnostic analysis 229
allele-sharing methods 333–34
AllTrials Project 203–4
alpha testing 9
AMSTAR 2 289*t*
analysis *see* data analysis
analysis of covariance (ANCOVA) 195
analysis of variance (ANOVA) 265
analytical studies 84
analytics 229
a priori hypothesis 260, 277
area under the ROC curve 15–16, 370–71
ascertainment 328
assent 63
Assessment Instrument for Mental Health Systems
    (WHO-AIMS) 416
association 255
  genetic 334–39
attitudes 7
attrition 176
attrition bias 294
autonomy 74
Avon Longitudinal Study of Parents and Childhood
    (ALSPAC) 87, 88, 391–92

backwards stepwise regression 310
baseline measurements 195
base population 128
Bayesianism 277
behavioural genetic designs 327–32
behaviours 7
beneficence 64, 65, 73
best interests 64
beta testing 9
between-cluster variations 123
bias 261
  attrition 294

confounding 286
critical appraisal 286
detection 294
ecological 120*b*, 263
inclusion 262
information 89–90, 157, 261, 286
interpretation 203–4
interviewer 289–90
observer 89–90, 157
performance 294
prevalence 263
publication 203–4, 240–43, 244
recall 89–90, 157, 261–62, 289–90
reporting 294
risk of 243
sampling 129
selection 89, 155, 262, 286, 294, 298
big data 228–31, 360, 427
binary variables 6
biobanks 430
bioethics 53
bio-informatics 359
Biomedical Research Centre (BRC) 79–80
birth cohorts 171–72, 391–94
Bland–Altman plots 18
blinding 90, 157, 198
bootstrapping 363
Bradford Hill criteria 275
British Child and Adolescent Mental Health
    Surveys 87–88
British Cohort Study (BCS) 391–92
British Paediatric Surveillance Unit 220
Broad Street pump 114, 363
burden of disease studies 373
burden of psychiatric disorders 373–74

CAMDEX 25
Campbell Collaboration 239–40, 241*t*
candidate gene studies 335, 352
capacity 55–58, 63
case–control studies 85*t*, 89, 145
  critical appraisal 289
  nested in cohort studies 158
  nested in cross-sectional studies 158
case-crossover design 160
case definition 151
case identification 151–52
case registers 222–27
categorical variables 6

category fallacy 37
causal criteria 275, 276t
causal pies 344
causation 267, 271, 310
censoring 328
central limit theorem 256–57
Centre for Epidemiological Studies – Depression
   (CES-D) 22
Centre for Evidence-Based Medicine 289t
Centre for Reviews and Dissemination
   (CRD) 239–40, 241t
chain sampling 104
Chalder Fatigue Scale 23
chance 165, 255–60
Child and Adolescent Psychiatric Assessment
   (CAPA) 25, 131–32
Child and Adolescent Psychiatry Surveillance System
   (CAPSS) 220–22
Child Behaviour Checklist (CBCL) 22
children
   capacity 63
   measurements for 21–22, 25–26, 131–32
Children of the 1990s 391–92
cholera 114, 363
classical cohort studies 88
classification 361
clinical heterogeneity 244
Clinical Interview Schedule – Revised (CIS-R) 21,
   131, 393–94
Clinical Record Interactive Search (CRIS)
   data 227–28
clinical trials 85t
   critical appraisal 293
   units 207
Clinical Trials Regulation (EU) 60, 61
Close Persons Questionnaire (CPQ) 27
clustering 123, 317–21, 364
cluster randomization 130t, 197
cluster randomized trials 90–91, 212
Cochrane resources 239–40, 241t, 243, 287, 289t
coding 105
coefficient kappa 19
coefficient of agreement 19
cognitive function measures 23
Cognitive Screening Instrument for Dementia
   (CSI-D) 23
Cohen's kappa coefficient 19
coherence assumption 248
cohort effects 179
cohort studies 85t, 88, 145, 146–47, 171
   birth cohorts 171–72, 391–94
   case–control studies nested in 158
   classical 88
   critical appraisal 290
   historical (retrospective) 88–89, 173, 290–91
   population 88
   prospective 174, 290–91
collinearity 308
combined emic–etic assessment 45
communication 203, 428
community prevalence and incidence 223

community trials 211
comparative psychiatry 36
complete ascertainment 328
complete case 202
complex interventions 198–99, 210, 425–26
complier average causal effect 202
Composite International Diagnostic Interview
   (CIDI) 13, 24, 131
compositional effects 121–22
computer-assisted personal interviewing
   (CAPI) 94–95
computer-assisted self interviewing (CASI) 94–95
computer-based data analysis 105
concealment of allocation 196–97
concurrent validity 11
confidence intervals 162, 257, 259, 260
confounding 154b, 164, 176, 263–67, 306, 312
   bias 286
   ecological 263
   residual 266
consensus 277
consent 55–63, 193
consistency
   assumption 248
   internal 19
Consolidated Criteria for Reporting Qualitative
   Research 107
Consolidated Standards of Reporting Trials
   (CONSORT) guidelines 193, 243, 431
construct validity 10
content analysis 106t
content validity 10
contextual effects 121–22
continued consent 63
continuous variables 6
controls 152–55, 198
   historical 212
convergent validity 11
conversation analysis 103, 104, 106t
cost–benefit analysis 382
cost-consequences analysis 381
cost-effectiveness analysis 377–78, 379b, 381
cost-minimization analysis 381
cost-of-illness studies 374
costs 382, 383, 384
cost–utility analysis 382
Cox proportional hazards models 265
critical appraisal 265, 285
   tools/checklists 287, 289t
Critical Appraisal Skills Programme
   (CASP) 289t, 295
   Qualitative Checklist 107
critical period 390
Cronbach's alpha 19–20
cross-cultural studies 34b, 35
cross-level inference 115b
cross-national studies 34b, 35
crossover trials 211
cross-sectional surveys 85t, 86, 127
   case–control studies nested in 158
   critical appraisal 288

cross-validation 363
cultural consonance modelling 40
cultural variables 39
culture 33, 430

data analysis
  case–control studies 154, 162–64
  cohort studies 178–81
  cross-sectional surveys 133
  life course epidemiology 394
  qualitative data 104
  randomized controlled trials 200–2
data availability 224, 227
data cleaning 360
data collection 94, 100–3, 359
data exploration 359
data extraction 243
data formats 359
data governance 227
data interpretation
  case–control studies 165
  cohort studies 178–81
  randomized controlled trials 203
data mining 229
data monitoring committee 200
data processing 94
data quality 226
data science 229
data value 428
data variety 228–29, 428
data velocity 228–29, 427–28
data veracity 228–29, 428
data visualization 428
data volume 228–29, 427
decision trees 367
deductive approach 99
dementia screening measures 23
demographic status 7
depression measures 22–23
descriptive studies 84, 223
detection bias 294
determinism 272
Development and Well-Being Assessment
    (DAWBA) 25, 131–32
deviant case analysis 106
diagnostic accuracy 13
diagnostic instruments 24–26, 40
Diagnostic Interview Schedule (DIS) 24
Diagnostic Interview Schedule for Children
    (DISC) 26, 131–32
dichotomous variables 6
differential misclassification 261
direction of causality 128
disability-adjusted life year (DALY) 373–74
discourse analysis 106t
discrete quantitative variables 6–7
disease risk factors 223–24
dissemination 137, 203
divergent validity 12
domains of measurement 7
double-blind study 90, 198

double-data entry 95
Downs and Black checklist 289t
Dunedin Multidisciplinary Health and Development
    Study 171–72, 391–92
Durkheim, Emile 114
Durkheim Project 231

ecological bias 120b, 263
ecological confounding 263
ecological fallacy 86, 114, 115b, 120b, 263
ecological studies 85t, 86, 113
  critical appraisal 292
ecological variables 119
economic evaluation studies 380–84
effectiveness 204
Effective Public Health Practice Project: Quality
    Assessment Tool for Quantitative Studies 289t
effect modification 280
efficacy 204
effort after meaning 89–90, 157, 261–62
electronic health records 223, 225–26, 232
emic 37
environmental exposures 353
EpiData 94–95
Epidemiologic Catchment Area (ECA)
    programme 134
epigenetic processes 346
ethics
  bioethics 53
  consent and capacity 51
  patient and public engagement 71
Ethiopian health systems 415
ethnicity 35
ethnography 103
etic 37
EURO-D 10, 13, 15–18, 19
Evaluation to Sign Consent (ESC) 58–59
evidence-based medicine 237
evidence-based mental health policy 405
evidence hierarchy 287
experimental studies 83
explanatory model 38
Explanatory Model Interview Catalogue
    (EMIC) 38b
explanatory trials 204
exploratory studies 150–51
exposure cohort 171, 174
exposure status 156
external responsiveness 16–18
Eysenck Personality Questionnaire (EPQ) 26

face-to-face interviews 93
factor analysis 322
factorial trials 211
factorial validity 13
fallacy
  category 37
  ecological 86, 114, 115b, 120b, 263
  individualistic 115b, 121–22
familial aggregation 328
family studies 328, 350

feature selection 361
financing of health systems 376
fixed effects model 319–20
focus groups 101*t*, 102, 103–4
follow-up 199
forward stepwise regression 310
framework approach 106*t*
Fraser guidelines 63
friction cost method 376

GBD Compare 418
gene–environment correlation 345–46
gene–environment interaction 35–36, 343
gene mapping designs 333–39
General Health Questionnaire (GHQ) 20
generalizability 108
generalized linear models 394–95
generation effects 181
genetic association studies 334–39
genetic epidemiology 327
genome-wide association studies 160, 335–37, 355, 356
genome-wide complex trait analysis 339
geographical ecological studies 114, 115, 116*b*
Geriatric Depression Scale (GDS) 22
Geriatric Mental State (GMS) 25
Gillick competence 63
Global Burden of Disease study 373–74
global guidelines and policies 415
globalization 430
global measures 7
global mental health 38
gold standard 13
governance 227
GRADE Pro – Guideline Development Tool 241*t*, 244–46
grounded theory 106*t*, 238–39

HapMap Project 335
Health and Social Care Information Centre 231
health economics 373
Health Inequalities Research Network (HERON) 76–78
health services need or use 7
health status 7
health systems 34–35, 38–39, 415
financing 376
healthy worker effect 175
heritability (h²) 330, 339
heterogeneity 244
hierarchical clustering 364
hierarchical data 122
hierarchy of evidence 287
historical (retrospective) cohort studies 88–89, 173, 290–91
historical controls 212
homogeneity 244
Hospital Episode Statistics (HES) database 232
human capital approach 376

Human Genome Project 335
hyper-plane 363
hypotheses 260, 273
a priori 260, 277
hypothesis-free research 229, 279
null 258–59
post hoc 260
primary 191

identity by descent 333–34
identity by state 333–34
imputation, multiple 308, 318*b*, 395
incident cases 152
inclusion bias 262
inconsistency 248
incremental cost-effectiveness ratio 384*b*, 384
individualistic fallacy 115*b*, 121–22
individually randomized trials 211
individual patient data meta-analysis 246
induction period 279
inductivism 99, 273
inequalities 75–76
inference 255, 271, 303–4, 310
Informant Questionnaire on Cognitive Decline in the Elderly (IQ-CODE) 23
information bias 89–90, 157, 261, 286
informative missingness 360
informed consent 58, 193
inheritance modes 328
intention-to-treat 201
interaction contrast ratio 348–49
interconnectedness 428
inter-interviewer reliability 18
internal consistency 19
internal responsiveness 16–18
International Pilot Study of Schizophrenia (IPSS) 34*b*
International Prospective Register of Systematic Reviews (PROSPERO) 240
Internet-based data collection 92–93, 104
interpretation bias 203–4
inter-rater reliability 18
interrupted time series 116–18
intervention group 198
intervention studies 90
economic evaluation of interventions 377–78
interviewer bias 289–90
interviews 92, 100, 101*t*, 103–4, 131
intra-class correlation 18, 320

justice 75

kappa coefficient 19
King's Centre for Military Health Research (KCMHR) cohort study 174
K-means 366
k-nearest neighbours algorithm 366
knowledge exchange 418
known-group validity 12
Kraepelin, Emile 36
Kreyòl Distress Idioms Screener 42–45

labelling 105
latent class analysis 322, 323, 395
latent class growth analysis 181
latent curve modelling 181, 324
latent growth modelling 398
latent period 279
latent profile analysis 322
latent trait analysis 322
latent variable analysis 322–24
lay interviewers 131
levels of measurement 6
liability-threshold model 328–29
Liaison and Education in General Practices (LEGs) study 380
life course epidemiology 389
life event measures 27
Life Events and Difficulties Schedule (LEDS) 158
lifestyles 7
Lind's scurvy study 189
linear regression 265, 304–5
linkage disequilibrium 334
linkage studies 333
List of Threatening Events (LTE) 27
literature review 191
locally developed tools 42
logarithm of odds (LOD score) 333
logistic regression 154b, 164, 265, 304–5
London Handicap Scale (LHS) 27

MacArthur Competence Assessment Tool for Clinical Research (MacCAT-CR) 57, 58–60
McGill Illness Narrative Interview (MINI) 38b
machine learning 361
    supervised 362, 366–68
    unsupervised 362, 363–64
MANAS trial 379b
matching 153, 154b, 154, 164, 264–65
Maudsley Biomedical Research Centre (BRC) 79–80
measurement 5
    clinical measures 20–28, 131
    copyrighted measures 20
    domains 7
    error 261
    invariance 40
    levels 6
    new measure development 8
    psychometric properties 10–19
    public domain measures 20
    selection 8
mediating factors 267
mediation 181, 310
Mental Capacity Act (MCA) 2005 56–57, 60–61, 62
Mental Health Action Plan 2013–2020 (WHO) 416
Mental Health Atlas (WHO) 416
Mental Health Gap Action Programme (WHO) 416
mental health policy 405
meta-analysis 107, 238, 243–44
    individual patient data 246
    multiple treatments (network) 248
meta-ethnography 107, 238–39

Methodological Expectations of Campbell Collaboration Intervention Reviews (MEC2IR) 241t
Methodological Expectations of Cochrane Intervention Reviews (MECIR) 241t
methodological heterogeneity 244
migration 430
Millennium Cohort Study (MCS) 391–92
Mini-International Neuropsychiatric Review (MINI) 131
Mini-Mental State Examination (MMSE) 23
minimization 198
misclassification 174–75, 261
missing at random 201b, 315–16, 360
missing completely at random 201b, 315–16, 360
missing data 200–1, 227, 314–16, 360, 395
missing heritability 339
missing not at random 201b, 315–16, 360
mixed effects models 122, 319–20
mixed methods studies 91, 100
model building 305–9
modified intention-to-treat 201
monoamine oxidase A gene (*MAOA*) 344–45, 352
MOOSE Checklist 241t
morbid risk 328
mortality data 84–86
multilevel modelling 113, 121–22, 317–21
multi-method studies 100
multiple imputation 308, 318b, 395
multiple incomplete ascertainment 328
multiple treatments meta-analysis 248
multi-strategy studies 100
multivariable analyses 265, 305–9, 394–95
multivariate models 332, 394–95
myhealthlocker 231

National Center for Health Technology Excellence (CENETEC Salud) 414
National Child Development Study (NCDS) 391–92
National Comorbidity Survey (NCS) 135
National Heart Lung and Blood Institute 289t
National Institute for Health and Care Excellence (NICE) 239–40, 413–14, 418
National Psychiatric Morbidity Surveys (NPMS) 135
National Service Framework for Mental Health (NSF-MH) 414
National Survey of Health and Development (NSHD) 171–72, 391–92
National Survey of Mental Health and Wellbeing 136
naturalistic research 102
natural language processing 225–26
negative predictive value 14–15, 370
nesting 122, 158
network meta-analysis 248
Newcastle–Ottawa Scale (NOS) 243, 289t
new cross-cultural psychiatry 37
New England Family Studies 391–92
new technology 428
NICE Pathways 418
N-of-1 designs 212
non-differential misclassification 261

non-maleficence 73
non-participant observation 102–3
non-randomized clinical trials 294
non-random misclassification 174–75
non-responders 94, 176
Nuclear Industry Family Study 172
null hypothesis 258–59
number needed to treat 203

observational studies 83, 84, 101t, 102
observer bias 89–90, 157
odds 148
odds ratio 148, 149, 162
ombudsmen 62–63
OneHealth 378b, 418
online communities 104
open science 431
open trial 198
opinions 7
ordered categorical variables 6
ordinal scales 6–7
Organization for Economic Cooperation and
    Development (OECD) 415–16
outcomes 175, 199–200, 224, 383–84
out-of-bag data 363
out-of-pocket payments 377
overfitting 362

panel design 146n
paper-based questionnaires 95
parameter tuning 366
Parental Bonding Inventory (PBI) 26
Parent–Child Joint Activity Scale (PJAS) 10, 11, 12
parsimonious predictive model 309
partial least squares 368
participant observation 102–3
path analysis 394–95
path diagram 331
pathway analysis 338
patient and public engagement 71
patient and public involvement 71–72
patient preference trials 213
PatientsLikeMe 231
peer review 429
perfect trial 190
performance bias 294
period effects 179, 392–93
period prevalence 133
per protocol 202
personality disorders assessment 26
person-years at risk 178
pharmaceutical trials 209–10
phase I–IV trials 209–10
PICO 240
pilot studies 94
placebo 90, 198
policy cycle 408, 409, 411t
polychotomous variables 6
polygenic model 328–29
polygenic risk scores 339, 355
Popper, Karl 273

population attributable fraction 178
population cohort studies 88
population registers 129
Porton Down cohort study 173
positive predictive value 14–15, 370
postal interviews 92–93
post hoc hypothesis 260
post-publication review 429
power calculations 192
pragmatic trials 204
precipitating factors 280
precision 83
Precision Medicine Initiative 430
predictive validity 12
predisposing factors 280
preference trials 212
pre-processing steps 359
Present State Examination (PSE) 24
prevalence 133
prevalence bias 263
prevalent cases 152
principal components analysis 364
PRISMA Statement 241t
proband method 328
process evaluation 91
Project Atlas (WHO) 416
propensity scores 264–65, 312
proportional hazards model 304–5
prospective cohort studies 174, 290–91
PROSPERO 240
protocol 240
provenance 226–27
psychiatric case registers 222–27
psychiatric disorder measures 20–23
Psychiatric Genomics Consortium 337–38
psychological autopsy 159
psychometric properties 10–19
psychotherapy, cost-effectiveness 378
psychotropic drugs, cost-effectiveness 377
PsyMaptic 418
publication 203
publication bias 203–4, 240–43, 244
purposive sampling 104
p-values 258–59, 260

qualitative research 91, 99
    critical appraisal 295
Quality Framework 295
quality of life measures 27
quantitative studies 91–94
quasi-experimental designs 91
questionnaire administration 95

race 35
random digit dialling 93
random effects models 122, 319–20
random forests 368
random intercepts models 122
randomization 90, 195, 265
    cluster 130t, 197
    stratified 130t, 196

randomized consent designs 212
randomized controlled trials 90, 187, 312
  case registers 224
  critical appraisal 293
  qualitative studies running alongside 107
random misclassification 174–75
rare disease assumption 148
rare disorders and events 220
rate 178
rate ratio 178
recall bias 89–90, 157, 261–62, 289–90
receiver operating characteristic (ROC)
    curve 15–16, 370
reciprocity 73
records-derived case registers 224
recruitment 193
recurrence risk 328
reference population 192
reflexivity 106
refutationism 273–75
regression 304–5, 361
  linear 265, 304–5
  logistic 154*b*, 164, 265, 304–5
  stepwise 310
relative risk ratio 328
relativist approaches 37
reliability 5, 18, 106
  inter-interviewer 18
  inter-rater 18
  test–retest 18
reporting bias 294
representativeness 130
reproducibility 361
research cycle 406, 409
research synthesis 237
residual confounding 266
resource utilization 382
respondent validation 106
response rates 130
responsiveness 16
restriction 154*b*, 264–65
retention strategies 177
retrospective (historical) cohort studies 88–89,
    173, 290–91
reverse causation 165
RevMan 241*t*
risk 147, 178
risk factors 223–24
risk of bias 243
risk ratio 148, 178
ROBINS-I (Acrobat NRSI) 289*t*
ROBIS 289*t*

sampling 104, 129
  bias 129
  distributions 256, 305
  error 256
saturation 104–5
scaling up services 378*b*
Schedule for Schizophrenia and Affective Disorder
    for children (K-SADS) 131–32

Schedules for Clinical Assessment in
    Neuropsychiatry (SCAN) 24
schizophrenia studies 34*b*
school-based research 63–64
science communication 428
scientific rigour 105
Scottish Intercollegiate Guidelines Network
    (SIGN) 289*t*
scurvy study 189
selection bias 89, 155, 262, 286, 294, 298
Self-Reporting Questionnaire – 20 (SRQ-20) 20
semi-structured interviews 100
sensitive period 390
sensitivity 14, 369
sensitivity analysis 384
SF-12 28
SF-36 28
Shona Symptom Questionnaire 42–46
Short Explanatory Model Interview
    (SEMI) 38*b*
Short Form-12 (SF-12) 28
Short Form Health Survey (SF-36) 28
sibling pair analysis 333–34
silhouette plot 366
similarity assumption 248
simple categorical variables 6
simple random samples 130*t*
simple variance components model 320
single ascertainment 328
single blind study 198
single nucleotide polymorphisms 335–36
Snow, John 114, 363
snowball sampling 104
social circumstances 7
social media 74
social network analysis 40
Social Network Assessment Instrument 27
Social Problems Questionnaire (SPQ) 27
social support measures 27
socioeconomic status 7
South East London Photography group
    (SELPh) 78–79
South London and Maudsley Clinical Record
    Interactive Search (CRIS) data 227–28
specificity 14, 369
spontaneous remission 90
stages heuristic model 408
standard error 257, 305
standardization 226
Standardized Assessment of Personality
    (SAP) 26
STARS study 90–91
statistical heterogeneity 244
statistical power 258–59, 354
statistical significance 258–59, 260
statistical techniques 303, 346
stepped wedge designs 212
stepwise regression 310
stopping trials 200
stratification 154*b*, 164, 265
stratified randomization 130*t*, 196

Strengthening the Reporting of Observational
    Studies in Epidemiology (STROBE)
    guidelines 162, 431
Strengths and Difficulties Questionnaire
    (SDQ) 21
structural equation modelling 324, 331, 394–95, 397
structural validity 13
study designs 83
    behavioural genetics 327–32
    economic evaluation 380
    ethics 54
    evidence-based policy studies 410
    gene–environment interaction 349–50
    life course epidemiology 391
study platforms 430
study population 192
sufficient causes framework 348
suicide studies 84–86, 114, 159–60
supervised learning 362, 366–68
support vector machines 368
surrogate decision makers 61–62
surveillance 219–20, 223–27
Swedish 1969 Conscription Cohort 391–92
symptom measurement 40
Systematic Assessment of Quality in Observational
    Research (SAQOR) 39–40
systematic reviews 237, 239–43, 244
    critical appraisal 296
    qualitative research 107

Telephone Interview for Cognitive Status
    (TICS-m) 23
telephone interviews 93
test–retest reliability 18
test set 363
thematic analysis 105, 106t
'thinking too much' 37
three Vs 228–29, 427–28
time trends 115, 116b
towards the null 261
training 363, 369
trait measurement 6, 26
trajectory analysis 181
transcultural translation and adaptation
    process 40–42, 42b, 43b, 44b
transitivity assumption 248
translational psychiatric research 75–76
triangulation 106
tri-partite consent process 62–63
triple-blind study 198
trust 73
twin studies 329–32, 350
two-phase surveys 132

two-tailed statistical tests 260
type 1/2 error 258–59

undercounting 129
unexposed cohort 171, 175
unit costs 383
unit non-response 176
universalist approaches 37
unstructured interviews 100
unsupervised learning 362, 363–64

validation set 363
validity 5, 83, 94, 106
    big data 232
    concurrent 11
    construct 10
    content 10
    convergent 11
    divergent 12
    factorial 13
    known-group 12
    predictive 12
    structural 13
variables 6–7
    binary 6
    categorical 6
    continuous 6
    cultural 39
    dichotomous 6
    discrete quantitative 6–7
    ecological 119
    ordered categorical 6
    polychotomous 6
    simple categorical 6
voluntariness of consent 60

waiting list control 212
wave non-response 176
Wellcome Trust Case Control Consortium 337–38
Whitehall I and II Study 172–73
WHO Assessment Instrument for Mental Health
    Systems (WHO-AIMS) 416
WHOQOL-BREF 27
willingness-to-pay techniques 382
with-in cluster correlation 123
World Health Organization (WHO) 415
World Health Report 2001 (WHO) 416
World Mental Health (WMH) surveys 137

Youden's index 15

z-score 259
Zung depression scale (ZDS) 22